WM 875

Worcs. Acute Hospitals NHS Trust

Therapy ﬃculties
Advocacy, Particip Partnership

D0337199

This book is due for return on or before the last date shown below.

-7. MAY 2003
-7. JAN 2003
19. MAR. 2003

-9 JUN 2011

1 9 DEC 2012

1 9 JUL 2013

Therapy and Learning Difficulties
Advocacy, Participation and Partnership

Edited by

John Swain BSc, PGCE, MSc, PhD
Principal Lecturer (Research) and Reader in Disability Studies,
Faculty of Health, Social Work and Education,
University of Northumbria, Newcastle-upon-Tyne, UK

and

Sally French Bsc, Msc (Psych), Msc (Soc), MSCP, Dip TP
Lecturer, School of Health and Social Welfare,
Open University, Milton Keynes, UK

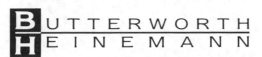

OXFORD AUCKLAND BOSTON JOHANNESBURG MELBOURNE NEW DELHI

Butterworth-Heinemann
Linacre House, Jordan Hill, Oxford OX2 8DP
225 Wildwood Avenue, Woburn, MA 01801-2041
A division of Reed Educational and Professional Publishing Ltd

A member of the Reed Elsevier plc group

First published 1999

© Reed Educational and Professional Publishing Ltd 1999

All rights reserved. No part of this publication may be reproduced in
any material form (including photocopying or storing in any medium by
electronic means and whether or not transiently or incidentally to some
other use of this publication) without the written permission of the
copyright holder except in accordance with the provisions of the Copyright,
Designs and Patents Act 1988 or under the terms of a licence issued by the
Copyright Licensing Agency Ltd, 90 Tottenham Court Road, London,
England W1P 9HE. Applications for the copyright holder's written
permission to reproduce any part of this publication should be addressed
to the publishers

British Library Cataloguing in Publication Data

A catalogue record for this book is available from the British Library

Library of Congress Cataloguing in Publication Data

A catalogue record for this book is available from the Library of Congress

ISBN 0 7506 3962 8

Composition by Genesis Typesetting, Laser Quay, Rochester, Kent
Printed and bound in Great Britain by Martins the Printers, Berwick-upon-Tweed

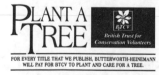

PLANT A TREE

British Trust for
Conservation Volunteers

FOR EVERY TITLE THAT WE PUBLISH, BUTTERWORTH-HEINEMANN
WILL PAY FOR BTCV TO PLANT AND CARE FOR A TREE.

Contents

Acknowledgements

We would like to thank all the authors who contributed to this book and Caroline Makepeace for her help and encouragement throughout the whole project.

Contributors

Dorothy Atkinson   Senior Lecturer, School of Health and Social Welfare, Open University, Milton Keynes

Jean Barclay   Author of *In Good Hands: The History of the Chartered Society of Physiotherapy 1894–1994*, Dunfermline, Fife

Ann Brechin   Senior Lecturer, School of Health and Social Welfare, Open University, Milton Keynes

Lindsay Brigham   Regional Manager, Health and Social Welfare, Open University (North Region), Newcastle-upon-Tyne

Hilary Brown   Professor in Social Care, School of Health and Social Welfare, Open University, Milton Meynes

Anne Chappell   Senior Lecturer in Social Policy, Department of Human Sciences, Buckinghamshire Chilterns University College

Jenny Corbett   Senior Lecturer in Special Education, Institute of Education, University of London

Mairian Corker   Senior Research Fellow in Deaf and Disability Studies, University of Central Lancashire; Research Associate on the ESRC-funded *Life as a Disabled Child Project* co-ordinated by the Disability Research Unit, University of Leeds, and the Department of Public Health Studies, University of Edinburgh

Sally Donati   Occupational Therapist, Service for People with Learning Disabilities, Camden and Islington Community Health Service (NHS) Trust, London

Caroline Downs   Teacher in Charge, Old Lodge Unit for Pupils with Autism, Old Lodge School, East Finchley, London

Sally French   Lecturer, School of Health and Social Welfare, Open University, Milton Keynes

Maureen Gillman   Principal Lecturer in Social Work, Faculty of Health, Social Work and Education, University of Northumbria, Newcastle-upon-Tyne

Elizabeth C. Handyside   Research Associate, University of Northumbria, Newcastle-upon-Tyne

Bob Heyman   Professor of Health Social Research, Faculty of Health, Social Work and Education, University of Northumbria, Newcastle-upon-Tyne

Margaret Hutchinson   Staff Tutor, Social Sciences Faculty, Open University, Milton Keynes

Phyllis Jones   Senior Lecturer in Education, Faculty of Health, Social Work and Education, University of Northumbria, Newcastle-upon-Tyne

Paul Lawrence   Senior Lecturer of Students with Learning Difficulties, North Tyneside College of Further Education, North Tyneside

Neil Palmer, Chris Peacock, Florence Turner and Brian Vasey, supported by Val Williams   Bristol Self-Advocacy Research Group, Bristol and District *People First*

Carol Potter   Research Fellow and Joint Director of the Joseph Rowntree Foundation *Communicative Empowerment in Autism Project*, School of Education, University of Durham

Frances Reynolds   Lecturer in Psychology and Rehabilitation Counselling, Department of Health Studies, Brunel University, Isleworth

Richard Servian   Service Manager, Resources for Children with Disabilities, Dudley Social Services, Dudley, West Midlands

Sue Standing   Superintendent physiotherapist for people with learning disabilities, Southampton Community Health Service (NHS) Trust

John Swain   Principal Lecturer (Research) and Reader in Disability Studies, Faculty of Health, Social Work and Education, University of Northumbria, Newcastle-upon-Tyne; Associate Lecturer, Open University, Milton Keynes

Carole Thirlaway   Deputy Headteacher, Parkside School, North Tyneside

Jan Walmsley   Senior Lecturer, School of Health and Social Welfare, Open University, Milton Keynes

Clare Ward   Speech and Language Therapist, Service for People with Learning Disabilities, Camden and Islington Community Health Service (NHS) Trust, London

Tricia Webb   Project Co-ordinator, Skills for People, Key House, Tankersville Place, Newcastle-upon-Tyne

Chris Whittaker   Research Fellow and Joint Director of the Joseph Rowntree Foundation *Communicative Empowerment in Autism Project*, School of Education, University of Durham

1

Introduction: changing reflections

Sally French and John Swain

Finding a viewpoint

We set the scene in this opening chapter. We aim to provide an introduction to and rationale for the approach taken in constructing this text for occupational therapists and physiotherapists working with people with learning difficulties. Therapy with people with learning difficulties is a complex arena of competing questions: what are the purposes of therapy; what is meant by 'learning difficulties'; what implications do learning difficulties have for the provision of therapy; and what implications does therapy have for people with learning difficulties. The first answer, as in all areas of social activity, is that it depends on where you are looking from. The perspective or orientation defines what is relevant, why it is relevant and how it is relevant. There are two related key questions to be addressed in setting the scene:

● What knowledge base do professionals require in their work with people with learning difficulties?
● How can professionals develop their knowledge?

Starting with the first question, there are two quite distinct standpoints. One would begin with the notion that different types of professionals intervene in different ways and have different responsibilities. Thus, each profession requires a specific knowledge base, often medical, to inform their work. This standpoint is expressed through the provision of separate training courses and separate bodies of literature, journals and texts.

An alternative view, which we are adopting here, argues that professionals are engaging in people's lives and require a broad-based knowledge of learning difficulties and what it means to be a person with learning difficulties at the change of the millennium in Western capitalist society. This standpoint does not deny that therapists require specific skills and techniques. Nor does it imply that therapists should conceive of their work as intervening in or delving into everything about the client and the client's life as a whole. This broad-based standpoint which we have adopted in editing this book addresses the human relations of therapy and learning difficulties. Therapy and learning difficulties are constructed within: the interactions and communication between therapist and client; the roles and expectations of the therapist–client relationship; and power relations and structures within which 'therapy' and 'learning difficulties' have meaning.

Reflections

How, then, do we begin to define and map this broad-based knowledge of learning difficulties? The past two decades have seen a period of social transition in the lives of people with learning difficulties. Though for some people with learning difficulties social change has not been reflected in personal change, for many it has, not least people moving out of large institutions. Again, how such changes are perceived, and indeed whether they are seen as cosmetic or substantial, depends on the viewpoint taken.

It seems to us that three related themes underpin this period of change: advocacy, participation and partnership. Under banners such as 'user participation' the three become integrated, as participation refers to a say in decision making (self-advocacy) in partnership with professionals and service purchasers and providers. In their most radical form and positive light they constitute a vision of full active citizenship for people with learning difficulties.

These three themes recur throughout *Therapy and Learning Difficulties*. They also provide a structure for the book in the three sections, each concentrating on one of the themes, as outlined below.

Towards advocacy

The focus of the first theme and section of the book (Part I) is *advocacy*, particularly in the form of self-advocacy. Many people would argue that self-advocacy has been the most significant development for people with learning difficulties (Ward, 1995), and there are now self-advocacy groups of different kinds across the country. Some are part of the People First movement which, for instance, runs national and international conferences and offers training and publications. Through the groups, people with learning difficulties, as 'service users' or 'clients', are having a say in what they need: what sort of services they require; the support they require; and whether the services and support are meeting their needs. Clwyd People First, for instance, is a group which has been consulted as a matter of policy by the local county council (Murray, 1991). Some groups, such as Skills for People, based in Newcastle, include people with physical or sensory impairments, while others have a more specific membership, such as the Black People First group.

Labelling has been an important concern for many self-advocacy groups, and certainly all have rejected the use of the term 'mentally handicapped'. A major campaign for People First has been for the acceptance of the term 'people with learning difficulties', as opposed to 'people with learning disabilities'. It is in this light that 'people with learning difficulties' is the preferred term within this book.

Independent or citizen advocates have also spoken and acted on behalf of some people with learning difficulties. Such advocates can help people who: have difficulties expressing their case; do express their case but are not listened to by service providers; are at risk of abuse; or who are vulnerable and isolated (Swain, 1993). Advocates can also help to promote self-advocacy, and Richardson and Ritchie (1989) found that some citizen advocacy schemes give much greater emphasis on helping people to have more control over, and make decisions about, their own lives.

Perhaps the most significant development in self-advocacy in recent years, is that People First joined the British Council of Disabled People (BCODP) in 1994, the key organization of the Disabled People's Movement. This has combined the strengths of two campaigning organizations, and has also meant changes from both sides to enable this merging (Campbell and Oliver, 1996).

The voices of people with learning difficulties, as expressed verbally, non-verbally or through mediums such as creative arts, are reflected upon throughout this book. Advocacy, in its broadest sense, is the specific focus for many of the chapters in Part I, and the section as a whole is an exploration of the social and historical context in which advocacy has meaning in therapy.

Towards participation

The second theme and focus for Part II is *participation*, and the support and intervention required to enable people with learning difficulties to live and participate as full and active members of the community. For many people with learning difficulties, being in the community is indeed a significant change. However, to be 'in' and to be 'a full active member of' a community are not necessarily the same things. A similar point can be made about the integration of young people with learning difficulties into mainstream school. It is possible to be isolated and, in a sense, segregated within a mainstream school. For this reason, the term 'inclusion' has been increasingly used to denote a process of changing every aspect of mainstream schools so that they truly provide 'education for all'.

O'Brien and Lyle (1987) have provided a framework, or working philosophy, for analysing community services and service plans under the guise of 'five accomplishments', as summarized below:

- The first is the physical presence and participation of people within community settings. This includes facilities which would be available to everyone: schools, workplaces, colleges, leisure facilities, pubs, churches, ordinary houses in ordinary streets and, of course, health care services including occupational therapy and physiotherapy.
- The second is opportunities to exercise individual choice and engage in particular interests.
- The third, contributing to the lives of others, runs counter to the dominant stereotype of people with learning difficulties as dependent on others. Jan Walmsley's (1993) study of people with learning difficulties acting in the role of carers underlined the importance of the 'accomplishment'.

- Next comes the more personal accomplishments of self-esteem, dignity and respect. The last of these returns us to the theme of self-advocacy, as respect is largely conveyed through having a say and being listened to.
- The final accomplishment is having relationships with others in the community, including sustaining and widening friendships. In the Booths' (1994) study of parents with learning difficulties, they found that one of the major obstacles to participation in family life was the discriminatory attitudes of professionals and, in particular, the widespread presumption of incompetence which so often marked the response of professionals to parents with learning difficulties.

The chapters in Part II reflect a broad range of areas of social life relevant to the work of therapists with people with learning difficulties, across institutions, social relationships, identity and social policy. The coverage of the social world is necessarily selective, but the section provides an overview of the challenges and barriers to be confronted in the inclusion of people with learning difficulties as full participative citizens in society.

Towards partnership

The third and final section and theme concentrates on *partnership*. Partnership and advocacy can be seen as challenging traditional relationships between people with learning difficulties and professionals, including therapists. A principle in recent policy changes has been the idea of partnership and, as mentioned above, partnership can be closely associated with advocacy (Whittaker, 1995).

There are different definitions and models of partnership. Dale (1996) has developed a 'negotiating model' through her work with families at the KIDS Family Centre in Camden, London. This model specifically relates to parent–professional relationships, but the principles are general. The negotiating model is based on the premise that both partners have 'separate and potentially highly valuable contributions' to offer. It recognizes that the two sides of the partnership can have different perspectives, different vested interests and different social roles and expectations. Thus, the decision-making process is conceived as one of a two-way dialogue and negotiation, allowing for the possibility of extreme disagreement or conflict as well as the development of shared understanding and consensus.

Elements of this model can be seen in the 'principles of practice' for partnerships which support self-advocacy put forward by Brechin and Swain:

1 be an entitlement rather than an imposition;
2 promote self-realization rather than compliance;
3 open up choices rather than replace one option with another;
4 develop opportunities, relationships and patterns of living, in line with individual wishes rather than rule-of-thumb normality;
5 enhance people's decision-making control of their own lives;
6 allow people to move at their own pace. (1989: 51)

Notions of partnership are examined in Part III in terms of the practice of therapy. Towell states:

> ... fundamental change in the position of people with learning disabilities in our society cannot be achieved by government on its own, by local agencies and paid staff on their own, by people and their families on their own, or by communities on their own. Rather progress requires all to become partners in informed action. (1998: xiii)

Therapists have a role to play in fundamental change, but, as explored in Part III, as partners in addressing the challenges of advocacy and participation.

Reflecting on reflections

We return to the second key question raised at the start of this chapter: how can professionals develop their knowledge base? Advocacy, participation and partnership challenge theory and practice in the provision of therapy. They have implications for:

- the organization of services;
- the aims of therapy;
- the role of the therapist;
- the client–therapist relationship;
- the evaluation of therapy.

It is in responding to and supporting advocacy, participation and partnership that therapists can develop their knowledge base. It is in this context that therapists can reflect critically on the provision of therapy.

Such a critical examination of professional practice underpins a 'reflective practitioner' approach to professional development (Schön, 1983). A more traditional approach to developing a knowledge base involves the therapist learning skills and strategies for achieving his or her own aims and objectives for therapy. The therapeutic context is designed and managed so that the therapist is in control of the factors he or she sees as relevant. The task of therapy is owned and controlled by the therapist. In contrast, a reflective practitioner approach involves the design and management of therapy in which all the participants have a say in controlling relevant factors. Learning is multifaceted and involves critical reflection on experiences, recognizing other perspectives and working with rather than on people. Williams captures the challenge to professionals as follows:

> 'To recognize clients' experiential knowledge as the foundation for learning, with the professional's expert knowledge at the *service* of the client. For professionals who have trained for many years to acquire a body of expert knowledge, who have passed examinations to gain qualifications and entry to the profession, to challenge the pre-eminence of their professional base constitutes a grave threat. It removes power from them and hands it over to the client; and locates their base of knowledge with their clients rather than with their professional body. (1993: 12)

From this critical stance it can be recognized that terms such as 'advocacy', 'partnership' and 'participation' can be used by professionals, service providers and purchasers to screen real conflicts of interest and a lack of real changes in power relations and structures. This is particularly apparent in the widespread use of the term 'empowerment' in conceiving changes in the approach of professionals. As Servian (1996) points out, it is a term that has different meanings to different people. In principle, it refers to a shift in power towards those who receive therapy, often involving, at its simplest, greater choice for clients.

The notion of empowerment is problematic in a number of respects, however. Oliver, for instance, suggests that empowerment is not something that is done by professionals to disabled people:

> It is often assumed that empowerment is a process by which those in society who have power can dispense some of their power to those who don't have any . . . However, it is more realistic to see empowerment as a collective process on which the powerless embark as part of their struggle to resist the oppression of others and/or to articulate their own views of the world. (1993: 24)

Gomm questions the reality of the supposed power shifts involved in empowerment:

> Those people who say that they are in the business of empowering rarely seem to be giving up their own power; they are usually giving up someone else's and they may actually be increasing their own . . . the term 'empowerment' designates many excellent practices, and some dubious ones, but exactly what they are, and who is doing what to whom, is hidden by its usage. (1993: 137)

Servian conducted a study of perceptions of power that carers, users, workers and managers have in health and social services for people with learning difficulties. The findings suggested that the exercise of power is characterized by contradictions and tensions, rather than the principle of empowerment being put into practice. He found, for instance, 'little evidence of a shared view of what empowerment is, or of a shared value of the importance of empowerment' (1996: 37)

Conclusion

This book, then, is for physiotherapists and occupational therapists who wish to review and develop their knowledge base in their work with people with learning difficulties. We have selected the content to offer a broad base of knowledge rather than concentrating on specific skills and techniques. We have, similarly, selected authors with a range of backgrounds. The voices of therapists are represented, but so too are the voices of other professionals (from areas such as education and social work), carers, researchers and people with learning difficulties themselves.

The last words of this introductory chapter are from a self-advocate:

Working with staff to change services is about people recognising our abilities and working with us as partners. It is about giving us choices. It is important to get our voice heard, to let the world know what we are all about and to get our messages across to purchasers and providers. (In Whittaker, 1995: 184)

References

Booth, T. and Booth, W. (1994) *Parenting Under Pressure: Mothers and Fathers with Learning Difficulties*, Open University Press, Buckingham

Brechin, A. and Swain, J. (1989) Creating a 'working alliance' with people with learning difficulties. In Brechin, A. and Walmsley, J. (eds), *Making Connections*, Hodder and Stoughton, Sevenoaks

Campbell, J. and Oliver, M. (1996) *Disability Politics: Understanding Our Past, Changing Our Future*, Routledge, London

Dale, N. (1996) *Working with Families of Children with Special Needs: Partnership and Practice*, Routledge, London

Gomm, R. (1993) Issues of power in health and welfare. In Walmsley, J. *et al.* (eds), *Health, Welfare and Practice: Reflecting on Roles and Relationships*, Sage in association with The Open University, London

Murray, N. (1991) In the driving seat, *Social Work Today*, 10 October

O'Brien, J. and Lyle, C. (1987) *Framework for Accomplishment: A Workshop for People Developing Better Services*, Responsive Systems Associates.

Oliver, M. (1993) *Disability, Citizenship and Empowerment*, Workbook 2 of the course (K665) 'The Disabling Society', Open University Press, Milton Keynes

Richardson, A. and Ritchie, J. (1989) *Developing Friendships: Enabling People With Learning Difficulties to Make and Maintain Friends*. Policy Studies Institute, London

Schön, D. (1983) *The Reflective Practitioner*, Basic Books, New York

Servian, R. (1996) *Theorising Empowerment: Individual Power and Community Care*, The Policy Press, Bristol

Swain, J. (1993) *Working Together for Citizenship*, Update Workbook of the course (P555U) 'Mental Handicap: Patterns for Living', Open University Press, Milton Keynes

Towell, D. (1998) Forward. In Felce, D. *et al.* (eds), *Towards a Full Life*, Butterworth-Heinemann, Oxford

Walmsley, J. (1993) Contradictions in caring: reciprocity and interdependence. *Disability, Handicap and Society*, 8(2) 129–141

Ward, L. (1995) Equal citizens: current issues for people with learning difficulties and their allies. In Philpot, T. and Ward, L. (eds), *Values and Visions: Changing Ideas in Services for People with Learning Difficulties*, Butterworth-Heinemann, Oxford

Whittaker, A. (1995) Partnership in practice: user participation in services for people with learning difficulties. In Philpot, T. and Ward, L. (eds), *Values and Visions: Changing Ideas in Services for People with Learning Difficulties*, Butterworth-Heinemann, Oxford

Williams, J. (1993) What is a profession? Experience versus expertise. In Walmsley, J. *et al.* (eds), *Health, Welfare and Practice: Reflecting on Roles and Relationships*, Sage in association with The Open University, London

Part I

Towards Advocacy: Differing Viewpoints and Changing Times

An old story

Dorothy Atkinson

Introduction

Why tell an old story? It is 'old' only in the sense that it goes back a long way in time. In many ways, and to many people, it is a *new story*. The history of learning disability is important to people with learning difficulties themselves, as it is their history. It is also important to people who live, or work, alongside people with learning disabilities, including therapists.

The history of learning disability is still to be told in all its complexity. Although the process has started in a small way, with some people with learning disabilities beginning to tell their personal stories, there is still a long way to go. This chapter looks at the history of learning disability as it is emerging through the life stories of people with learning disability. The message which comes from these stories is that history matters. It matters both at a personal and a social level. It brings understanding to all of us, but, to the people most centrally concerned, it brings a sense of personal and group identity.

How do life stories come to be told? It is not easy for people without ready recourse to the written (and sometimes the spoken) word to tell their stories. People with learning disabilities need support, practical and emotional, in order to do so. There is a role here for therapists, and other practitioners, in recognizing that everyone has a story to tell and in *listening* to that story. Being listened to may be the first step in the telling of the life story and the reclaiming of identity.

Searching for the past

Some of it, like the names they called you in them days, that hurt a little bit, but otherwise I think it was great.

This is Mabel Cooper talking about her quest to uncover her past. Like many other people with learning difficulties throughout this century, she has spent much of her life in a long-stay hospital. She remembered those days only too well – but what had gone before? Who was she? And how did she come to live in a large mental handicap hospital? The quest to find out more has taken Mabel and myself into the offices of the Lifecare Trust, the London Metropolitan Archives and the Bedfordshire County Record Office in search of the documented past.

The search has been revealing. It has disclosed the names used in the past, many of which have now passed into everyday use as terms of abuse. It was a salutary moment for Mabel to find in her records that such terms had been applied to her younger self. The story itself, of loss, separation and segregation, represents the history of exclusion of people with learning difficulties, particularly in this century. The overriding view from Mabel, however, is that it is 'great' to know about oneself, and to know about the past – in spite of the words used and the messages they conveyed.

This chapter will look at the history of exclusion of people with learning difficulties. It takes many forms, not least the exclusion of people from their own life stories. Many (if not most) people with learning difficulties who have lived in long-stay institutions have little if any access to, or knowledge of, their prior lives. This leaves people vulnerable to having their history told for them by others, including therapists (Gillman *et al.*, 1997). The 'case history', as it then becomes, may be built on myths and hearsay, and may perpetuate reputations best forgotten. A good way to counteract any such misrepresentation is through the telling of the story by, and with, the person concerned. All people working in the field, including therapists, have a potential role in this process.

The life story may be told entirely from memory. This was the case in my oral history project, where a group of older people with learning difficulties came together to tell their individual and shared stories. (I return, below, to this project, and the stories which emerged from it.) This was also Mabel Cooper's starting point and her (then) life story was published in a book on the history of learning disability (Cooper, 1997). Now she is reviewing, and revising, that version of her life in the light of our subsequent findings from contemporary written records. There is no doubt that the two approaches of oral and documented history, separately or together, could enable many more people – with support – to tell their life stories and, in the process, to help reveal the largely 'hidden history' of learning disability (Atkinson, 1997).

Revealing the hidden history of learning disability

The all-pervasive exclusion of people with learning difficulties from everyday life has meant that they have been silent, or in effect *silenced*, for much of the century. They do speak now and, to an ever increasing degree, they are heard, but this is a late twentieth century phenomenon. They were, until recently, silent and, in their silence, other people spoke for – or against – them (Ryan and Thomas, 1980).

In the early years of this century, people with learning difficulties were thought to be a threat to society. They were viewed as a main source of poverty, crime, drunkenness and other social ills of the time. Not only this but, if they were not stopped, they were seen as likely to produce subsequent generations of similarly afflicted people. These views were based on the arguments of the eugenics movement, and were influential in the fate of many people with learning difficulties who found themselves segregated from everyone else in society until they were literally out of earshot. They were thus effectively silenced. As 'deficit' theories (the measurement of differences) came into vogue first in medicine and psychology, but later in education, people were seen as cases to be treated or specially trained. The voices of people themselves were replaced by their case histories, prepared by others on their behalf (a situation which still persists in learning disability practice, according to Gillman *et al.*, 1997).

As social theories came into fashion from the 1960s and 1970s onwards, people with learning difficulties were represented not as the perpetrators of social problems but as the victims of societal oppression. Now at the end of the century their own voices are increasingly being heard. Neither 'villains' nor 'victims', in their own accounts they are each individuals with a personal history, a culture, a class and a gender (Atkinson and Williams, 1990).

Some of the earliest opportunities to speak out came with the CMH-sponsored participation workshops in the 1970s (CMH refers to the Campaign for People with Mental Handicaps; now known as Values Into Action, or VIA). These gave at least a few people with learning difficulties the chance to speak of their experiences, including the segregated lives they had led in the long-stay hospitals. The 1980s saw the formation of self-advocacy groups, People First organizations and groups/committees in day and residential services. These developments were given a further boost with the National Health Service and Community Care Act 1990, with its emphasis on user participation and involvement.

Self-advocacy has encouraged people to 'speak up' about their experiences; not as villains, cases, victims, burdens or joys but as *people*, with a whole range of experiences, views and characteristics. Clearly people with learning difficulties are not a homogeneous group. Individual lives and experiences reveal differences between people in terms of their gender, class, and social and cultural background. And yet people also have a lot of things in common too – with each other and with all of us. Bogdan and Taylor (1982) have written passionately about that common humanity which links us all, including people with learning difficulties.

One important link which people with learning difficulties share together, and which links them with people from other social groups, is the labelling process by which they are seen, categorized and treated as different from 'ordinary' people. This is a social process which operates in relation to other marginalized groups too – other disabled people, black people, women and mental health service survivors, for example. On this basis, people with learning difficulties can be seen as an oppressed group in society – one which has things in common with other oppressed groups. The 'converging stereotypes' which cut across these different oppressed social groups mean that they come to be seen – perhaps at different moments in time – in very similar ways (Williams, 1993). Not only people with learning difficulties, therefore, but also black people and working class women, have been seen as irrational, volatile, irresponsible, excitable, childlike and possessing a hidden but dangerous sexuality.

One way of countering such stereotypes is to encourage the development of people's own life stories, as they can act very effectively as a counterbalancing force to the generalizations which otherwise persist. It is through people's own accounts of their lives and histories that an overall history can start to be written about the oppression and exclusion of people with learning difficulties. If written from their point of view, such a collective version of a shared history could do much to counteract the prevailing official accounts.

In the meantime, however, individual life stories remain important. They can enable us to get to know people with learning difficulties from 'the inside' (Bogdan and Taylor, 1982). The developments in self-advocacy, and life story work, have shown that people have the capacity to express themselves and to make sense of their lives. When people tell their stories, they allow us to look at life through their eyes, as people who have been labelled, and to see their world as they see and experience it. The individual life story, and the collections of various life stories (see, for example, in this context the anthology *Know Me As I Am*, Atkinson and Williams, 1990) can begin to challenge the many myths which surround people with learning difficulties.

Words which exclude

This chapter adopts the terms in current use; thus 'learning disability' is used instead of its forerunners 'mental deficiency', 'mental subnormality' and 'mental handicap'. And the phrase 'people with learning difficulties' replaces the designations used throughout the course of this century: 'idiot', 'imbecile', 'feeble-minded', 'moral defective', 'subnormal', 'severely subnormal' and 'mentally handicapped'. The terms have supplanted each other in rapid succession in what Joanna Ryan suggests is 'an illusory search for a designation that is neutral or euphemistic' (Ryan and Thomas, 1980: 11). The search is illusory because the process of labelling itself identifies and creates social distance between people. As learning disability is usually seen negatively, so people themselves come to be viewed and treated negatively, whatever the terminology used; except, that is, where they speak for, and represent, themselves in their own words and through their own stories. The history of changing terminology is, however, one important aspect of the history of exclusion of people with learning difficulties.

The terminology of 'learning difficulties' emerged from self-advocacy groups and is the term preferred and most widely used by people who call themselves *people with learning difficulties* (or a person with a learning difficulty). This term has been quite widely adopted, for example in the 1995 Open University course, 'Working with Equal People' and by organizations such as the Central Council for Education and Training in Social Work (CCETSW) and Values Into Action (VIA). However, in recent years the alternative term of *learning disability* has emerged from government guidelines and policy documents. This lends itself to the phrase *people with learning disabilities* (or a person with a learning disability). The terminology of 'learning disability' has found favour in professional circles in particular, but it is also beginning to find some acceptance in People First circles.

In a sense, both terms are problematic. They both locate 'the problem' as being in the person, rather than being socially constructed. They both suggest that 'the problem' will be resolved only through enhanced learning on the part of the individual and not by changes within a wider social and political framework. This is in contrast with the wider disability movement which reverses the order of words to 'disabled people'. This is intended to emphasize that, whatever the nature of the original impairment, people are effectively 'disabled' by a society which not only fails to include them in the mainstream of everyday life but actually excludes them through social and physical barriers.

Whatever their limitations, though, the terms 'learning difficulties' and 'learning disability' represent a major advance on what has gone before. For the first time in history, the language of policy makers and practitioners is acceptable to those whom it seeks to describe. Both terms coexisted for a while with the terminology of 'mental handicap'. This lent itself to the phrase 'mentally handicapped people' (or even 'the mentally handicapped') but this was later softened to 'people with mental handicap(s)' (or a person with a mental handicap). In the 1970s and 1980s 'mental handicap' was the official medical and administrative term and was widely used. It is still sometimes added in parentheses to people with learning difficulties/disabilities (mental handicap) to clarify the group being referred to. Other than that, the term has largely disappeared from everyday use, though with two notable exceptions. The major national charity MENCAP still reflects the term in its title, and RESCARE, an organization of parents which seeks to halt the hospital closure programme and the resettlement of people with learning difficulties in the community, still pointedly refer to their sons and daughters as 'mentally handicapped'.

The Mental Health Act 1983 coined the phrase 'mental impairment' but this never found general favour. One of the problems with this term was that it continued the use of the word 'mental'. This has been largely rejected by the people to whom it referred and most agencies and organizations acting on their behalf. The use of the word 'mental' has also tended to reinforce the general public confusion between mental handicap and mental health/illness.

In its time, mental handicap was seen as an advance on earlier terminology. It was introduced in 1971 to replace the widely discredited term 'subnormal' or 'mentally subnormal', with its connotations of people who are somehow seen as 'subhuman' or less than human. 'Subnormality' became the official medical and administrative term following the Mental Health Act 1959. It, in turn, replaced the terms 'mental deficiency' and 'mental defective' (and the sub-categories of 'idiot', 'imbecile', 'feeble-minded' and 'moral defective') which had been introduced by the Mental Deficiency Act 1913, and which had prevailed until then – terminology which had remained unchanged for almost 50 years.

Mabel Cooper was admitted to St Lawrence's Hospital in Caterham, under the terms of the Mental Deficiency Act 1913. She had no idea of this at the time, and it is only through our search for her recorded history that she has found this out. It was the terminology of this legislation which she said had 'hurt a bit'. Terms can and do become labels which group people together. And yesterday's labels can all too easily become today's terms of abuse. The following poem by some people with learning difficulties (their term) graphically illustrates this point:

Tell them the truth

There goes the mongol up the street
Getting on the looneybus
The schoolbairns call
Making funny faces at us
Calling us names
Headcase, spassy, wally
Nutter, Dylan, Twit!

There goes the dumb-bell into the nuthouse!
The schoolbairns are all daft themselves
They should see a psychiatrist
About their brains
It makes you mad, it boils up your blood
Their wooden heads are full of nonsense.

They've got nothing else to do
Except make fun of us
We are human beings
And should be treated as equals
Treated as adults
Tell them the truth.
    (St Clair Centre, Kirkcaldy: from the anthology, *Know Me As I Am*,
                                    Atkinson and Williams, 1990)

This poem makes important points. It is a statement by people with learning difficulties about how, in reality, they are seen and treated, and how they want to be seen as human beings, equal to and respected by other people. The reclaiming of people's life stories is one way of demonstrating their equality and gaining the respect of others.

Stories of exclusion

The Mental Deficiency Act 1913 established the basis of a separate and unified service which was intended to exclude mentally deficient people from other welfare and social agencies, and to bar them from the general educational system. The policies of exclusion thus set in train have operated, one way and another, for much of this century. An energetic nationwide crusade for most, it not all, mental defectives to be institutionalized for life – 'for their protection and the protection of others' – had been influential in the passing of the Act. As a result, the Act required local authorities to certify all mental defectives and set up special certified institutions. The drive to institutionalization was based, according to Fido and Potts (1989), on the overriding fear that the feeble-minded would 'repeat their type', resulting in the 'propagation of a degenerate stock'. There was a particular concern about young feeble-minded women, as they were presumed to be more immoral and fertile than other women (Atkinson and Walmsley, 1995; Digby, 1996).

The first step to detainment and institutionalization was certification, involving the assessment of people according to three levels of defect: idiot, imbecile and feeble-minded, together with a catch-all category of moral defective. This latter category was used to detain many people, often adolescents, on account of minor offences, like petty thefts or having an illegitimate baby. Many thousands of lives were touched, and changed, by the Mental Deficiency Act 1913. They included the nine older people with learning difficulties who joined my oral history group to share their experiences of those past times.

The group members told many stories of exclusion. Such stories often started, though, as personal accounts of separation or loss in someone's life. Often the loss, whatever it was, proved to be the turning point which determined that, sooner or later, that person would be labelled as 'mentally detective', and would pursue a separate path though life. Although that separate path could well lead someone into 'institutional care', this was by no means a universal experience. Even at the height of institutionalization most people with learning difficulties continued to live in the community. Two members of my group had lived with their families well into adult life. Even so, they too revealed their own stories of exclusion; from school, work and parenthood, for example.

Most people in the oral history group, though, had experienced exclusion from the community through incarceration in a long-stay institution. George Coley, for example, remembered how, as a young man, he was taken early one morning to Bromham Hospital in Bedfordshire. This was a move which was to change his life completely. His immediate losses were considerable. As well as losing his home and his father, his photographs and his cigarette card collection, he lost his girlfriend, Gwendoline, and never saw her again. This is how George portrayed these momentous events in his life:

> My mother died, then later on I went into hospital. I had bad nerves. I had St Vitus's dance. I'm better now. I was in Bromham Hospital, between Northampton and Bedford. Then we went to Hasells Hall. From there we went to Fairfield Hospital.
>
> I was in Bromham 20 years. I went there in 1938, March 3rd.
>
> I ain't got any photos. I had ever so many at home before I went to Bromham but, you know, I didn't have time because the people who came to fetch me came so bloomin' early in the morning. I wasn't ready to go!
>
> When I was at home, of course, I only smoked tobacco. I hadn't many fag cards at home. My tin wasn't very big – I used to put them in a tin – and I said to my father, when I was going to Bromham, I said, 'I'll take them to Bromham with me, I might get something for them'. But of course the person that took me to Bromham, he came early...

> I used to have a girl, a nice girl, Gwendoline. She lived not far from my mother and father, in one of the council houses. I lost her when I went away.

George's life changed dramatically on 3rd March 1938, a date he has remembered all his life. He had lived, until then, with his father in the village in which he was born. He has, therefore, a wealth of memories of the very different life which he had led before he went to hospital. The lives of some of the other group members, by way of contrast, had sometimes taken a different course. Bill Baker, for example, lost his home and family as a child. His life changed when his mother died. He was 10 years old, and he was sent to a residential school. This is what Bill told us in the group:

> My mother died when I was ten, it was a shame. It was her chest. She was an old lady, getting on. We had a big family. I have three brothers and a sister, Nellie, but I don't worry about them. I lived at Kingsmead School. I got visited once a month. Dad was in the army, then he was a car park attendant. He used to come and see me once a month. I had to work hard. My sister Nellie came and told me when Dad died. I was at Kingsmead School then.
> In 1934, I went to Cell Barnes. I was 14. I left Cell Barnes in 1954, then I went to Hasells Hall.

Unfortunately for Bill, his father died during the time he was away at school. Not only did he lose his surviving parent, and his only visitor, he lost the possibility of ever returning home. He went instead to Cell Barnes, the first of several long-stay hospitals in which he was to spend much of his life (this later included Hasells Hall, an annexe of Bromham Hospital, Bedfordshire). He lost touch with Nellie and his brothers from that point on, a loss he still feels keenly even though he says 'I don't worry about them'. In their oral history of 'The Park' colony in the north of England, Potts and Fido remark on how often people who had lost touch with their families would say 'I'm not bothered about them' or 'I'm not worried about them'. They suggest this is a way of coping with a loss which actually does matter and *is* a worry (Potts and Fido, 1991).

What happened when group members entered the enclosed world of the long-stay hospital? Here Margaret Day recalls what it was like for her following her admission to Bromham Hospital at the age of 16, in 1938:

> I thought how big it was, and they were building a lot of new wards. I was on F1 and then I moved to F2. I ran away from there. The sister on the ward didn't like me and I didn't like her. I was there 20 years and I was always scrubbing. After 20 years we changed over. I went to F4 the children's ward, the babies' ward. We had a sister down there who I used to get on with,
> Sister Smith was on F2. When I was in the stores one day, there was a lot of mats and Smith said I had to clean 'em all. So I threw 'em at her! And she fell over! She put me in punishment there. I ran away from F2. We hid in a haystack and got frost-bitten feet. I ran away with another girl and caught yellow jaundice.

> The sister would keep on at me, saying my work wasn't done properly. She was being horrible. I'd scrubbed the ward and she said I had to do it over again! I said, 'Well I aren't going to do it over again!' I told the doctor. He come round and he wanted to know what I was doing on the stairs again. I said, 'I've been told I've got to do it again, it wasn't done properly'.

As well as recalling particular incidents, such as throwing the mats at Sister Smith, rescrubbing an already well-scrubbed ward and talking to the doctor on the stairs, Margaret's story ranges over many years of misery. This was not just an odd unhappy week in her life, this *was* her life. She was at Bromham for 36 years in all, but spent 20 years on a ward where she, and the all-powerful Sister Smith, did not get on. Margaret spent 20 years of her life scrubbing floors, a job which she hated. Each act of defiance on her part led to being 'put in punishment', which meant yet more scrubbing.

The story was told in the oral history group, so at least it was told to a sympathetic and supportive audience. Other people listened with respect and shared some of Margaret's sadness. After the telling it was written down in the group's own private publication, *Past Times* (Atkinson, 1993). It has appeared elsewhere (Atkinson, 1997), as well as here, the overall effect being that this story, and others, will be heard more widely. This is what the group intended; that other people would know what an institutional regime, in all its harshness, really meant for the person who had to endure it.

Reclaiming the past

People with learning difficulties are, of course, much more than the victims of oppression and the policies of exclusion. In the telling of their stories they also reclaim a past which is shared with the rest of us; memories, for example, of family life, of friendship, of period dress, popular songs and the major events of the twentieth century. The oral history group talked about their schooldays, and shared their memories of parks, picnics and fairgrounds. Marbles and mangles, catapults and cigarette cards, and many more rich details of the past, were revealed in the group. This was where their memories came close to mine, where our experiences were shared and differences ceased to matter.

In the telling of her life story, Mabel Cooper talks about the difference between her life and the lives of others. But she also talks about the similarities. Her life now, in the community, stands in stark contrast with her life in hospital. She is reclaiming the past and, in so doing, is also claiming the present. Her life revolves around family and friends, the joys of travel and the everyday business of living a full life. As she says at the end of her published life story: 'A lot of people might not like it, some of them not at all, but I'm quite happy as I am' (Cooper, 1997: 34).

Mabel Cooper enjoys her life now. She is 'quite happy', not only because her life has been transformed in so many ways – materially, socially and emotionally – but also because she now knows who she is. She has found out about her family, including her parents and grandparents; and she knows now how she came to be certified under the Mental Deficiency Act 1913 and to spend 20 years of her young life in St Lawrence's Hospital. The telling of her story from memory was an important milestone in reclaiming the past, as Mabel has elsewhere explained:

> I think it was nice for me to be able to do something, so that I could say 'I've done it'. It made me feel that it was something I had done. You've got something so that you can say, 'This is what happened to me'. Some of it hurts, some of it's sad, some of it I'd like to remember. My story means a lot to me because I can say, 'This is what happened to me', if anyone asks. So it's great, and I will keep it for the rest of my life. I will keep the book. (Atkinson *et al.*, 1997: 11)

The subsequent finding out about the documented past from case records, institutional diaries, history books, press cuttings and the like has proved at times to be an upsetting experience but one which nevertheless was an enlightening and empowering process. Reclaiming the past means more even than claiming the present – for Mabel Cooper it has meant claiming her identity. It means in effect that she can not only know the past, and understand it, but she can challenge it. This is how Mabel put these points to me during one of our discussions about the past:

> It was something I needed to find out. And I'd rather know than not know. I think if you don't know then it isn't fair, it's not the same as knowing. So, for me, I'd rather know. I went to St Lawrence's and went through their records, to see how I was put in St Lawrence's and all the rest of it, and then going to the archives, that was great again, that was somewhere I'd never been.
> For me, it did upset me for them to say I wasn't teachable. I think if someone goes around and says something like that, are you going to learn? You're not because they're still going to say, 'Oh, you're not teachable'. And for them to say, you know, I needed to be looked after, trained for life, I don't know who made that decision. Who makes those assumptions?

Conclusion

It is good that Mabel Cooper has had the opportunity to describe her life, to reflect on it and to think about it in relation to other lives. With this has come her own developing historical awareness of how past ideas and policies (and labels) impinged on her and changed her life. In the telling and the retelling of her story, Mabel has demonstrated how important it is for people with learning difficulties to have and to own a history which is theirs.

There are, however, 'many more stories still to be told and voices yet to be heard' (Atkinson and Williams, 1990: 244). The challenge is for people, including therapists, who work with those with learning difficulties to play their part in the telling of more stories. What is that part? Therapists are well placed, through their work and in their relationships with people with learning disabilities, to play an active part in the telling of stories.

This starts with recognizing that everyone has a personal past, and acknowledging and respecting that past. It goes further: it means listening to the life story when it is told; helping, where possible, with the telling and the researching of that story; and recording the present sensitively, so that today's stories are recorded for the future in ways that people themselves approve.

The process of life story-telling may hurt a bit, as Mabel has warned, but ultimately it is a great thing to do.

(For further information on the history of learning difficulties the reader is referred to Chapter 3.)

References

Atkinson, D. (1993) *Past Times*, Milton Keynes, private publication.

Atkinson, D. (1997) *An Auto/Biographical Approach to Learning Disability Research*, Ashgate, Aldershot

Atkinson, D., Jackson, M and Walmsley, J. (1997) Introduction: methods and themes. In Atkinson, D. *et al.* (eds), *Forgotten Lives. Exploring the History of Learning Disability*, British Institute of Learning Disability Publications, Kidderminster

Atkinson, D. and Walmsley, J. (1995) A woman's place? Issues of gender. In Philipot, T. and Ward, L. (eds), *Values and Visions. Changing Ideas in Services for People with Learning Difficulties*, Butterworth-Heinemann, Oxford

Atkinson, D. and Williams, F. (1990) *'Know Me As I Am'. An Anthology of Prose, Poetry and Art by People with Learning Difficulties*, Hodder and Stoughton, London (in association with the Open University Press)

Bogdan, R. and Taylor, S.J. (1982) *Inside Out: The Social Meaning of Retardation*, Toronto, University of Toronto Press

Cooper, M. (1997) Mabel Cooper's life story. In Atkinson, D. *et al.* (eds), *Forgotten Lives. Exploring the History of Learning Disability*, British Institute of Learning Disability Publications, Kidderminster

Digby, A. (1996) 'Contexts and perspectives. In Wright, D. and Digby, A. (eds), *From Idiocy to Mental Deficiency. Historical Perspectives on People with Learning Disabilities*, Routledge, London

Fido, R. and Potts, M. (1989) 'It's not true what was written down!' Experiences of Life in a Mental Handicap Institution. *Oral History*, **17**(2), 31–34

Gillman, M., Swain, J. and Heyman, B. (1997) 'Life' history or 'Case' history: the objectification of people with learning difficulties through the tyranny of professional discourses'. *Disability and Society*, **12**(5), 675–693

Potts, M. and Fido, R. (1991) *'A Fit Person to Be Removed': Personal Accounts of Life in a Mental Deficiency Institution*, Northcote House, Plymouth

Ryan, J. with Thomas, F. (1980) *The Politics of Mental Handicap*, Penguin, Harmondsworth

Williams, F. (1993) *Social Policy, Social Divisions and Social Change*, unpublished PhD thesis, Open University

3

A historical review of learning difficulties, remedial therapy and the rise of the professional therapist

Jean Barclay

Introduction

This brief professional history aims to give occupational therapists and physiotherapists an insight into the roots of one aspect of their work – remedial therapy for people with learning difficulties. The chapter covers the terminology of learning difficulties; hospitals and remedial therapy; the move to community care and the rise of the physiotherapy and occupational therapy professions. Only in recent years have numbers of remedial therapists entered the learning difficulty field and the chapter ends by discussing the possible reasons for this.

Physiotherapy is the treatment of disease, injury, deformity or disability by such physical methods as massage, heat, exercise, hydrotherapy and electrotherapy. Occupational therapy is the treatment of disease, injury, deformity or disability by regulated courses of work or training. Although physiotherapists have traditionally treated bodily ills and occupational therapists have had a larger psychiatric component in their training and routine, both work in either field today, often as colleagues in multidisciplinary teams providing clients with individual packages of care.

The terminology of learning difficulties

The term 'learning difficulties' is the latest manifestation of an ever-changing terminology, which includes many words that sound stigmatizing today but were once common parlance. The terminology reflects the perceptions of successive generations, which have ranged from believing that 'simple' people were in the grip of demons to seeing them as children of God – hence the name 'cretin' from the French for Christian (Hallas *et al.*, 1982).

Historically, the difference between the various types of learning difficulty or even between learning difficulty and mental illness was far from clear, and the words 'idiot', 'imbecile' and 'lunatic' tended to be used indiscriminately. The Idiots Act 1886, which allowed local authorities to set up special asylums, clarified an old misunderstanding by stating categorically that 'idiots' and 'imbeciles' were not 'lunatics'. The Mental Deficiency Act 1913 identified and defined four classes of 'mental defective'. Idiots, imbeciles and the feeble-minded formed three grades of rising intelligence, while the fourth category was the 'moral imbecile' who had 'some permanent mental defect coupled with strong vicious or criminal propensities on which punishment had little or no effect'. The Mental Deficiency Act 1927 replaced 'moral imbecile' with 'moral defective'.

In the wake of local government and mental health legislation in 1929–30, 'asylums' became 'hospitals' and 'lunatics' became 'persons of unsound mind', but the term 'mental defective' survived until the end of the 1950s, as did the official terms 'idiot' (IQ below 20–25); 'imbecile' (20–50) and 'feeble-minded' (50–70) (Bone *et al.*, 1972). The Mental Health Act 1959 used the term 'mental disorder' to cover both mental illness and learning difficulties and replaced the four mental deficiency classes of earlier legislation with 'severe subnormality', 'subnormality' and 'psychopathic disorder'.

Following the Government White Paper 'Better Services for the Mentally Handicapped' of 1971, 'mental handicap', which might be mild, moderate or severe, came into use, while the Mental Health Act 1983 introduced 'mental impairment' and 'severe mental impairment'. In the early 1990s, in keeping with the community care and 'people first' ethos of official publications and of the Community Care Act 1990, the term 'mentally handicapped' was rejected in favour of 'people with learning disabilities' or, as is preferred in this book, 'people with learning difficulties'.

The founding of institutions

In pre-industrial Europe most people with learning difficulties lived at home in the rural community, where some were lovingly cared for like Wordsworth's 'Idiot Boy' but many were badly treated. A number lived in poorhouses or in religious houses, where the more able people could work for their keep.

The development of therapy went hand in hand with the spread of institutions, particularly training schools for so-called 'imbecile children', who might be in their teens or twenties. In 1828 the first such school was opened in Paris by Dr Ferrus, chief physician at the Bicêtre Asylum, and others followed, not only in Paris but in Berlin, Leipzig and near Interlaken in the Swiss mountains (Hallas *et al.*, 1982).

In early-Victorian Britain, large numbers of 'imbeciles' were accommodated in the new public lunatic asylums, in Poor Law workhouses or in prisons. The first special accommodation appears to have been a small private home in Bath opened in 1846 by the Misses White. Park House Asylum was founded in Highgate, London, in 1847 and moved to Surrey in 1855 where it was relaunched by Prince Albert as the Earlswood Asylum (Brady, 1865).

Earlswood was one of five regional asylums, each accommodating about 500 patients in the early years but growing to more than twice that size. In 1850 the Park House committee opened an institution in Essex Hall, near Colchester, which became the Eastern Counties Asylum. The Western Counties Institution followed at Starcross near Exeter in 1864; the Midland Counties Institution at Knowle near Birmingham in 1868; and in 1870 the Royal Albert Asylum for the northern counties at Lancaster, which accommodated 600 young male patients whose fees, like those at the other institutions, were paid by family or by their Poor Law union (Douglas, 1899, 1910).

Voluntary effort in Scotland led to the founding of several asylum-schools, including the Baldovan Institution near Dundee in 1852 and The Scottish National Institution for the Education of Imbecile Children at Larbert near Falkirk in 1863. In the wake of the Lunacy Act (Scotland) 1857, which covered all types of mental disorder, several institutions (like Larbert) were founded and a system of supervised 'boarding-out' with relatives or responsible strangers began. Although this system was widely used on the Continent, notably at Gheel in Belgium, in Britain only Scotland used it to any extent and in 1907 maintained about 20 per cent of its dependent 'insane' population in this way (Cunyngham Brown, 1908).

The first public (rate-supported) institution was the Darenth Asylum for Idiots in Kent, which was opened in 1877 by the Metropolitan Asylums Board as training schools for 500 children. Blocks for adults followed and by 1900 there were 2260 inmates. In 1911 the name was changed to the Darenth Colony for the Industrial Training of Improvable Imbeciles, 'colony' being the buzz-word of the era. Like the colonies overseas, the new institutions were intended to be self-contained, self-supporting communities where people with a shared problem could work together for the common good (Spensley, 1913; Korman and Glennerster, 1985).

The nineteenth century movement to institutionalize children and young people with learning difficulties prevailed throughout the Western world. Eugenic theories in Britain influenced the founding of the National Association for the Feeble-Minded in 1896 which had the twin aims of protection and control, including the control of reproduction. In 1902, at the instigation of Miss Mary Dendy, a Manchester educationalist, the Lancashire and Cheshire Society for the Permanent Care of the Feeble-Minded opened the Sandlebridge Colony, in Cheshire – soon renamed the Mary Dendy Homes – where more than 400 patients could stay for life (Jones, 1960).

The Mental Deficiency Act 1913 led to increased provision and by the end of 1914 there were 38 certified institutions, the largest being the five regional asylums. But demand still exceeded supply and of an estimated 175 000 mentally deficient adults in Britain in 1929, only 10 per cent were patients in mental deficiency hospitals, while 25 per cent were in mental hospitals and 39 per cent in workhouses. More hospitals and colonies were added in the interwar years and by 1950 there were 53. A peak of 61 439 patients was reached in 1955 but further peaks were to follow as patients were admitted for short-term care (Jones, 1960).

Isolated in the country and surrounded by their farms, the large institutions became 'worlds on their own' within which the more able patients worked in strict sexual segregation to produce much of their food and clothing (Humphries and Gordon, 1992). As late as the 1960s hospitals were still being built, including three in Scotland with 1200 beds between them. Although 80 per cent of patients were fully ambulant and most could wash and dress themselves, 42 per cent had been institutionalized for 20 years or more and 25 per cent for 10 years (National Society for Mentally Handicapped Children (NSMHC), 1969; Kirman and Bicknell, 1975).

During the 1960s severe criticism of mental and mental handicap hospitals appeared in the reports of committees of enquiry into the treatment of patients and in books like *Asylums* (Goffman, 1961) and *Put Away* (Morris 1969). The institutions which had been greeted with such enthusiasm in the nineteenth century were increasingly seen as dehumanizing as well as expensive to run, and the movement to close them gained momentum.

Therapy for people with learning difficulties

The nineteenth century institutions were built on the hope that therapeutic care, treatment and training in a protective environment would make the best of whatever facilities people with learning difficulties possessed. If we take 'therapy' in mental disorder to mean systematic treatment by techniques other than medication or surgery, we can trace its origins to early nineteenth century Paris, above all to the work of Jean Itard and his pupil Edouard Séguin. In 1800 Itard, physician to the National Institution for Deaf Mutes, began working with Victor, the 'savage of Aveyron', who had been found living wild in the woods. In his attempts to socialize the boy and teach him to speak, Itard devised a variety of training exercises but, meeting with only limited success, he concluded that some people had an innate defect that could be minimized but not eradicated with training, and that they required care and protection (Hallas *et al.*, 1982).

Edouard Séguin opened a school in 1837 that was so successful that he was asked to work with the retarded patients at the Bicêtre and at the Paris Hospital for Incurables. In his book *Traitement Moral, Hygiène et Éducation des Idiots et des autres Enfants Arriérés* of 1846, Séguin recommended pleasant and stimulating surroundings, a large hall for social activities, singing and drawing classes to develop the senses and exercises to correct contractures and physical deformities. According to Esquirol, the noted alienist (asylum doctor), Séguin had 'removed the mark of the beast from the forehead of the imbecile'. In his second major work, *Idiocy and its Treatment by the Physiological Method*, of 1866, which was published in the USA where he had settled, Séguin stressed that training was a work of love 'not for one individual, but for the teacher, the nurse, the physician, the philosopher, physiologist, psychologist, and moralist all to work as a team . . .'. The multidisciplinary approach is not as new as it sounds (Hallas *et al.*, 1982).

In 1839 Dr J. Guggenbuhl, a Swiss authority on cretinism (a thyroid deficiency which caused retarded growth and learning difficulties), opened an alpine hospital for people with the condition, where he introduced a wide range of occupations and exercises to improve their condition. Dr Saegert of Berlin built on the work of Séguin and Guggenbuhl by developing new techniques which he described in *The Treatment of the Blunt Mind in a Scientific Way*, (circa 1840). Saegert observed that whether the defect was due to heredity or disease, mental improvement would only occur if the underlying physical problems were addressed in special institutions providing a healthy environment, humane nursing, exercise, education and training (Hallas *et al.*, 1982).

The medical men in charge of British homes and asylums also recognized the importance of physical therapy. At Park House, Highgate, steam baths and other treatments were tried, while at Essex Hall medical galvanism was applied to patients whose muscular powers were defective, although no real benefit occurred as there was 'so little vital energy in Idiots upon which to work'. Essex Hall was set in six acres of grounds, which provided plenty of space for 'healthful exercise', and had a large gymnasium and a pheasant house where the pupils could enjoy tending living things (Millard, 1864).

Occupation and training were also regarded as being therapeutic as well as essential for the running of the asylum. Dr Langdon Down (after whom Down's syndrome is named) claimed that of every 100 mentally defective patients admitted to a properly equipped hospital, 10 per cent could be trained to be self-supporting, 40 per cent would improve to a point where they would no longer need a carer, and all but 6 per cent of the remainder would improve in their habits and become less of a burden (Rhodes, 1888).

Training and occupation were controlled by the medical superintendent and his colleagues and managed by a subsidiary staff of teachers, nurses, attendants, craftsmen and 'workwomen' or 'work mistresses'. At the Royal Albert Asylum (opened 1870) in the early decades, 'highly certificated teachers' had taught the young patients, but by 1910 'intelligent nurses' and attendants did most of the teaching. The occupations offered were much the same as at all institutions and included woodwork and joinery, shoemaking, basket work, bookbinding, printing, tailoring, brushmaking, upholstery and labouring on the asylum farms (Douglas, 1910).

The Darenth Colony, in Kent, offered 22 types of training for males and six for females, and in 1913, 835 of the 1064 adult patients were undergoing industrial training. The income from sales of work had increased from £4138 in 1907 to £12367 in 1912. Nearly all the patients did drill and other exercises (Spensley, 1913).

The work carried out at a mental deficiency hospital in the 1930s was described in 1934 by Thomas Lindsay. Founded as a public asylum for chronic lunatics and imbeciles in the late nineteenth century, Caterham had 2000 patients, of whom nearly all were mentally defective and 573 had epilepsy.

There were seven medical and 500 other staff. Of the nursing staff, only 79 of the 160 males and 74 of the 188 females were trained. A few nurses supervised the adult patients in the routine work of the hospital, and a former charge nurse was employed as an 'occupation supervisor' to teach crafts. In one section, about 100 patients worked at shoemaking, tailoring, basket weaving and mat-making; in another, 38 women with severe learning difficulties did simple crafts, while ward-bound patients were provided with materials.

The occupation centre at the school was the responsibility of the medical officer in charge of the psychological department. The supervisor had taught herself a range of handicrafts and, with a staff of seven or eight nurses, gave lessons in crafts and physical drill as well as the usual classroom subjects to 80 boys under 16. Unusually for this period, a masseuse was about to join the staff and Dr Lindsay hoped that remedial exercises would become a feature of the training (Lindsay, 1934).

Occupational therapists had worked in British psychiatric hospitals since the 1920s but, like physiotherapists, they were rarely employed to work with people with learning difficulties. One problem was finding a niche in an established order. This was highlighted in an article in 1948 by Miss Enid Chorley, MAOT, who taught crafts to patients of all abilities in a 'mental deficiency colony'. Miss Chorley observed that many prejudices would have to be overcome before the trained occupational therapist could have a say in work placements and be able to cooperate between the doctors and the tradesmen for the welfare of the patients. She suggested that the occupational therapist should be in charge of country dancing, indoor and outdoor games, gymnastics, eurhythmics and guiding and scouting, much of which sounds like physiotherapy (Chorley, 1948).

At a conference which was reported in the journal *Occupational Therapy*, in 1951, an occupational therapist from Rampton Hospital described how she coped with people of different abilities. She kept a large class of patients busy with sewing, painting and toymaking, always with plenty of music and bright colours, and taught some patients imaginative crafts like pottery and puppetry. She claimed that maladjusted young women, like those at Rampton, might be difficult to control in the laundry and other workplaces but they often had a latent artistic sense and enjoyed coming to her department.

Several hospitals made improvements in the wake of the Royal Commission on the Law relating to Mental Illness and Mental Deficiency of 1954–57 which paved the way for the Mental Health Act 1959. In September 1959 a patients' club was opened at Brockhall Hospital, Lancashire, where 2000 people with learning difficulties lived in overcrowded conditions with little mental stimulation. Run by the headmaster of the hospital school, the club initially offered 40 young people music, dancing, arts and crafts on one evening a week, but grew into an evening centre run by Lancashire Education Authority, providing 450 patients with a choice of 70 classes, covering literacy and numeracy and nearly every type of hobby and craft (Bland, 1970).

Many improvements were piecemeal and an enquiry carried out by the DHSS in 1972 showed that overcrowding and understaffing meant that some 39 per cent of patients were not occupied in any way and, adding to their boredom, was the fact that more than half were never visited. Work or industrial therapy increasingly involved carrying out contracts with outside firms and factories but, although patients had the benefit of a small wage, the work could be hard to obtain and its repetitive nature sometimes made it more boring than working around the hospital.

The development of community care

Change was needed and throughout the 1970s demands grew for the spread of community care. Community care for people with learning difficulties has always existed in some families and, as we saw, was part of official policy in Scotland in the nineteenth century. And although the main thrust of the movement belongs to recent decades, the beginnings of a systematic approach can be traced to the interwar years.

In 1922 the Central Association for the Care of the Mentally Defective and other voluntary bodies were offering a range of crafts and activities in 20 day centres; by 1927 there were 99 centres attended by over 1250 people daily (Jones, 1960). Progress was relatively slow until the 1960s when, in the wake of the Mental Health Act 1959, Adult and Junior Training Centres (ATCs and JTCs) were set up by hospital management committees and local authorities, and discharge to community hostels began in earnest. The therapeutic community and the open-door model of care that evolved in psychiatric hospitals in the 1950s and 1960s had repercussions in hospitals for people with learning difficulties and the more able patients began to be discharged on license to hostels and outside employment.

In 1960 there were 19 000 local authority training places and 1700 places in hostels for people with learning difficulties; by 1968 the numbers had risen to 42 000 and 3492, respectively, with an additional 1599 in other homes and hostels. Between 1974 and 1984 ATC places increased from 32 000 to 47 000, and the places in Special Care Units for profoundly disabled people from 600 to 2800. In 1975 49 000 patients (83 per cent of the total ascertained) were in hospital; by 1982 this had fallen to 41 700 and by 1989 to 39 000 (NSMHC, 1969). ATCs offered work, exercise and a social life and great hopes surrounded their setting, but the King's Fund publication *An Ordinary Working Life*, of 1984, questioned their usefulness and stressed that disabled people had a right to work in the ordinary community unsegregated from others (Myers and Heron, 1985).

The Riding for the Disabled Association (RDA) provides 'hippotherapy', particularly to children and young people. Publications of the Association of Chartered Physiotherapists in Riding for the Disabled (ACPRD) describe how the modern phase began with the rehabilitation of people affected by the polio epidemics in the 1940s and 1950s, and the example of Liz Hartel of Denmark, who was crippled by the disease but won a medal for dressage at the 1952 Helsinki Olympics. Groups began in the 1950s and the RDA was founded in 1969. By 1991 there were over 700 groups attended by some 26 000 people, of whom more than half have a learning difficulty. In addition to the general benefits that stem from communication and exercise, hyperactive children become absorbed and calmed, children with physical problems like cerebral palsy improve in balance and control, while autistic children often relate better to the horses than they do to people. Some adults and children take part in the riding and driving events at the Paralympic Games which began in the late 1940s. Physiotherapists were involved from the start and in 1970 they formed the ACPRD as a specific interest group of the Chartered Society of Physiotherapy, with its own conferences and examinations.

De-institutionalization is without precedent and alternatives to the old hospitals have been observed with interest. A concentrated effort to explore the various options was made in Sheffield in the 1970s when DHSS and local money funded the closure of old hospitals; the building of 24-bedded hostels; expansion of a child development centre; and the setting up of an assessment centre for school leavers and of a computer case register. The scheme was adjusted after it was judged too piecemeal and building-centred.

A radical scheme launched by parents in Omaha, Nebraska, enables young people with learning problems to live with two or three others in homes with 24-hour staffing. The King's Fund publication *An Ordinary Life*, of 1980, advocated that the Nebraskan scheme be introduced elsewhere (Myers and Heron, 1985).

Professional organizations

Against this changing background of care, professional bodies for physiotherapists and occupational therapists *had* been founded and consolidated. The Chartered Society of Physiotherapy (CSP) was founded in 1894, as the Society of Trained Masseuses, by four nurse-masseuses who were anxious to improve the reputation of massage. Examinations in anatomy, physiology and massage were held straight away; examinations in Swedish remedial exercises followed in 1909 and in medical electricity in 1915. The status of trained masseuses was enhanced during and after the Great War of 1914–18 when their skills were much in demand. Initially for women only, the society began to train male masseurs in 1905 and admitted them to membership in 1920. The number of training schools grew from a handful in 1895 to 35 in the 1980s, but decreased as schools amalgamated and joined higher education colleges. Each year about 950 students qualify in physiotherapy which is now an all-degree profession.

Having merged with rival organizations over the years, in 1986 the CSP amalgamated with the Society of Remedial Gymnasts and Recreational Therapists which had been formed in 1946 by army drill instructors who had retrained in remedial work. In 1994, its centenary year, the CSP had a membership of 26 000, many of whom belonged to one of 25 occupational or clinical interest groups. Having previously been a regional group in Trent, the Association of Chartered Physiotherapists in

Mental Handicap (now for People with Learning Disabilities) was founded with 26 members in 1985; by 1989 its membership had reached 215.

Occupational therapy has its roots in the arts-and-crafts movement and began to emerge as a profession in the USA in the early years of this century. Like physiotherapy, its status was boosted during the Great War. The first British occupational therapist began psychiatric work in Aberdeen in 1925, after training in Philadelphia, and the first school, Dorset House, was opened in Bristol in 1930. The Scottish Association of Occupational Therapists was launched in 1932 by 11 women, most of whom held art college diplomas and worked in psychiatry. The Association of Occupational Therapists for the rest of the UK was founded in 1936 and the first diploma examination was held in 1938. The Scottish and British organizations merged in 1974 to become the British Association of Occupational Therapists (BAOT). In 1978 the College of Occupational Therapists was formed as a subsidiary of the BOAT with responsibility for educational and professional affairs. By 1993 there were 11 000 members, 3000 registered students and 28 training courses, including a handful of degree courses. Occupational therapists working in the field of learning difficulties form the third largest group within the BAOT – only mental health and geriatrics employing more – and their interests are represented in the Association of Occupational Therapists in Learning Disabilities.

Why were there so few remedial therapists?

Physiotherapists and occupational therapists were slow to enter the field. At Larbert Hospital, formal physiotherapy was in place by the 1950s but this was unusual, as a report *Helping Mentally Handicapped People in Hospital*, of 1978, stated that there were only 80 full-time physiotherapists in mental handicap hospitals in the whole country, and as recently as 1984 a medical witness to the Social Services Committee on Community Care reported a shortage of physiotherapists, a considerable shortage of occupational therapists and a very big shortage of speech therapists.

One reason for the shortage before 1948, when mental handicap hospitals joined the new NHS, may have been the way in which medical superintendents controlled all aspects of the patients' lives. It has been suggested that by the 1960s the 'Chief' in psychiatric hospitals had lost some of his power because of the improved status of nurses and other professionals, the advent of a multidisciplinary approach, and his/her increasing involvement in bureaucratic affairs (Smith and Swann, 1993). If this was also true for mental handicap hospitals, remedial therapists may have found a new opportunity for work which would not involve taking orders from medical staff and jeopardizing their growing professional autonomy.

In an article of 1983 entitled 'Mental handicap: why are there so few occupational therapists?' a clinical tutor observed (as Miss Chorley had in 1948) that it was not easy to fit occupational therapy into a system that had functioned for generations – sometimes adequately, sometimes not – without it, especially as the duties of the various professions were not always well defined. In addition, there was too little coverage of the topic during training; prejudice and nervousness; and mental handicap's perceived position as the 'Cinderella of the NHS' which could mean a continual battle for funds and assistance (Candlish, 1983).

Fear of the unknown and inadequate coverage of learning difficulties during training were also mentioned at an interview in 1995 by a physiotherapist who worked for an inner-city NHS trust. In her experience the specialism had much to offer physiotherapists, particularly in a dynamic community care setting with its holistic approach that involved clients, parents, teachers, social workers and other health professionals. In the same interview the superintendent physiotherapist of the Learning Disability Service of Plymouth Community Services NHS Trust admitted that the work was not always seen as 'proper physiotherapy' and that recruitment was difficult, but felt that things were improving. Ten years ago no physiotherapists worked with adults with learning disabilities in Plymouth, but now there were one full-time and six part-time posts (Friend, 1995).

Another possibility is that in the heyday of the large hospitals, funding agencies felt that there was little point in paying professional therapists to work with people who were deemed 'incurable'. Only in the 1970s and 1980s when Darenth, Brockhall and the other hospitals began to discharge large numbers of patients was rehabilitation for a more independent life given the attention it deserved.

Conclusion

In all but name, occupational therapy and physiotherapy have long been part of the treatment of people with learning difficulties, especially hospital patients, but have involved doctors, nurses, artisans and drill masters rather than trained remedial therapists. The reasons for this include medical autonomy and a staffing system that was difficult to break into; lack of impetus for change; poor funding for patients who were thought unlikely to improve; and, on the therapists' part, inadequate coverage during training, preconceived ideas and a lack of awareness of how satisfying the work can be.

References

Bland, G. (1970) The Brockhall Evening Centre, pamphlet, Brockhall, Lancs.

Bone, M., Spain, B. and Martin, F.M. (1972) *Plans and Provisions for the Mentally Handicapped*, George Allen and Unwin, London

Brady, C. (1865) *The Training of Idiotic and Feeble-Minded Children*, Hodges, Smith and Co., Dublin

Candlish, E. (1983) Mental handicap: why are there so few occupational therapists? *Occupational Therapy*, October, 282–283

Chorley, E. (1948) Occupational therapy with the mentally defective. *Journal of the Association of Occupational Therapists*, **31**, 14–16

Cunyngham Brown, R. (1908) The boarding out of the insane in private dwellings, *Journal of Mental Science*, July, 533–550

Douglas, A.R. (1899) The Royal Albert Asylum, a Training Institution for the feeble-minded of the Northern Counties, booklet, printed in Lancaster

Douglas, A.R. (1910) The care and training of the feeble-minded. *Journal of Mental Science*, April, 253–261

Friend, B. (1995) Dispelling the Cinderella image: focus on learning disabilities. *Physiotherapy Frontline*, 3 May, 16–17

Goffman, E. (1961) *Asylums: Essays on the Social Situation of Mental Patients and other Inmates*, Anchor Books, New York.

Hallas, C.H., Fraser, W.I. and McGillivray, R.C. (1982) *The Care and Training of the Mentally Handicapped*, Wright, London

Humphries, S. and Gordon, P. (1992) *Out of Sight, the Experience of Disability 1900–1950*, a Channel Four Book, Northcote House, Plymouth

Jones, K. (1960) *Mental Health and Social Policy*, Routledge and Kegan Paul, London

Kirman, B. and Bicknell, J. (1975) *Mental Handicap*, Churchill Livingstone, London

Korman, N. and Glennerster, H. (1985) *Closing a Hospital. The Darenth Park Project*, National Council for Voluntary Organisations, London

Lindsay, T. (1934) Mental deficiency practice at Caterham Mental Hospital., *Journal of Mental Science*, April, 397–401

Millard, W. (1864) The Idiot and his helpers, Including the History of Essex Hall, booklet, printed in Colchester

Morris, P. (1969) *Put Away: A Sociological Study of Institutions for the Mentally Retarded*, Routledge and Kegan Paul, London.

Myers, M. and Heron, A. (1985) Concepts about 'mental handicap'. *Physiotherapy*, **71** (3), 103–104.

National Society for Mentally Handicapped Children (1969) The Road to Community Care, conference report, 3–4

Rhodes, J.M. (1888) Pauper Lunatics, North Western District Poor Law Conference Report, 207–208

Smith, I. and Swann, A. (1993) Medical officers and therapeutics, 1814–1921. In Andrews, J. and Smith, I. (eds), *'Let there be Light Again' – A History of Gartnavel Royal Hospital*, Greater Glasgow Health Board

Spensley, F.O. (1913) A brief account of Darenth and its industrial training. *Journal of Mental Science*, April, 305–311

4

Telling people what you think

Neil Palmer, Chris Peacock, Florence Turner and Brian Vasey, supported by Val Williams

This work was researched and transcribed by the Bristol Self-Advocacy Research Group, which are people with intellectual talent.

Doing our own research

Research is when you join up and talk about different things. It's about finding things out, and getting other people to listen to you. We are a group of four self-advocates, and we got interested in research in different ways. One of us said:

> I got interested in it when I went to a meeting of People First. And I saw this video of Gary, and I thought he was rather nice, I did, and I thought what he's doing – if Gary Bourlet's doing it, and he's disabled, I don't see why I can't do it. Then I thought, I went home, and I thought I'd like to work with Gary, so I thought I'd go to one of the meetings in Bristol, and from there that's how I think I joined it. That's my story.

We think we've got on quite well. What research does, is that it takes you outside yourself, and you think about other people more than you do about yourself. We do research because it's interesting to get people's opinions, like people who go to day centres, and at college. We find out what their ideas are, how they cope when they get angry and how they go about things.

Where did our ideas come from?

What we wanted to find out, was whether other people are banging their heads against a brick wall like we are:

> I felt the one thing that really sparked it all off was people's ideas, experiences and also how people respond to you.

A lot of the questions that we wanted to ask came from our experiences with other groups. For instance, one of our members went to college courses, and he was the Disability Officer in the Student Union. This meant that he started to think about what 'disability' means, and what it means to people who are in wheelchairs, and who have visual impairments, as well as people with learning difficulties:

I think that's what started me off, the Student Union bit, related to disability. That is why I wanted to do more research on this. I felt it affected a lot of people at college, and all these day centres people go to.

The pilot project (it is a pilot project because we are hoping to go further with it!)

Back about a year ago, we put some ideas down about what we wanted to do, and applied to the National Lottery for a small grant. We were delighted when we got some money from them to actually do our research, and then we had to start working. Our plan was to visit other groups and ask them questions. We have been to visit five other groups so far, and we tape record and make videos of our research interviews with them.

We found the groups to visit by going through the list of people who had come to a seminar we did for the Norah Fry Research Centre in Bristol in December 1996. Everyone we wrote to invited us to come and see them. These are the groups we have visited so far:

In all, we have talked to 47 people, and this chapter is based on what they said to us. We made our own list of research questions, about all sorts of subjects which interested us. The ideas came to us at different times; one of our members gets her ideas in bed! So we went off on our research visits, with one supporter, a tape recorder and a video camera:

Visiting other places, and talking about different things, I quite enjoyed it you know.

Our feelings about doing research

We've all really enjoyed the research visits, meeting new people and making new friends:

I was looking at my photographs yesterday when I was at home, and all the different places I've been. And I've got all the photographs in my photograph album at home. I'm quite proud of what I did. And you feel very important. People say: 'You do do a lot'. They're quite impressed with what I do. I've achieved a lot – too much!

Doing research is not always easy, and we have learnt a lot of things. One of our members, Neil Palmer, has been the chairperson at the research interviews, and this is what he has to say about it:

From the chairing point of view, I felt probably nervous at first. Not nervous, but the atmosphere of the other People First group, how they reflected on us, how they felt about us. I thought that was important, very important I think.

Doing research can be really hard going, and really tough too. That's because you're meeting new people all the time, and we did find that they might not always understand our questions in the way we put them. After our research visits, we tried to look back at the videos, and think how we could make the questions better, how we could listen to people better, and encourage them to say things.

Most of our work has been very enjoyable:

To tell you the honest truth, I think it's been a wonderful project, the research mainly. Not only – the thing what I really like about it is the actual atmosphere, the reactions people have (about) things like transport, jobs and money and disability. I reckon all of those come together into one thing.

We reckon we've learnt to work together as a team, and we all have patience with each other now. Even people who didn't really know what they were doing at first, have done a brilliant job.

Why is it important for self-advocates to do our own research?

Everybody's got power in their own right, and research gives us more power. It means people will listen to us. This is better than being a politician, in the Government:

> I don't think you're going to get as much information from an MP as you do from a researcher.

Some of the things that are happening at the moment about benefits cuts do affect us, and we are also concerned about people being bullied. These are the important things that we must stand up and talk about and it's good to do it through research, not just by saying what we ourselves think. It was quite nice actually to hear people's opinions about the subjects we were doing:

> I hope we can continue to actually produce more information for people. The more we do that, the better understanding other people will have of actually listening to us.

It's a good job, doing research. It takes determination, but you do get a feeling of achievement out of it. What we hope is that we can go further with this, and that more people can join in:

> Do you know what I hope to see happening really, is to get more people involved in research. The more we do that, the better chance we have of actually producing more booklets, whatever, getting people like us known to the public.

What is disability? Cutting out all the labels

Edited by Neil Palmer

We are people who have often been labelled, in different ways. This is something that we feel very strongly about, and we decided to ask people about it. We asked them: 'What do you think about people being labelled?'

This was quite a difficult question to start off with, and sometimes we had to explain a bit about what we meant, but nearly everyone we met had some very strong views. Lots of people said that they were against all kinds of labelling, and wanted to throw out all the words which people use about us. For instance, one person told us:

> I don't think it's a very good thing, people being labelled myself, being labelled 'disabled' or anything like that. I don't think it's a very good idea, because people who don't understand you, or don't spend time to get to know you, don't really understand about it, you know.

When people get labelled as 'disabled people' or 'people with learning disabilities', then other people probably think of us as all the same. We get put in a box, and stereotyped. People should take the time to get to know us.

Someone in a different group told us:

> I'm thinking 'disabled' is not the right word, I'm thinking that you're still a human being, that . . . we are put here on this world to be loved and be cared for, not to be called names. And that's what I'm saying is, labelling should be banned completely, right off, and scrub it right in the bin, the scrap heap.

Feelings

Being labelled makes many people feel very low. It does not help at all. These were some of the things people said about their feelings:

> I think it demoralizes what you're like as a person, because if people get to hear that you're learning disabled, they automatically think you're not capable of doing what they're doing, you know.
>
> I think it's a bit of a cruel one, don't you, because it doesn't – it makes the people feel, it makes their problem worse, the learning difficulty. It doesn't break down the barriers, it makes it bigger, doesn't it – learning difficulty?

But labels are everywhere. You find it on anything, like a newsletter, or a college course on the prospectus. You're going to find it anywhere, and it isn't changing.

Who really has 'learning difficulties?'

Nobody does. Everyone is their own individual, and has something to offer the world. In another way, as someone said in one group: 'Everyone in the world has a learning difficulty.'

It is true that everyone has a problem with something or other. But they should not get labelled for that reason.

There were some people who said that 'learning difficulties' or 'disabled' were words that they might use about other people, who had more problems than they themselves did. But the People First groups who were most experienced included people who had physical problems, who could not talk, or who were blind. They had all sorts of people, and they all found that labelling did *not* help them. Lots of people talked about the problems for someone who uses a wheelchair. Those people may need ramps, or special access to buildings, and they have problems with transport, and getting to People First meetings. But that does not mean that we have to label them as 'disabled'.

Which words are the worst?

Some people we talked to picked out particular words, especially the ones they thought were the worst. Most of these words aren't used now, but you still hear some of them sometimes. This is what people said:

> I don't like the term 'mental handicap'. I prefer the term 'learning difficulty' or 'learning disability' myself, only I don't like the term 'mental handicap'. I was labelled myself some years ago until my mother spoke up for me, as a 'mentally defective.'
>
> I don't like 'mentally handicapped' or 'spastic' at all. It's a horrible word, I want to destroy it altogether.

Some of these people picked out the word 'learning difficulties' as the only word which was OK. They hated all the other words which were used about them, but if they had to be called anything, then they thought 'learning difficulties' was probably the best:

> I prefer being called 'people with learning difficulties'. I don't know about other people. I don't want 'disabled people' or 'handicapped', I don't want that.

We got into a couple of discussions about the difference between 'learning difficulties' and 'learning disability'. One man told us that the word 'learning disability' had been chosen by the Government – but it is better to have a word which is chosen by us, by ourselves. That is why 'learning difficulties' is probably better for most people.

Sometimes a label can get you somewhere

One person in one of the interviews told us that she was pleased to use the words 'someone with Down's syndrome'. This was because 'it's all part of acting'. She had got a job on a film, which she had really enjoyed, because she was someone who had Down's syndrome.

Joining a self-advocacy group is something good about being someone 'with a learning difficulty', because we can get together and have power to do things for ourselves. Meeting with other people who have the same sort of life as ourselves, that's good because we can all help each other: 'We look forward, and enjoy meeting with enthusiasm.'

Mostly, though, it's other people who do the labelling to us. They do it so that they can put us all together in one place.

Having special services for people with learning difficulties

Being called 'people with learning difficulties' is sometimes more than just being called names. It does sometimes mean that you get the support that you may need. It also means that lots of other things happen to you – like day centres, and being sent to live in houses you don't like. Nearly all the people we spoke to in the interviews did use services that were 'special services' for people with learning difficulties. Lots of people talked to us about these, and how they felt about them. Some people thought that people with learning difficulties should get special help, and that day centres are a good part of this help:

> Where I work at X, it is for people with learning difficulties, it is. It's called a Resource and Activity Centre, and it's based *on* people with learning difficulties – like me, for instance. I think it's a very good place where I work in.

But other people thought that day centres were not always good. People get mixed in together, just because they happen to have the label 'learning difficulties', and then other people, from outside, think that everyone who goes to the day centre is the same, and can't do anything useful. That is the trouble with labelling people and putting them all together in one place.

What support would be better?

If we didn't have any labels put on us, then people might think of everyone as an individual. Just because people need help, you don't have to put them all in one box. One of our members said that she has a problem crossing roads, but that doesn't mean that she has to live with lots of other people who can't cross roads. It also doesn't mean she should be called or thought of as a 'bad road crosser'. We all have things that we need help with, and the services should think about what help they will offer, not spend time trying to say it's only for one group of people or another.

Jobs and work

Edited by Brian Vasey

One of the questions we asked people in the groups was about the work they had done. The jobs that people did were things like gardening, shop work, care work with children, and lots of other jobs. Nearly all these jobs were things people had done in day centres, or as work placements. There were 10 people who said they had jobs, but this was nearly all voluntary work. What did people think about voluntary work? Well, it's better than nothing:

> I'm working in a place called Scrabble, refurbishing old furniture. I'm enjoying it, you know, it's a good thing to do, and it's like in a little factory. What I've always wanted.
>   Is it like a day centre?
>   Not like a day centre, no, a warehouse, a proper warehouse.

People often like doing the work, because it's getting them out of the day centre. But in the end we all need money to live. You've got to get a lot of money to be able to buy things, haven't you? You've got to get food and clothing to live in. This means that we should get real jobs, like the new Government has promised. Most of us would like real jobs.

Benefits

One of the problems in getting real jobs is that our benefits get stopped. Most people need money from benefits, because it costs a lot to have the support that we need. But if we get money from a job, this may mean that we lose our benefits, and this can be a problem – especially if we then lose the job too. It's too risky for most of us:

> I used to work in a hotel two years ago now. Chamberperson I was, changing the beds I used to do, changing all the towels and all that. But I blew it, a bit of a problem. I had to see the boss then of the hotel like, because the point was, my benefits, it was. I had to pack it in.

In our position, most people do get entitlement to certain benefits, like Income Support and DLA, which is disability living allowance:

> Because I'm working, I'm not allowed to earn over £15. If I earn over £15, my benefit gets stopped.

This is why so many of us end up doing voluntary work. It is safer for us, because we know then that we are going to get the money we need.

Problems in jobs

Jobs are very hard to find nowadays. Some of the problems people talked about were to do with getting jobs. There is discrimination against us, and this is to do with labelling:

When you get labelled it affects you as regards getting a job, and everything. And there's too much discrimination against disability people, I think.

If someone has a problem with reading and writing, sometimes this stops them from getting a job. A few people talked about this, and said that they had worked at getting better at reading and writing. But it is very hard, if people expect you to be able to read everything, and fill in forms too:

I've been discriminated against because of my reading difficulty, because I couldn't read or write, they said, 'Oh, if you could read or write you'd have this job'. So that to me was a type of discrimination because I couldn't read or write properly. Of course I've improved now, but it's amazing because I've proved a lot of people wrong you see.

Support in work

People often have problems in finding a job, and we may also need help once we're in a job. This is where support workers can really help. Support workers can come through college, through a scheme like Pathway, or something else. It doesn't matter, as long as they know how to support you.

It is important to help people at work in the right way. Most of us do *not* want a support worker there all the time:

I didn't want her in the daytime, only at 4 o'clock, if she came in before the taxi came, to see how you did. She did that for a long time.

Some people, though, might need more help, and that's fine. If someone needs more help, then they should get it. That way, they can still go out to work and do a job.

One person thought it was very important that you should learn the skills and confidence, when you're on the job, and that the support worker can then withdraw his or her help altogether:

What it is, is we've had these few monthly meetings, going on to last year, when I started in December because it was like a review meeting to see how I was getting on. And Carol Green said to me, 'How would you feel if I didn't come to the office any more?' And I said to her 'I think it's time for me to do it myself'. And I did, and from that day on, I have been so confident in what I was doing, and that's why Carol Green hasn't continued. Because I've learnt from her support how to do the job, and since then, I've gone from strength to strength.

If your supervisor at work also learns how to support you in the right way, then you can gradually get more independent. Some people can learn how to really take responsibility, and the only support they then need is for other people to value what they can do:

What I'm trying to do now is to do with prioritizing, like. Which my supervisors have noticed quite a lot about me. . . . And there was one thing that I done on my own, which my supervisor couldn't believe I had done. When he was out, on – in job training thing, or whatever – I said to him, no he said to me, 'How did you get on while I was away that week?' 'Very well, I've got on with the filing work, and I saw people.' 'Did you use your initiative? You found the work that had got to be done, and made the time to do it.' And I felt quite happy.

Working in day centres

All the people who went to day centres said that they went to work at the day centre. Lots of things go on at day centres, and people told us that they did things like do-it-yourself groups, shopping, gardening, assembly work, and other things like self-advocacy groups and line dancing!

Some of these things are more like 'work' than others, but no one gets paid for contract work any more. A lot of people talked about this, and about the work they used to do:

> We used to do contracts, but it all came to an end. And we didn't know why it all folded like. But that's what we done. And they let all our contracts drop flat. It used to be our work before. And they won't come back and do any more.

People ought to ask us before they make changes like this, although we know that in some places, people were asked, and we also think that getting £2 for a week's work is an insult. But some of the people we talked to would like to do contract work, even if they just get a small salary from it. It's better than being bored:

> We did have lots of work at one time, didn't we? Now it's nothing for us.

Working for People First

Our interviews were all with self-advocates, or people in Speaking Up or People First groups. Some of these people did paid work for People First, and some of them just got involved as volunteers. One person talked about doing a job which was training professionals. This was a paid job, which was offered to the People First group where she was a member:

> I represent People First, and I do training of nurses, in self-advocacy, to stick up for themselves. Listening as well. And I enjoy the work. Get paid for it as well.

Absolutely everyone who did this kind of work really loved it:

> What I'm saying is what I've achieved for a long time is, is being in the office and working very hard and I'm going to stick like that for a time. But what I'm thinking is all I've achieved for a long time is going to be there. For a long time.

It is really important to have a job which you enjoy, and that you can feel good about doing. We have lots of things to offer, and doing work as a self-advocate makes us more confident.

One man told us that he represents his People First group on the consultation group for Social Services. This can be very hard work:

> And it's two meetings in one, sometimes, isn't it Julia? You go into one meeting, and one meeting ends, and then you go into another one. And the other Friday we were so cosy me and Julia, that we were nearly falling asleep, and Julia said to me, 'If I go to sleep, you nudge me', and

I said, 'You nudge me too', and it was a really long day. It was a really long day.

In this sort of work, people are interested in doing the job because it is important work. It's not just for yourself, it's helping other people:

> And what we underlined, was issues to do with the hospital, and the problems they have there, and what will happen to the money when they pull down the hospital, and we said the money's got to be used to house them and all the problems they have there. So we are involved with people's problems, although it doesn't personally affect us.

This shows that people can do a lot more than they are often given credit for. It's not just the ordinary jobs doing trolley-pushing and washing up, although these are important too. Nowadays, people are doing different and exciting work, like we do as research workers. There ought to be more chances like this for people to get paid for doing things which are important.

The staff who support us

Edited by Florence Turner

Everyone we spoke to had support from staff – at home, in day centres, at work, or in college, and even in People First groups. These staff people do different jobs, and most people said that they thought their staff were very good:

> So, the staff who's very good, and they're excellent, and they do their job very well. So if, say, all of us or me had a problem we'd go straight to the staff, and see what we've got to do. And they do try to help us.

It's important to have staff people who are there to listen, in case you have a problem, and will put themselves out to do something for you. Whatever job the staff person is doing, there are some things which we want from all our staff. This is the same, even if they are the 'top snobs'. However high up they are, staff people should be there for you, and ready to help.

The sort of person who's best to support people is someone who's good at listening, will have time for a chat, and can offer friendship too. This is what one person said about his ideal support person:

> There's one person I get on very well with. He's the sort of person who, I always look forward to seeing him. I've got a good relationship with him. . . . He's a good support person, who you can get on well with. He's very understanding, and he's the sort of person you can chat about things, and you can tell him things.

Unfortunately, there are lots of problems people have had, and some of these are to do with things staff do, and attitudes they have. These are the things we *don't* like.

Being treated like children

Lots of people talked to us about problems they have had at home, or in day centres, when they are bossed around by staff. Some staff are a bit bossy, and they make rules and treat people like children. For instance, one person said:

They treat us like children, some of the staff do up there. Oh, you're not allowed to do this. If we go out, we have got to be signed out or signed back in.

It might not be a bad thing to tell people where you are going, because this is to do with fire regulations, but it is still bad if staff boss you around, and give you punishments like staying in your room or not going out somewhere. If you want someone to do something, you should *ask* them politely, and not tell them what to do. We are all equals, and we want to be treated like equals.

Being forced to be independent

Staff people always think that we all want to be more and more independent. This can be wrong, because they expect us to do too many things ourselves. It should be our choice, not theirs.

if you're married, you've got to give and take. One person does one thing, and people help each other out. It's the same in any house – I don't want staff to keep on forcing me to be independent. How would they feel?

Another person told us about being forced to do her own shopping, when she found this really hard. She would have liked someone to go with her.

Talking behind your back

This happens all the time. We meet people who are very nice to us when they are with us, but they talk about us behind our backs, or ring people up without our permission:

I'm not going to say her name, but she's horrible. She's nice and friendly when she feels, but she talks behind your back about you, and says nasty things about you.

We do not want to be talked about when we are not there. We are human beings, and if someone has got something to say to us, then they can say it to our face.

Poking their nose into our business

There are some things which are private, and are our own affair. For instance, one person told us about a member of staff where he lives, who wanted to know everything about his money:

I don't want to mention people's names, but I get so fed up with people, like I've got this money here, and my carer found out about it, and she says, 'Where are you getting it?' And I say, 'It's none of your business, it's my business, not yours.'

We know that staff people do this sort of thing, perhaps, because they are worried we can't cope, or will lose things. But it is very annoying to have someone who pokes their nose into your business all the time. Everyone needs a bit of privacy and respect.

Support staff in self-advocacy

In the People First groups, we also have support staff. This is a different job again, and the support person is there only to help the self-advocates do their own job. This means that they must not take over the show, or start saying things which are their own ideas and not the self-advocates' ideas. Usually we all get on very well together, and we are friends, as one person said: 'I think we're like a family, aren't we?'

But we don't want to be like a family where we are the children, and we are told what we can think and say. In the interviews we did, the support staff tried to keep quiet, and to let people have their own say. This is hard, but some of them did it very well, and we are very grateful to them.

Some people in self-advocacy groups were doing paid work in helping to train staff, and this seems to be a very good thing. Everyone enjoys it, and it should be done more, so that all staff training includes self-advocates.

Transport

Edited by Chris Peacock

People told us that they used lots of different kinds of transport: buses, taxis, minibuses and trains. The reason people need to use transport is to go to work, or to go out in the evening, or to go shopping. That's why it's so important.

Some bus drivers are all right, and some are not. The good drivers talk to people on the bus, and would help you out if you had a problem. Some people told us about problems they had, like one person whose bag had got caught in an automatic door. When she went to talk to the driver about this, he called her stupid and silly. This is not good. Another group told us:

> The only problem I have come across is bus drivers' attitudes, you know, the attitudes are sometimes a bit off, they don't want to know.

If you go to work on a bus, the bus driver should stop the bus when you put your hand out. But some of the drivers are a bit rude, and when you're standing at the bus stop they go straight past without stopping:

> I was mucked about one night. The bus went past, and I had my hand up, and it zoomed straight past, and they said they couldn't see me, because I had a big jacket on. Not – they took it up with the Parish Council, and I didn't say anything to them. But we thought it was rather a bit silly, because we'd have thought they'd have automatically stopped. That's the situations I've had with them, there was just nobody there to write off to and tell them, it's either ring them up – it's just breaking the barrier of responsibility. And getting it off your chest.

Transport is by train, buses, anything really. It would be very difficult if we couldn't use the bus to get to work. Some people walk to work, or go in a car. People in wheelchairs have the biggest problems of all, because they can't get the wheelchair on the bus. Lots of people in People First groups told us about this problem.

When you live in a city like Bristol, you can get from one place to another on the city buses. But when people live in the country, they find it very hard to get buses. Then it makes it difficult to go out at night, because you can't get back. This is what people said:

> The only trouble I had with the council is whether or not you can go out in the evenings. You know, the last bus only goes to a certain time, and

we have trouble with, you can get to town, but you can't get back to where you're living. That's a difficulty, if you live in a rural area, you can't get from A to B unless it's at a certain time when the buses go through.

Because of all these problems, sometimes people need to use taxis. Taxis should really help you out, because they're expensive. But we have also had some problems with taxis. For instance, they should go to where you want to go, but somebody we spoke to said that they had ordered a taxi to go home, and the taxi didn't come. When she phoned up, they still didn't come, and she had to get a taxi from another firm. Taxi drivers sometimes think they know best, or they treat you badly:

Yeah, you know that . . . on a Friday, that we gone to, right, the Centre? He [the taxi driver] turned up, and I said, 'You taking me?' And he said, 'Excuse me, I don't know where to go'. So he went, so I goes home. So my worker phones him up and says, 'Why didn't you take her?' And he turns round and says, 'Because I was ill', and it wasn't, because he saw me. Then he came back the following Monday, and he asked for his money, and I told him to get stuffed.

Some people can use buses, some can't. But there are more people who could use the bus if they had some training. Also, bus drivers could have training, so they know how to help people without being rude. Then we could all get around better.

Self-advocacy – what does it mean?

Edited by all of us

Self-advocacy is important because you achieve a lot by talking to people. It's speaking up for your rights.

We asked people in the groups what it meant to them, and everyone thought self-advocacy was brilliant:

Self-advocacy is a special word. Because the special word is, everybody is working together like a team, because we do lots of advocacy, we do a lot of things, we go to self-advocacy groups, we run groups, we does a lot of groups. But I'm finding is, we work hard. I think if I didn't have that, we wouldn't have a word. So what we do, we arrange, we think of it ourselves. Like the self-advocacy groups. I'm thinking it's a better way for I'm thinking, it's ace. I think it's great. I think we're working hard for people. But I'm thinking, we don't have enough of it, we want more of it

Self-advocacy is people doing it for themselves, and it's not supposed to be the supporters organizing things. People like Gary Bourlet started it all off in this country. It's important for people that it is something they organize themselves. This is what Gary Bourlet said in a speech in the European Parliament in Brussels on 4th December 1997:

For the first time, people with learning difficulties are being listened to, and consulted. We are learning the confidence to stick up for our own rights, rather than have other people always doing things for us.
    People First groups should be run by and for people with learning difficulties, who may be supported by a paid person, or a volunteer. In

some countries, these groups work together with parent's groups. But parents and carers have a different agenda.

We all need to talk about this together, and share our views in a round-table discussion.

Self-advocacy must not be tokenism.

Things you learn from self-advocacy are: listening to people and not butting into conversations, being tolerant, having patience with other people, and being confident in your own opinions. Many people talked to us about things they had learnt, especially how to listen:

I would say that advocacy's being a good listener, and listening to people and listening to their problems.

Self-advocacy is about discussing your feelings, and making your own decisions, and being sure people don't boss you about. This is what someone from a People First group said:

It can help you to make up your mind. You can sit and discuss things, how you feel about things.

Our research group works together as a team, and everyone thinks this is important. Some people picked this out as the best thing about self-advocacy groups – the team work. Other people even said it was like a family, but we think it's probably more like a team, because people don't always get on with others in their family!

Question: You can't do it on your own, can you?

Answer: Because actually Ben's been there for me, and I've been for him, because we've been running the group together.

Question: You work like a team, do you?

Answer: I work like a team, yes. . . . So we've got lots of people running like clockwork.

In People First groups especially, we don't just talk to ourselves and go there to get educated. We discuss things with each other, and then other people must listen to us. It wouldn't really be People First if others didn't listen. This is how one person put it:

It's saying what you want, and hoping that you'll get it. You can say what you like, and put the points of view to them, and let them know what you want.

More and more People First groups are now working to let the authorities know what services they need, and to help in projects – like telling Social Services whether things are good or bad. But the people who should listen to us are also our parents and our families, all the different groups, and researchers. Staff people sometimes listen to you, but they don't always understand what you are saying. This might be because they don't understand what we are doing when we go to do self-advocacy.

Social Services should be helping people, and they ought to listen to us too. One member of our group is very good at politics, and he voted in the Election in 1997. We think Tony Blair is a very good prime minister, and it was the British people who put him there. But it's important for him to go on listening to people like us. We hope he will read this book.

For the future we need money to keep groups like this going, and to do European work. We are a part of Europe People First, which is a project started by Gary Bourlet. Lots of self-advocates are trying to work at this project, and it is to encourage people to speak up for themselves throughout Europe. The aim is to speak up and get rights for ourselves throughout Europe. We're trying to do more European work – for instance, the research we have done in this country would be very good to do in other countries in Europe too. So, if you've got any ideas or information, do contact us at:

The Bristol Self-Advocacy Research Group
c/o Val Williams
Norah Fry Research Centre
3 Priory Road
Bristol BS8 1TX

Acknowledgements

We would like to thank the National Lottery Small Grants Team (SW) for funding this research project. We are also very grateful to all the groups who took part in it: Frome Education and Resource Centre, Hilltop Resource and Activity Centre, Cardiff People First, Swindon People First and Barnstaple People First. We would also like to thank Bristol and District People First, of which we are a part, and the Norah Fry Research Centre for supporting us, especially Karen Gyde for her help during group meetings, and Oliver Russell for supporting our grant application.

5

Voices of people with learning difficulties

Tricia Webb

Introduction

Those of us who work with people with learning difficulties tend to assume that we know lots about their lives and we like to see ourselves as something of an expert. After all, if you spend much of your working life with something, you get to understand it quite well. This is, I think, especially true of those of us who work for the more 'right-on' agencies. I am currently Project Co-ordinator at Skills for People which is a small voluntary organization based in the north-east, well respected both locally and nationally. We support people with learning difficulties to speak up for themselves by running short courses and support groups. The majority of our work is planned and presented by disabled people themselves and we have a huge team of disabled volunteers (Wright, 1995).

We are proud of what we do and, of course, we *know* about people with learning difficulties. I am confident of this because my opinion is often asked, particularly by other people working in the field. I enjoy heated debates about people's right to choose the path of their own life, the dilemmas of advocacy and the eternal problem of how to genuinely empower people. Best of all, I can set people straight when they are obviously wrong. I am writing with my tongue firmly in my cheek but perhaps it is nearer the truth than I would like to admit?

This chapter is about the lives of people with learning difficulties and I decided to talk to three of our volunteers whom I felt I knew relatively well. I wanted to use their experiences to explore issues important to disabled people. I have changed the names of all people and places involved. At the initial interview, we talked about their lives and their experiences of services, both good and bad. Looking at my notes afterwards, there seemed to be something lacking, something rather impersonal and even clinical about what I had written. I realized that I had managed to confine all three people to talking about the things I felt confident that I already knew about people with learning difficulties. My paper was full of comments like, 'people don't listen to what I want', 'professionals never have the time for me', 'I had to do what they thought was best for me', 'they try and run my life for me', 'speaking up for yourself can be really hard'. I had unconsciously set myself in the role of expert – leading rather than following – and in some ways the people themselves need not have been there. I had created a caricature of a person with learning difficulties and learned nothing new.

Luckily, I was able to stop at this point and step back. I began to think more deeply about the people I had chosen to talk to. They were three people who I felt had really fought the system. Strong individuals who had, against the odds, created the lives *they* wanted. Sarah has spent time in both children's homes and long-stay hospitals and is now mother to two children. Daniel was one of the first people to be resettled from Newlands Hospital and spent several years living alone in his own flat. Elizabeth has spent time in hostels, long-stay hospitals and group homes and is now married and lives with her husband in their own flat. I know their stories well; they are powerful and often disturbing. I wanted them to be told but it was almost as if I was not prepared to hear anything new.

My own challenge then in writing this chapter was to give these three people I know so well the opportunity to tell their stories, yes, but also to help me understand some of the things that I might usually miss, or not want to hear because of who I am – a professional working in advocacy and committed to the cause! When I began to listen, each one of them told me things I had not heard before and did not always feel comfortable with. I gained a new insight into their lives. The result is, I hope, a slightly different slant and a chance to look a little more closely at the things we sometimes miss because we are too busy gazing at a beautiful wood we have created to see the trees.

Relationships and friendships

Most us would agree that friendships and relationships are pivotal to our happiness; the people we have around us keep us centred. Over the years my observations have been that people with learning difficulties do not always have the same network of people that I certainly take for granted, or at least their network does not operate in quite the same way. This seemed an appropriate place to start and I was interested in finding out what Sarah, Daniel and Elizabeth felt. I began by asking them about the people in their lives and their friends. Elizabeth said:

> I've got a lot of friends. I'm close to Julie. I go shopping with her and I help with the trolley when she's on the Metro. We've been going to her house, playing dominoes, me and Clive and Billy, we took a bottle of wine the other day. I've got Terry and Marjorie. He goes to Smith Hall [a club], he's a youth leader, they used to live near my Mam and Dad. I've got Emma, I go and see her and have a cup of tea, it's through 'Goodcare'. I've got Gemma, I used to live with her, I've got Eric, but he's a pain in the bum, he winds us up. I've got Mrs Davidson, she knew my Mam. Lots of people really. . . . Julie buys me dinner and she bought Clive his dinner the other day. She's just got Billy and Alison but I don't bother with Alison. I met Julie in London, we went on a weekend together to see 'Grease', that's where I met her. They took us to her house and from there I just kept going down.

This seemed wonderfully ordinary. Elizabeth obviously does have a very real network. I wondered how she had built this up and whether she felt that making friends was hard:

> No, I've got a load of friends. You've got to get out and see friends, haven't you, because your friends don't just come to you if you don't make an effort. If you sit on your bum in the house, you can't get friends that way, I've always known that. When I was little, my Dad bought us a pram for the dolls, you know, and I used to put all the bairns in, when I was little in The Ridings [where she grew up], and I was wheeling it around. I used to play with the other bairns in the street.

Daniel does not feel the same way,

> I had one or two friends but not a lot of friends when I was in there [hospital], you know, I'm a bad mixer, friends you know, particularly in hospital. It was very hard to start up with friends in hospital, your friends were very difficult. Difficult to make a friend, to have a friend and, you know, if you went anywhere you had to go with them [the staff].

I asked him to tell me more about living in Newlands:

> Well Newlands was, the bit about Newlands would be that I was in the house all the time and you couldn't go where you wanted to. If you had to go to the dentists always someone had to go with you if you had to go to the barbers someone had to be there, if you went to the shop there had to be somebody. They were nice to you, some staff were nice and some were not nice to you, you know. There could have been a bit better way of doing things, helping you. When I first came into the ward I was in a room, I shared a room and then I got a little room to myself, but you had to tell people not to go in it, it's private. If people went in they would steal or go for things. You had to say, 'No, I'm sorry, you can't come in to watch the telly'. . . . They put a tag in your clothes all the time, I didn't like the labels. I hate being labelled. They used to label all your clothes, your name in your shirt and your trousers, you know. When you used to put your clothes away at night time or they'd put them away for you, and there used to be labels on you, you were labelled. It was funny being labelled. I mean we don't want to be labelled at Skills for People, we don't like labelling people.

We talked about how things have changed for Daniel. He moved from long-stay hospital to a flat on his own on an estate. As he says:

> I lived on my own for a while, for a lot of years and I think I did very well for myself. John [Daniel's support worker] used to come and I saw my Mam. I didn't have lots of people but I was OK. . . . when she died, when my mother died I think I got very lonely in that house, in that estate with no one around me. I met this friend and I didn't know about this friend, what he was like, you know, 'til the end of it. People told me what he was like but I didn't take notice of people, you know I thought he was doing a good turn for me. He was telling me. 'Oh come for your dinner' and then he was charging me for a meal! Not like when you go and see your friends, they don't charge you. He would charge you for every meal you had, even if you weren't that fussed on the dinner, he'd charge you! I think it was odd, but I was

very lonely and I wanted some company then. That was the only time I would get company.

Daniel eventually moved on and now lives with a family. I asked him how things have changed and he told me about the people he now has in his life. In particular, the grandchild of the family he lives with:

The first time I saw Clare she took to me no bother. She treats you like you're normal. She doesn't treat you like the other bairns, she treats you like *you*, and she looks after you and she won't let anyone else look after you. She's only six years old. Not many six year olds would do that, would they? We have our arguments sometimes, but not many, just over little things. I want to be in my room on my own sometimes you know, that's the only thing. But she looks after you, she cares for you. She's like a grandbairn. She's not, but it just feels like that to me. I've got family again now, not friends really but family.

How people make friends

It seems that Daniel and Elizabeth's early experiences of making and having friends is very different and I wondered how significant this is. When I think of my own life and early childhood I am aware of how important my early friendships were. I asked Sarah about her experience. Sarah is a woman I had always thought of as having many people in her life and I was interested to hear about her friends:

I don't have any. I have a relationship with Doug [father of Sarah's second child] but that's as much as it is, it's nothing, it's not even love I don't think. It's just what he wants sort of thing, but as for friends, I don't have friends. I have Jane, but she was actually a nurse in the hospital. We're still friendly but she's quite, you know, she's all right, she's nice but it just depends on her. But I don't really have friends, I can't make friends because I don't know how to. I mean, even going on courses and making friends, you know, doing it that way, it wasn't right. Because what sort of people do I meet? Other people with learning disabilities or who have problems that I have to look after, so that is not a friend. And I can't be a friend to people like Liz [Project Co-ordinator at 'Skills'] and you know, I couldn't make friends with them because it's their job. Can't make friends with nurses because that's their job; can't make friends with teachers because that's their job, they're normal people. Right? And outside? I don't talk to people because of the way they do things. You know, the way you see them. People around the doors, the way they deal with their children? I wouldn't lower myself to speak to them. It's hard to make friends, I'd rather be without. I've got Jane and I think that's enough. I mean she's hard to deal with sometimes.

I wasn't quite sure what to do with this and I thought back to the first time I met Sarah. She came to a course at Skills for People called 'Making Friends' which I was helping to run. At that time I was also a volunteer. During the course we talked about what having friends means, about good and bad friends and about the different types of relationships in our lives. We focused on the difference between people who are our friends and those paid to be there for us and I am now struck by how completely

Sarah took this on board, or perhaps how well it reflected her own life. We talked about why she finds it so hard to have friends:

> I think it's the fact that when you're in hospital, you're not allowed to be friendly with anyone. Everyone you see you're not allowed to be friends with because they're professionals, they're this or that and you get this thing where you don't make friends with people. It's not an issue, you don't need friends. You know what I mean, friends are nothing, friends are people you can do without. It's not really. It's nice to know that you can speak to someone in a friendship, relationship sort of thing and where you can have a coffee and not talk about problems you've got, you can talk about everyday things when you can have a really good laugh about them. That sort of thing, that's what I would like to do. I can't because, I don't know. If I go out with anyone, right, if I went out with you, I wouldn't know what to say to you, I don't do anything. The only thing I could talk about is the kids and that's the truth. That's the only thing I can talk about and people get pissed off listening about your children. They think that's all I, you know they say, 'Is that all you can talk about, the kids, forget the kids man' . . . and I don't know what else to talk about. I'm stuck and I start stammering and I think I'm nervous again, so it's a waste of time.

Elizabeth was also aware that making friends is not easy for everyone:

> Alison has just got Julie, I don't think she's got a lot of friends. She talks too much and different things. We get a bad head with her talking too much. She maybe can't help it. Her sister has told her to find new friends, more friends to go out with, but she's not, I don't think she knows how to.

Professional distance

Sarah had touched on the role professionals play in her life and she went on to talk about our relationship and the whole issue of relationships with people she sees as professionals:

> Now I've found it really hard with you, now I'll tell you this because you're here. When you were at 'Skills' at first and you were doing, what was it, when you first started, when you first come and you were just a voluntary like me, you come just like us did, but you came to help, didn't you, you didn't come like as me, you did come to help out. But at the same time it wasn't basically a job as in full, right? Now we made friends, we did, didn't we? and that's all disappeared, 'cos now it's your job. It's gone. I looked at you as a friend and I used to think, 'I really like Trish', and I used to think you can talk to me, I can talk to you, because you had problems as well, and I always remember. I even dreamed about you once. Something happened and I come and rescued you and all sorts in my dream. But then I couldn't be that close anymore. I wasn't your friend anymore because, it was your job. I didn't want you to get the job and that was the truth, it's just the way it works . . . you get a friend and then they disappear, you know, you used to think they were a nice person and you really got on and used to see each other and then all of a sudden he's gone. . . . That's why I

just give up, give up the friends [laughs and shrugs] but it must be. I do understand on your point of views as well, making friends with people, you know, that may have a learning disability, that they may bother you, you know because it can be an issue, people do do that sort of a thing, and they do and I know they do and you know I've had people, people with learning difficulties come to my house and bothering me, you know, all of the time. . . . I know how you must feel, but, I mean, there's a lot of people who wouldn't bother you. There's no way I would come all the way up to yours or Liz's house to bother you. I couldn't be bothered. By the time I've seen to my kids I'm knacked! [laughs]. I haven't got the time, it's like, giving someone your phone number, now it's like, 'Should I, should I? I hesitate about giving people my phone number because they'll be phoning me all the time, I'll never get anything done or have a chance to talk to my friends. I don't phone people all the time. I had your number once and you know I thought 'I'll give Trish a ring just to let her know I'm all right', you know. Or I'll give this one a ring, or that one but, it would be no good for me all the time, I couldn't be bothered, because I know how people must feel, do you know what I mean? I feel as if they give you their number and you're bothering them all the time, that's what they feel and that's why it's best not to. . . . Does anyone else feel that way about friends? I think a lot of people are frightened to say it in case they upset you, they are, because every person with a disability thinks that you're their friend, they do, they really think, until you go and then it hurts, it does hurt. . . . [Talks about Christine, a social worker]: now she's lovely, I really like her, yeah but we used to do loads and loads together. We were working up to be friends but she wasn't even allowed to be my Key Worker because she liked us, and that really hurt me. It just tore me, pulled me apart and I just, like a lot of people like Elizabeth would fight for it, but I just couldn't. It was killing me, I just didn't want to know. They were saying so many things to me that really hurt, not Christine of course, but other people, but Christine had to say them to me as well, in that room. She had to say how she felt, that it wasn't right. It made me feel as if I was just a bit of muck, you know what I mean and it really hurt. I just didn't know what was going on and I saw her the other day in the street and I just didn't know what to say to her. I mean she asked about the kids and I told her that the bairn's been really bad, but I didn't know what else to say and I wanted to go. It was like I should have had a bit of paper and say, 'Yes, I'm allowed to talk to you today because you're not at work'. You just don't know whether you should or not. Do you know what I mean? I might be thingying her job or something. I don't understand it, Trish, I must admit, I still don't understand it. Even though I do stand up for my rights, sometimes I find it very very hard. I still find it very hard and I end up crying and hurting, and some days it's just as easy to pretend.

Listening to Sarah tell me these things was one of the hardest things I have had to do and it really challenged the way I view the 'professional' relationship I have with volunteers at 'Skills'. It is almost as if we create relationships that will confine people by our fixation with the need for boundaries. Sarah was right, we *were* friends and it *did* change. Perhaps I moved on, perhaps I hid behind my job. Professional boundaries are a wonderful concept that we have created which effectively prevent genuine relationships. Elizabeth told me about her experience:

> They come and told us I had to change my keyworker and I says I didn't want that, I wanted Kate. They said I was getting too friendly with her, too. . . . I don't know what word they used. Too . . .?. You've got to have a change. Me and Julie, they did the same to Julie. So we wrote letters, 'Skills' helped us. They came to my house and had a meeting. I just says I wanted Kate, no one else. I won in the end and Julie won as well, I helped her.

We also change the goalposts:

> They says, can I have your diary Elizabeth, I'm going to cross the number out. They give us it in case I wanted her through the night, in the beginning. Then I rang her on a Saturday night, I think I was agitated, she said, 'Why are you ringing me at home?'. I'm frightened to ring her now, 'cos they've got two little bairns, you see and it was late at night. I've got the emergency number and if it was an emergency they could get in touch with them straight away. They said if you need anybody, just ring the emergency number.'

So, if we are not allowed to get too close to people, what type of relationship are we trying to create? I asked Sarah to tell me about her current social worker:

> She's very nice, she listens to me, and I mean she's the one who helped us get the kitchen done, so I mean she's good, you know what I mean? Other than that she's got nothing to do with the kids. I mean it's just me, on my terms. I phone her and tell her that I need her. She doesn't come looking for me, you know. . . . She's different from most social workers I've ever had. She listens. She listens and she understands it all. There are some social workers who always think that they know it all. This one, she listens to you and that's all she wants. She doesn't want to be . . . pushy or anything.

That sounded like the perfect social worker–client relationship; genuinely empowering, friendly, open, warm and yet completely soulless. How does Sarah see the relationship?

> Well there's really no relationship there, it's just that she's such a nice person and you can talk to her. When she's not there you just get on with it, like everyone else.

And we think we are so indispensable!

This made me really interested in hearing how people with learning difficulties perceive our relationships with them. Daniel talks a lot about Bob, his social worker, and obviously feels very cared for and supported by him but I wondered if he felt *liked* by him?

> No, I don't think he likes you, he gets on with all his people but I wouldn't say he likes you, he just treats you like anybody. Treats you all the same.

I asked if Daniel would count him as a friend?

> No, not a friend, like a social worker I would say. That's different.

Professionals in control

Sarah said earlier that she felt disabled people generally think of workers as friends, but everything she, Daniel and Elizabeth had told me contradicted this. All of them have a far clearer idea of the nature of the relationship than we give them credit for. I think we have need both to control the relationships we have with people with learning difficulties and to rule and govern the relationships they have with other people. It is part of the historical desire to control their lives. This is no great revelation. Much has been written about how, as professionals, we struggle to empower people with learning difficulties, but there seems to me to be a fundamental flaw in how this works that is to do with who we are as people. We tell ourselves that we really do have people's best interests at heart when the reality is that we just want people to do it *our* way or to cover our backs. We have a fixed idea of how people with learning difficulties should live their lives, based on our (often white, middle class) notion of normality. Sarah talks about her experiences of pregnancy and being a mother:

> Well people's reaction to that [being pregnant] was that I should have had an abortion. They said that I was going to be incapable of looking after a baby because of my learning difficulties and I have fits. People like me don't have babies. So the best thing to do is take the baby away and let me get on with my life. They even mentioned hysterectomy at one stage, because they were going to put me on the pill and I turned round and said, 'No'. The pill makes me too big, I mean I'm big as it is and I don't want to be bigger, and I hate it because it's drugs. And I said to them, 'No, I don't want tablets 'cos they make me sick', and they said, 'Right, the next thing's a hysterectomy' and I went 'What on earth's one of them?' and it was my Mam that explained. We went home and my Mam said 'What do you want then?' and I said 'I want it, I want my baby', and it was the next day my Mam went and got us a blanket and a pair of booties and brought them in and put them on the side. She said, 'Well that's a start' and to her, well she'd made her own mind up. If I wanted the baby, it's my baby, you know, I do what I want. She wasn't going to make us do that.

Elizabeth had a similar experience when she wanted to move in with her boyfriend:

> You know when I moved in with my other boyfriend? She kept saying are you sure you want to move . . . my sisters didn't used to like it . . . they didn't used to come around because I was with him . . . she just says 'Are you doing the right thing? Why are you moving in with him?' . . . when I was getting the furniture in the wagon, Kate was helping us and she said, 'Are you sure you want to do this?' because they know what this lad was like. I kept saying, 'I want to move, I want to move'.

Because we cannot be sure that people will do something the right way on their own we set up services that attempt to *make* them. We create 'halfway houses' so that people can practice living independently, sex education programmes so that they are safe to have relationships (presumably we have some measure for when this has been achieved?) and a whole system of hoops to jump through for every decision people need to take: case reviews, meetings, risk assessments, monitoring. We require tangible proof that people are not going to make a mistake when most of *us* learn by our mistakes.

Sarah said:

> When I was in the hospital, I remember this, there were like loads of babies crying and my baby wasn't, well I didn't know where he was. The nurses came in and I was up at the bed of the Mam whose baby was crying. I said, 'You're baby's crying, it needs to be fed', and the Mam's like 'Oh na', and I said, 'No, come on, you can't do that when you've got a baby', and the lass, she was just a young kid, she'd never ever had a baby before, she heard all these babies crying and assumed it wasn't hers. I woke up for everyone else's baby and the nurse in the end brought my baby in for me . . . but I had to prove to her . . . and then they said, 'I think we'll have the Health Visitor to visit you every day – every day you know.'

Elizabeth felt that she had to earn the right to get married:

> Well I was living with Clive and we decided we were going to get married. Kate said, 'What do you want to do that for, you're happy as you are!' I just said, 'Well we do.' We had a meeting about it and talked about it and that and in the end they said it was OK. They just wanted me to be sure.

Sarah talks about being taught to bath her new baby when she was well able to do it already:

> . . . Then they said, 'We're going to teach you to bath the baby', and I says, 'Can I show you?' and they says, 'No we have to show you' and then she says, 'We'll bath him today and tomorrow and then you can bath him'. And the next day I bathed him and I said, 'Let me do it myself, I know, I seen you do it yesterday so I have remembered', you know, so it's a big game, a game for copying. Kate Copy Cat sort of thing. Right, and I did everything I was supposed to do, do his hair, wash his face and stuff and then get another sponge to do the other parts of his body, and I was doing that and they just watched us and I impressed them and they said, 'I don't think she needs practice'.

Sarah describes it as a *game* which is a wonderful analogy. I am, however struck by the fact that sometimes it is a game of Russian roulette. Daniel endured a terrible few months living in an almost empty block of flats on a decaying estate while the people who supported him decided what should be done. As he says:

> When John retired I got Dennis. Dennis was a bit, he wasn't as nice as, he was all right but he didn't come as much as John used to come in the car. You'd get a phone call from him to say, 'I'm sorry I can't come today, I'll come tomorrow, I'll come next week', you know. That's when things started to go down hill. . . . I knew what I wanted to do and the care workers said they'd see to it, but they didn't. They wouldn't rush into things but Bob did. He found this lovely family and they're lovely people and that's it. I love it where I am. If I'm in a mood I know she thinks about us, but I if I wanted to move again I would have to be really, really sure. Well I'm happy.

Sometimes the rules of the game are just impossible to figure out, as Sarah explains:

> When I was in hospital I had to prove I was a good person before they let me out on the outside, and I didn't know how to be good, because I was being good anyway. I wasn't doing anything that to me would offend anybody or hurt anybody. It was really hard to prove. How can you prove something like that? Do you know what I mean? I mean, I didn't know how, I didn't know what they meant by being good because I thought I was anyway. If I was doing anything wrong, well there was nothing to do wrong there, do you know, and as much as you could do wrong was to say that you didn't like something. So you can't cope, you know, it was really hard. That's why I was in so long, I think [laughs] I never got it right, well it never worked.

If people fight our control and the games we play we do not like it. As Sarah says:

> Well it's still a bit hard now, because a lot of people think 'Skills' has gone to my head [laughs]. They do, you know what I mean! But at the same time they say I'm a nastier person. I'm not. I just know that when something's not right there's no way I'm going to let them walk all over us. Do you know what I mean? I'll put it to people and if they don't like it. . . . it is hard, because I mean I just don't like, wish to think people can just walk all over us no matter what. I think that people with learning difficulties, like I've been in the past, you just sit there, take what comes to you and accept everything that happens and do as you're told, basically. That's the way they see you. They won't expect you to back chat or say, 'I'm not doing that, no way'.

I imagine that many professionals would feel quite uncomfortable with this observation and would even deny it. I know how I felt when Sarah told me how she felt about our relationship and I think we have too much invested in our role to let ourselves be completely honest. At the end of the day we need people to need us or we are out of a job!

How people survive

I wanted to end on a positive note and this happened during a conversation I had with Elizabeth about how she 'manages' her support workers and doesn't allow them to rule her life:

> I borrow the TV money, and the video money, and the phone money sometimes and then I've got to put it back . . . then we're short of pocket money and Kate will say. 'Oh, how are you short of pocket money?' and I just tell her I've been spending it. I'll say on the bingo or something. The other day she says it's gambling, playing on bingo. I says we've been going to Julie's, playing dominoes, she says it's gambling, playing bingo, but it's our money, isn't it, that we're spending?

What a wonderful strategy for dealing with our inadequacies! I realised that Elizabeth, Sarah and Daniel all cope with the way they are treated far better than I would. At first I thought it was acceptance but now I believe it is far more active than that. All three of them are able to see a way through that works for them and keeps us happy.

Sarah told me:

> After I'd had him, they says to us that they're going to take him into a nursery sort of thing to let me sleep, because I was on too many drugs and I wouldn't wake up for him. I thought, 'Oh no, leave him with me, he's my baby.' They said, 'No, wait 'til you're at home with your Mam and your Mam can get up to him', and I thought, 'But he's mine', you know. To myself you know. I never used to say anything to them, I used to just sit there and accept everything they say because it's easier and they wouldn't take him away sort of thing. I wouldn't have spoken up for myself then because if I did, they might have thought they would do it anyway. If I played at what they were saying I was being a good girl and my Mam was getting up to the baby, yeah, like a hide and seek sort of a thing. Seek it out later and I won!

Conclusion

In our professional training we are taught that we are 'givers' and that the people we support are 'disabled' and need help. How then can we ever have genuine relationships with people with learning difficulties? Our challenge, surely, is to turn this way of thinking around and remind ourselves that if we really do stop and listen with an open mind, the two roles can be reversed.

The last word goes to Elizabeth:

> She [Kate] came round the other day and Clive says, 'Do you want a cup of tea?', and she says 'Yes', and before she left she was spilling [pouring it away] it in the kitchen. She didn't drink it and she was looking in the kitchen. I says, 'It's nice and tidy, isn't it?', and she stood up like this [draws herself up to full height!]. She went like this and had a good look round, I just seen her, I seen her eyes, the eyes were all over. I just laugh at it!

Reference

Wright, L. (1995) Take it from us: training by people who know what they are talking about. In Philpot, T. and Ward, L. (eds), *Values & Visions: Changing Ideas in Services for People with Learning Difficulties*, Butterworth-Heinemann, Oxford

6

Understandings of learning disability

Ann Brechin

Introduction

With some trepidation, the term 'learning disability' rather than 'learning difficulties' is used here in the title and for the most part in the discussion which follows. There are two reasons for this, despite accepting the strong preference among those most closely involved to be called people with learning difficulties.

The first reason is that there are some very important and relevant debates about disablement more generally, which it is helpful to connect with. The term 'disabled' is used extensively in arguing that it is our social world that disables people. The challenges raised mainly in relation to physical and sensory disablement need to be recognized also in relation to learning disability. Equally, though not often acknowledged, some of the debates from learning disability can challenge thinking in relation to broader concepts of disability. Using a common language helps to facilitate this process, although that is not to make the mistake of assuming that using the same words automatically makes the meanings the same.

The second reason is that to think in terms of people with learning difficulties risks short-circuiting any attempt to understand disability in broader terms. It is welcomed as a term which at least allows that people *can* learn and which sounds more specific and less all-embracing than terms such as 'mentally handicapped', 'mentally deficient' or even 'disabled'. It also puts 'people' first; a powerful emphasis.

At the same time, and more problematically from the point of view of a discussion such as this, it locates the 'problem' in the individual: people *with* learning difficulties. In this sense it is the equivalent of the notion of physical impairment used to make a distinction between physical impairment and disablement. If 'disability' is disallowed in favour of 'learning difficulties' it then becomes quite difficult to find the language to raise questions about the enabling or disabling processes in society which may be at work in 'constructing' learning disability – questions which are at the heart of discussions about social models of disability more generally. If the whole problem, *by definition*, lies *with* the individual, then our understandings and our interventions start and stop with the individual.

It remains fundamentally important to pay attention to the views and experiences of people with learning difficulties. As people have begun to find a 'voice' which can be heard, it becomes possible for them and others to understand more about such experiences. It also gradually becomes possible to understand more about how such experience is constituted; the ways in which the lived experience emerges within the particular current and historical contexts; the ways in which the category of learning disability is itself created. Social disablement or individualist impairment models may increasingly come under pressure from clearer analyses of the meanings and politics of experience.

This chapter will explore meanings and understandings of learning disability in relation to broad implications for therapy in practice. It will consider how changing models impact on the assumptions made about the purposes and processes of therapy. The work of physio-therapists, occupational therapists, speech and language therapists and others is built upon detailed theoretical analyses and knowledge and skill bases. As these underpinning formulations shift and change and the ground, as it were, shifts beneath our feet, keeping a sense of direction and a sense of where the boundaries lie can become very challenging. This chapter will consider some of these changes and their implications.

Why try to understand?

That the chapter is called, 'Understandings of learning disability', rather than just 'Understanding learning disability', is quite significant. It confronts us immediately with the problem that there is not just one simple, and right, way of understanding disability. What it signals, rather, is that there may be more than one way of looking at things. What may have seemed a question of simply getting to the bottom of it once and for all, may actually become a matter of discovering that quite different and sometimes conflicting accounts of learning disability exist.

Understandings of learning disability are built upon a host of assumptions which will have a fundamental effect on relationships between individuals and therapists, the communications that take place between them, the approach to understanding needs and options and the kind of strategies that are adopted. Theoretical debates about meanings can be interesting in their own right, but the purpose here is to to go beyond that to consider meanings and understandings in relation to their implications in practice.

The chapter title is about 'understandings', but it might easily have been about theories, models, definitions or concepts of disability. The debates are all interrelated and 'understandings' serves as a useful umbrella term to encompass them all. I will refer to 'understandings' as incorporating both formal and informal ways of thinking and talking about disability. 'Theories', I will take to mean more detailed frameworks which include explicit explanatory and predictive elements. 'Models' seem to serve as a useful halfway house between understandings and theories; semi-formal in that they are the focus of much discussion and debate, but without necessarily being formulated into a predictive theory. Models will be the main medium for discussion and exploration here. Models can help:

● to achieve explanatory and predictive power;
● to facilitate administrative decisions, for example about financial eligibility, the targeting of resources, or access to certain facilities or services;
● to assist in the planning of support or intervention.

The most powerful models this century have come first from an identification of the 'otherness' of people with learning disabilities as akin to disease and sickness, leading to the medicalization of the problem and the inevitable imposition of a 'sick role'. Secondly the model of people as essentially childlike brought with it the need for both 'protective' care (although in practice it seldom was experienced as protective) and latterly a recognition of the value of education. With advances in educational techniques combined with a strong push for the rights of such children, legislation eventually allowed full rights to education in the UK for such children only in 1970. Now instead of the sick role, people with learning difficulties found themselves in another role – that of 'learner', perhaps for life (Tomlinson, 1985).

Because models are bound up with our images and experiences of disability, they will have influences of which we are less consciously aware. For example, they will play a part in negative labelling and discriminatory processes in society. Stereotyped images abound, stemming from deep-seated fears and past attitudes. People with learning difficulties are still frequently seen as sick; as the eternal child; the holy innocent; an object of dread and so on (Wolfensberger, 1975) and such feelings are at the root of the models which emerge.

Models of disability

Models emerge as part of a process of trying to make sense of things; trying to understand better, in order to be in a better position to predict or intervene. About 10 years ago, before Alzheimer's disease was widely known, a woman in her sixties wandered in through my kitchen door and made herself at home, alternately admiring my house and asking for sweets. Gentle questioning about who she was, where she lived and so on got nowhere. I was completely at a loss. I knew enough people with learning disability and mental health problems to feel sure that this pattern just did not fit. Looking back now, I can remember the sense of inadequacy and almost paralysis that came with having no model in my mind that I could draw on to make sense of what was happening. I could neither predict what she might do next nor feel any confidence about what I should do.

Later on I discovered who she was and what was happening to her and then I 'understood'; then I could make some kind of sense out of this unfamiliar pattern of behaviour. Years later, with increased familiarity with Alzheimer's disease through books, workshops, television programmes and journals, as well as through personal experience with my own father, my model is detailed and comprehensive. It may not necessarily be 'correct' or the best or only way of understanding what is happening, but it provides me with a measure of confidence about what to expect and how to respond.

The kinds of models primarily under discussion below are relatively formal, theoretical models; the kind drawn up by professionals, written about in books and journals and taught to successive generations of physiotherapists, occupational and speech and language therapists. It is worth remembering, though, that it is not only scientists and professionals who develop models to try to get to grips with the world. Trying to understand is something fundamentally human, something we all do. Irrespective of formal theories, people have always had ideas and beliefs about why other people behave in certain 'unfamiliar' or 'different' ways. Professional theories and models have emerged from these same human processes of trying to understand.

There is no one simple way to frame and present models of disability. For the purposes of this chapter and in the hope of clarifying what may be some of the key issues as far as therapists are concerned, I have divided existing models notionally into three categories as illustrated below. These vary according to where the primary focus of interest is located:

● *Individual deficit/malfunction models* (Figure 6.1) tend to focus on the individual and the nature of any impairment or functional problem within that person's make-up. Such models may recognize the way in which that individual learns and develops through interaction with the world around, but the 'problem' remains located with the individual.

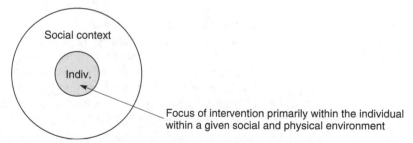

Figure 6.1   Individual deficit/malfunction model

● *Social models* (Figure 6.2) focus on the nature of the social world which impacts on people. The 'problem' is identified as arising from the disabling nature of the social and physical environment, developed to suit the needs of an able-bodied majority.

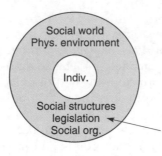

Focus is on the structures and organization of the social and physical environment and the oppressive forces ranged against disabled people

Figure 6.2   Social model

● In *Social interactionist models* (Figure 6.3) the focus shifts more explicitly onto both the individual and the nature of his or her social and physical environment and the processes of interaction between them.

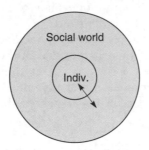

Focus on both the individual and the social world and the interaction between them

Key question is how far the individual and the social world are taken as given; how far the concepts are problematized and politicized

Figure 6.3   Interactional model

There is another dimension on which such models vary and that is the extent to which different elements in the models are assumed to be known and fixed as opposed to being 'problematized'. If we assume that someone simply does or does not have 'learning difficulties', then we are assuming it is a fixed and knowable entity about which every reasonable person should agree. Questions about how notions of learning disability come to be constructed, of how some people in some settings, or at different times in history, or with different colour skins, are more, or less, likely to be labelled, simply do not arise. If we ask questions about how it comes to be understood in these various ways, why there are such conflicting views and experiences, then we are recognizing the 'it' as a social and political construction arising out of social, cultural and linguistic processes; we are problematizing it.

If we generalize about these models, we might suggest that the individual models tend not to analyse the meaning of disability, whereas the social models are predominantly analytical models; the interactional models vary enormously, but tend, perhaps surprisingly, not to problematize. This chapter will be suggesting that a problematizing interactional model might well offer a more constructive way forward and will be making some suggestions about what that might entail. First we can look in a little more detail at some of the existing models.

Individual deficit/ malfunction models

In such models the focus is on the difficulty or impairment in the individual, whether this is the absence of a limb, the presence of cerebral palsy, a spinal injury, a genetic abnormality or a pattern of delayed development and difficulty with learning which appears intrinsic to the individual. Attempts will be made to identify or diagnose the source and nature of the problem, to predict likely outcomes and to suggest the kind of interventions that may be possible. The focus of research will also be primarily on the medico-physiological aspects of the problem, including genetics, often with a view to prevention rather than cure. Therapeutic assessment and intervention will also be appropriate within this focus.

The 1980 World Health Organisation International Classification of Impairment, Disabilities and Handicaps can be seen as such a model. It offers the following definitions:

- *Impairment*: 'Any loss or abnormality of psychological, physiological or anatomical structure or function.'
- *Disability*: 'Any restriction or lack (resulting from an impairment) of ability to perform an activity in the manner or within the range considered normal for a human being.'
- *Handicap*: 'A disadvantage for a given individual, resulting from an impairment or disability, that limits or prevents the fulfilment of a role (depending on age, sex and social and cultural factors) for that individual.'

The focus and modelling implicit in these definitions suggests an individual, whose impairment is fixed, and whose functioning or degree of disability or handicap will arise directly from this impairment. It takes account of, but is not primarily involved with, the role and nature of the physical and social world into which the individual is expected to fit (or from which they may be excluded if they do not). That world, however, is taken as a given; it may be seen as a major factor, but not as a focus for intervention or change, and certainly not as a causative factor. The same applies to the handling of 'psychological problems'. How individuals cope with the emotions surrounding impairments (or the subsequent difficulties and stresses); how they feel about themselves and approach relationships with others – are seen as significant factors, but consequent upon their impairments, rather like side effects.

Rather surprisingly there have been few attempts to develop more explicit psychological models. A recent attempt to extend models of disability within a psychological framework (Johnston, 1996) argued that the WHO model fails to explain discrepancies in the predicted relationship between impairment and disability, including variations in therapists' ratings of the same people's level of disability. Explaining these by recourse to 'coping' theory, which might suggest variation in the extent of 'disabled behaviour' according to the success of coping strategies, still fails to tally with observations. The intervening factor which Johnston proposes as significant is that of 'mental representations'. It may be, she suggests, that people develop certain expectations about themselves and what they will be able to do, and that these affect directly what they then can and do do.

Champions of the social model are quick to point out the failure of Johnston's paper to take account of the extensive literature and well-constructed arguments which exist about the role of the social and physical environment in the creation of disability (Shakespeare and Watson, 1997, leading to a defence from Johnstone (1997) and Pinder (1997). Indeed her analysis does fail to incorporate the implications of this wider framework of understanding. Hers remains a theory with a focus in individual behaviour, although one obvious question to ask could be what a social model perspective might have to say about likely influences on such mental representations of disability. Asking such questions would lead into the interesting realms of identity and self-esteem and the interrelating physiological, psychological, social, cultural, environmental and political influences.

Social models

The assertion of social model theorists is that it is the way the social and physical environment is constructed and controlled by able-bodied people which disables physically impaired people. The development of such ideas has been well recorded, emerging largely through the political movements of disabled people as they organized into pressure groups and established a social identity (e.g. Oliver, 1990; Davis, 1993; Finklestein, 1993).

A shift of perception onto the disabling and discriminatory processes and structures embedded in society is fundamental to a social model of disability. The Union of the Physically Impaired Against Segregation (UPIAS) defined disability as

> The disadvantage or restriction of ability caused by contemporary social organization which takes little or no account of people who have physical impairments and thus excludes them from participation in the mainstream of social activities. Physical disability is therefore a particular form of social oppression. (1976: 14)

The developments of thinking and organization by disabled people went hand in hand and has shifted from a dawning awareness of social injustice at an *individual* level, leading to calls for more and better welfare provision, to a recognition of social injustice to disabled people as a *social group* (Davis, 1993). He describes what was needed to underpin this shift as, 'a vision of unity to help clear the fog of separate identities, single issues, contradictions and general fragmentation' (Davis, 1993: 288). The fog-clearing process culminated, in a sense, in the formation of the British Council of Organisations *of* Disabled People in 1981, which has acted since as the coordinating and campaigning focus both nationally and internationally.

It is important to recognize this history and to understand the political context of the social model of disability. The resistance to fragmenting issues such as separate identities may play some part in the difficulties of connecting the social model with the experience of people with learning difficulties. Their trajectory of development and organization as well as their issues have been different, allowing different, often personal and individual, kinds of story to emerge. Any such challenge to hard-won unity could be seen as very risky.

The major conflict with the learning disability field has, however, stemmed from another kind of social model, rather than from individualized accounts. Normalization, or social role valorization, is described elsewhere in this volume, but in essence it suggests the creation of support structures and opportunities to enable people to have access to ordinary lifestyles and patterns of living (Nirje, 1980; Wolfensberger and Tullman, 1989). It has been a powerful force for change.

It focuses primarily on the social environment and argues that people with learning difficulties are excluded from valued social roles. This, it suggests, severely limits the quality of their lives and, if oppressive and discriminatory practices are removed, their lives can be immeasurably improved. The emphasis is also on playing down any differences, which translates into seeking to make people behave and appear as 'normal'.

Given that normalization recognizes how malleable people and circumstances can be, it shows surprisingly little inclination as a theoretical framework to problematize concepts. Everything is taken as a given. This is where the two social models part company. 'Normal life' here is assumed to be agreed and something to which all will aspire, rather than arising from social constructs, social structures and physical environment, all powerfully under the control and influence of able-bodied people, largely white, middle class and Western. Gender issues, race issues, etc., have been largely ignored. Even disability issues are ignored in the sense that, rather insultingly, it is suggested that it is not a good idea for people with learning difficulties to mix together, because the association will have a devaluing effect. Those who occupy the 'normal world' are deemed to know best and to be the best models for people with learning difficulties.

Others (Brechin and Swain, 1990; Brown and Smith, 1992; Chappell, 1997; Walmsley, 1997) have pointed out some of these contradictions and clashes of value base between normalization and the social model advanced by disabled people. Chappell, in particular, highlighted some of the confusions, raising also the question of how people with learning difficulties can more fully engage with and influence key disability debates and models. (For further information on 'normalization, the reader is referred to Chapters 8 and 10.)

Social interactionist models

Social interactionist models overlap with the individual and social models, but the emphasis shifts towards a focus which encompasses both the individual and the environment (social and/or physical) and the interactions between them. It can be argued that much of the work of therapists is focused on such interactions between people and their physical and social environments. The emphasis is far more on repairing the capacity to function. Disability becomes framed in an interactional model, rather than with an impairment focus. The issue is then not how well someone can, for example, walk, or hear, or reason, but how best to enable them to get about, communicate or manage their life. Various combinations of aids, adaptations and support, combined with appropriate and sensitive educative therapy and practice opportunity, will form the basis of such an approach.

Within such an interactional model, however, a range of very different assumptions can be made. The assumptions vary largely in the extent to which the individual and his or her social world are taken at face value or analysed. The frequent absence of recognition in such frameworks of the need to analyse and reflect upon the social environment leads to challenges from social model theorists (e.g. Finklestein, 1993). One analysis of someone's problems may, for example, talk in terms of poor motivation, failure to adjust, the importance of having realistic expectations given the nature of his or her housing or work opportunities; another may seek to understand issues of motivation, adjustment and expectations in quite different terms, as arising from a complexity of social and personal experiences and constructions. Thus lack of job opportunity, or innaccessible public transport, or public prejudice may be seen as primary sources of limitation and frustration.

In the former, the view reflects the therapist's version of reality – it assumes this is how things are. The latter therapist makes no such assumptions about realities, but assumes multiple influences on how understandings, experiences and feelings may evolve. One powerful consequence of suspending judgement in this latter way is the space it opens up for trying to understand the views and experiences of the individual more directly. It also politicizes the relationship by allowing the relevance of wider questions about benefits, housing, unemployment, poverty, attitudes to disability, scarcity of resource and so on, to be acknowledged.

An interactional model is not in itself enough, therefore, to encompass a broader analysis of the constitution of disability in society. A mapping of psychological models which suggests the kind of terrain that might be covered in a broader analysis (Finklestein and French, 1993) tracks through issues of both impairment and disability, and is essentially embedded in an interactional social analysis:

> We have suggested that both impairment and disabling physical and social barriers can impact on individuals to create psychological differences and psychological reactions. There is a dynamic relationship between impairment and disability which we believe provides the starting-point for the construction of a new approach to the psychology of disability. (1993: 32–33)

The concept of a dynamic relationship is a helpful one and, as a model, this kind of conceptualization could clearly be relevant to more than just a psychology of disability. An interactional model seems to offer the possibility of integrating social and individual models, but that may not be sufficient in itself unless it can hold onto this sense of dynamic process through which disability is constituted in individual and social experience in the broadest sense.

Combining a social model and a politics of experience

Other voices have questioned whether the social model deals adequately with people's experience of impairment (Morris, 1991; French, 1993; Crow, 1996). Such critiques argue the value of recognizing individual experience within the social model, but as Shakespeare and Watson (1997) point out, this has been resisted as watering down the social model (Oliver, 1996).

This other kind of theorizing, grounded in the stories and experiences of individuals, has emerged not only from disabled people as above (and also Campling, 1981; Saxton and Howe, 1988) and from people with learning difficulties (Deacon, 1977; Atkinson and Williams, 1990; Atkinson, 1994; Barron, 1996) but also from women, from people with mental health problems (Harding, 1985; Millett, 1990) and from Black people, Black women in particular (Grewal et al. 1988). As understanding has developed, gradually the issues around the nature of such experiential testimony have been better understood.

The danger of one unified voice representing group identity proved a major challenge for women, as it was recognized that, for example, Black or third world or working class or lesbian women had been left out of account. From this recognition, however, grew a new strength as more groups claimed 'a voice'. The category of 'experience' was seen as a source of information about 'the ways in which social categories and the social/psychic selves which inhabit them are constituted' (Lewis, 1996: 25). In other words, it is not the experience itself which provides direct access to some absolute form of first-hand knowledge, rather the key is coming to understand the processes by which those experiences come about. Stories of individuals have to to be understood as 'deeply embedded in a web of social and cultural relations' (Lewis, 1996). This goes some way to addressing the concern among disabled activists that social group unity should not be lost amid a plethora of individualized cases.

Hence the need to understand the context within which experience arises (Lewis, 1996); to develop a 'politics of experience'. Put the other way round, this could be seen as an argument for holding the experiential face of the social model of disability more clearly in the frame. Rather than seeing individual accounts as risking dilution and fragmentation and as a challenge to the social model of disability, this suggests they could indeed become part of a more coherent and integrated set of understandings, leading to a more comprehensive model.

A related challenge to the social model to find ways of encompassing individual experience more explicitly has called for a sociology of impairment (Hughes and Paterson, 1997). They suggest that the separation of body from culture or impairment from disability is an untenable position for the social model theorist to adopt. What is called for is, they suggest, an expansion of the social model to encompass an embodied, rather than a disembodied, notion of disability:

> A formulation of identity which recognizes a sentient being and a lived experience allows for both an analysis of disabling social process and an acceptance of the 'lived body'. (1997: 337)

The notion of embodiment is grounded in physical and sensory impairment. Can such ideas apply in relation to learning disability (or cognitive impairment)? Unless we return to untenable debates about mind/body dualities, we have to accept that our sense of ourselves is an embodied sense and that personhood and embodiment are inseparable (see, for example, Thornquist, 1994; Wendell, 1996). Hughes and Paterson themselves see their framework as tied up with a broader sense of identity:

> . . . the social model of disability embodies an adequate theoretical basis for emancipatory politics but not for an *emancipatory politics of identity* [my emphasis]. (1997: 337)

There is not space here to explore such similarities and differences as might exist between a politics of identity and a politics of experience. For our purposes here, we can assume that they have a similar focus. The People First movement of those with learning difficulties is essentially an assertion of the right to a positive identity emerging through increasing awareness of shared experience. Although there is still a strong resistance to labelling stemming from the normalization model (Walmsley, 1997), the movement is beginning to embrace an acceptance of an impairment defined in terms of 'having learning difficulties' and from that embodied position to stake a claim to equal rights in the face of social oppression.

Exclusion to engagement

Experientially-based accounts of social oppression and discrimination convey the critical importance of participation by such groups in the shaping of society. It is not enough to enhance an individual's access to a 'normal life', although preventing discriminatory exclusion and increasing life choices may in itself be highly desirable and appropriate. The recognition that is forced if our model incorporates both a social model and a politics of experience, is the need for ongoing political as well as personal empowerment. Personal empowerment alone is not only not enough, it is not appropriate if it is based on a model that involves simply shaping people to fit into, cope better with or adapt to a damaging and discriminatory status quo.

In trying to think about the implications of any of these models, it seems useful to think in terms of a dimension or scale. Exclusion, passivity, dependency and barriers to valued social roles would form one end, or pole, of such a scale. We might expect to find a reasonable level of consensus from disabled people that the aim of any action, service or support should be to facilitate movement towards the positive end of such a scale. This is a different way of approaching it from starting with impairment and asking questions about where that might lead and what might be done about it. It recognizes essentially the dynamic relationship between impairment and disability (Finklestein and French, 1993).

Identifying what might lie at the positive end of such a scale, however, is problematic. 'Exclusion to inclusion' is the obvious choice, but 'inclusion' carries connotations of passive incorporation into a pre-determined (and still discriminatory) society. It also seems to portray society doing the including, rather than the individual playing an active role in creating terms for engagement. Widening the definition to include engagement, activity, autonomy, health and wellbeing, interdependence, the creation of positive roles in society as well as inclusion is one possible response. This would mean a dimension from *exclusion/alienation* to *inclusion/engagement* to encompass the role of society and the individual at both extremes.

What this does is to draw into the model, at least potentially, theoretical frameworks from psychology and sociology. Alienation and engagement reflect experiences, relationships and individual behaviour patterns at the level of personal and political experience; exclusion and inclusion focus attention on the societal processes at work which may be seen as powerful contexts for such experiences. It may be more appropriate to envisage these as two separate, but interrelating dimensions, and renaming the social dimension poles as shown in Figure 6.4.

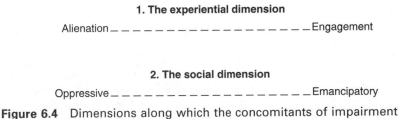

Figure 6.4 Dimensions along which the concomitants of impairment (rather like any form of difference) may vary

The social model of disability creates a sense of separation between the disabling process and the bodily impairment, making it hard to see how to model any dynamic interaction between the two. Perhaps the impairment/disablement split has only a limited value and is ultimately misleading. There is a continual problem of seeming to slip from one paradigm model to another: talk about the individual and the impairment and you lose sight of the social dimension; talk about the social dimension and you lose the individual and the impairment. Yet what happens to and for people is multidimensional. Perhaps by recognizing at least two different but interrelated and interacting dynamic dimensions, it becomes possible to find new ways of understanding or modelling what is happening. In a sense this is not to suggest anything new, rather it is to suggest a way of looking at some complex and interrelating sets of ideas and models which already exist.

If such a suggestion were to prove helpful, then one measure of helpfulness might be whether it sheds light on the kinds of roles different people might play: what it might mean, for example, for our understanding of learning disability and consequently for therapists in relation to working with people with learning difficulties.

Conclusion

The social model as it stands is arguably difficult for therapists to embrace. The implications seem to be, either to become political allies and support the struggle for anti-discriminatory change; or to stay with the impairment focus and work within that narrowly conceived frame. Yet therapists work primarily in an interactional frame, seeing their skills and analysis rooted in an understanding of the interrelationships, both psychological and physical, between individuals and their psychosocial environment. This is the very territory which the social model challenges, seeing it as complicit in accepting an undesirable status quo.

What happens to and for people is multidimensional. The model depicted in Figure 6.4 attempts to recognize this and to hold it all in the frame. On such a model, the role of therapists can be seen as engaging with disabled people's capacity to function at an individual level while concurrently supporting greater social and political emancipation and challenging oppressive attitudes and practice. Essentially, therapists are then grappling with both the experiential and the social dimensions of the model, promoting movement from 'alienation' to 'engagement' and from 'oppression' to 'emancipation'. There may be disagreement over how best to achieve this, or where the focus should lie, but this at least would suggest a coherent value base and purpose, embedded in a coherent model.

References

Atkinson, D. (1994) I got put away. In Bornat, J. (ed.), *Reminiscence Reviewed: Perspectives, Evaluations, Achievements*, Open University Press, Buckingham

Atkinson, D. and Williams, F. (1990) *Know Me As I Am, An anthology of prose, poetry and art by people with learning difficulties*, Hodder and Stoughton, London (in association with the Open University Press)

Barron, D. (1996) *A Price to be Born*, Mencap Northern Division, Harrogate

Brechin, A. and Swain, J. (1990) professional/client relationships: creating a 'working alliance' with people with learning difficulties. In Brechin, A. and Walmsley J. (eds), *Making Connections: Reflecting on the Lives and Experiences of People with Learning Difficulties*, Hodder and Stoughton, London

Brown, H. and Smith, H. (1992) *Normalisation: A Reader for the Nineties*, Routledge, London and New York

Campling, J. (ed) (1981) *Images of Ourselves: Women with Disabilities Talking*, Routledge and Kegan Paul, London

Chappell, A.L. (1997) From normalisation to where? In Barton, L. and Oliver, M. (eds), *Disability Studies*, The Disability Press, Leeds

Crow, L. (1996). Including all of our lives: renewing the social model of disability. In Barnes, C. and Mercer, G. (eds) *Exploring the Divide: Illness and Disability*, The Disability Press, Leeds

Davis, K. (1993) *On the Movement*. In Swain, J., Finkelstein, V., French, S. and Oliver, M. (eds), *Disabling Barriers: Enabling Environments*, Sage, London.

Deacon, J. (1977) *Tongue Tied*, National Society for Mentally Handicapped Children, London

Finklestein, V. (1993) Disability: a social challenge or an administrative responsibility? In Swain, J. *et al.* (eds), *Disabling Barriers: Enabling Environments*, Sage, London (in association with The Open University)

Finklestein, V. and French, S. (1993) Towards a psychology of disability. In Swain, J. *et al.* (eds), *Disabling Barriers: Enabling Environments*, Sage, London (in association with The Open University)

French, S. (1993) Disability, impairment or something in between. In Swain, J. *et al.* (eds), *Disabling Barriers: Enabling Environments*, Sage, London (in association with The Open University)

Grewal, S., Kay, J., Landar, L., Lewis, G. and Parmar, P. (1988) *Charting the Journey: Writings by Black and Third World Women*, Sheba Feminist Publishers, London

Harding, L. (1985). *Born a Number*, Mind, London

Hughes, B. and Paterson, K. (1997) The social model of disability and the disappearing body: towards a sociology of impairment. *Disability and Society*, **12**(3), 325–340

Johnston, M. (1996) Models of disability. *The Psychologist*, **9**(5), 205–212

Johnston, M. (1997) Integrating models of disability: a reply to Shakespeare and Watson. *Disability and Society*, **12**(2), 307–310

Lewis, G. (1996) Situated voices: black women's experience and social work. *Feminist Review*, **53**, 24–56

Millett, K. (1990) *The Loony Bin Trip*, Virago, London

Morris, J. (1991) *Pride against Prejudice. Transforming Attitudes to Disability*, Women's Press, London

Nirje, B. (1980) The normalisation principle. In Flynn, R.J. and Nitsch, K.E. (eds), *Normalisation, Social Integration and Community Services*, University Park Press, Baltimore

Oliver, M. (1990) *The Politics of Disablement*, Macmillan, London

Oliver, M. (1996) *Defining Impairment and Disability: issues at stake*. In Barnes, C. and Mercer, G. (eds). *Exploring the Divide: Illness and Disabilities*, The Disability Press, Leeds

Pinder, R. (1997) A reply to Tom Shakespeare and Nicholas Watson. *Disability and Society*, **12**(2), 301–305

Saxton, M. and Howe, F. (1988) *With Wings: An anthology of Literature by Women with Disabilities*, Virago Press, London

Shakespeare, T. and Watson, N. (1997) Defending the social model. *Disability and Society*, **12**(2), 293–300

Thornquist, E. (1994) Profession and life: separate worlds. *Social Science and Medicine*, **39**(5), 701–713

Tomlinson, S. (1985) The expansion of special education. *Oxford Review of Education*, **11**(2), 157–165

UPIAS (1976) *Fundamental Principles of Disability*, Union of the Physically Impaired Against Segregation, London

Walmsley, J. (1997) Including people with learning difficulties: theory and practice. In Barton, L. and Oliver, M. (eds), *Disability Studies*, The Disability Press, Leeds

Wendell, S. (1996) *The Rejected Body: feminist philosophical reflections on disability*. Routledge, London

Wolfensberger, W. (1975) *The Origin and Nature of Our Institutional Models*, Human Policy Press, New York

Wolfensberger, W. and Tullman, S. (1989) A brief outline of the principle of normalisation. In Brechin, A. and Walmsley, J. (ed) *Making Connections: Reflecting on the Lives and Experiences of People with Learning Difficulties*, Hodder and Stoughton, Sevenoaks

7

Learning difficulties: a biological perspective

Sally French

Introduction

The aim of this chapter is to reflect critically upon the influence of biological factors and medical diagnoses in the lives of people with learning difficulties. It will be argued that, although this knowledge can be of value to therapists as they plan interventions to improve their clients' lives, it will only be useful when viewed within a broad social context. The behaviour of all human beings is determined, at least in part, by the physiological processes of various biological structures, especially those of the central nervous system and the endocrine system. These processes and behaviours are, however, greatly influenced by the external world. As Toates states:

> Behaviour is controlled by the nervous system but activity within the nervous system is itself dependent upon, amongst other things, the external environment. Therefore there is a cycle of causes. (1996: 37)

This is apparent in seemingly basic biological sensations such as pain. It is now recognized that pain is dependent upon a wide range of biological, psychological, social and cultural factors, such as the meaning the pain has for the individual, how other people react to it, the social context in which the pain is experienced, past experiences of pain and the degree to which the individual's mind is occupied in other ways (French, 1997). Pain can also be abolished or made tolerable by psychological interventions, such as the administration of a placebo, behaviour modification, counselling, hypnosis and relaxation (Melzack and Wall, 1988). Pain can also cause anxiety and depression which in turn can heighten the experience of pain, creating a vicious circle.

In a similar way, 'challenging behaviour', which is sometimes displayed by people with learning difficulties, is likely to have a multitude of causes relating to biological, psychological and social factors. These may include damage to those areas of the brain that control emotion, the inability to express feelings, the hostile or inappropriate reactions of other people and an unstimulating or hostile environment. (For further information on challenging behaviour the reader is referred to Chapter 18).

For many years the problems which people with learning difficulties experienced were defined and explained predominantly in biological and medical terms. This was made explicit in 1948 when the National Health Service took over the administration of the mental handicap institutions. These institutions were renamed 'hospitals' and the inmates were defined as 'patients' in need of medical care although, in reality, little care was given. Indeed, Ryan and Thomas (1990) describe people with learning difficulties as being, at one and the same time, defined and abandoned by medicine. Not only was the care inadequate, it was also dehumanizing and abusive. A woman interviewed by Potts and Fido explains:

> They used to make you scrub from one end t'other. And if you didn't do it proper, you had to do it over. Sometimes, if we didn't do it, we didn't get anything to eat. They once put me to bed without any tea. (1991:60)

This situation has led to an understandable reluctance to focus on the part that biological and medical factors may play in the creation of learning difficulties and in the health and illness patterns of people with learning difficulties. There is a very real danger that an overemphasis on biology will lead to a return of the damaging influence of the medical model. An emphasis on biological factors, together with an intolerance of difference, can also lead to an uncritical doctrine that the lives of people with learning difficulties (as well as other disabled people) are of limited value and should, therefore, be prevented. This judgment is often fuelled by the unthinking assumption that disabled people will inevitably be unhappy and have a poorer quality of life when compared with non-disabled people (Swain and French, 1997).

The growing sophistication of genetic engineering and prenatal screening during pregnancy is of growing concern to many disabled people. Bailey states:

> Disabled people ... have taken issue with the feminist defence of selective abortion and raised a number of concerns about the growing use of prenatal testing facilitated by the new genetics. In short, they see prenatal testing and selective abortion as being rooted in and perpetuating the oppression of disabled people. (1996:144)

Biological factors should never be viewed in isolation from social, environmental, psychological and cultural factors and yet for therapists, who are medically educated professionals, some understanding of the biological and medical issues are of importance in their role (Watson, 1997). It is within the context and spirit of a broad definition of learning difficulties, encompassing psychological, social, environmental and cultural factors, that biological and medical factors will now be discussed.

The incidence of learning difficulties

It is estimated that 20 people per 1000 in the UK have a learning difficulty and that 3–4 per 1000 have a severe or profound learning difficulty (Sperlinger, 1997). An estimated 22 per cent of people with severe and profound learning difficulties are under the age of 16 (Sperlinger, 1997).

This is because more severely disabled infants are surviving and many people with severe and profound learning difficulties have a shortened life expectancy (Walker and Walker, 1998).

About 85 per cent of people with learning difficulties have mild learning difficulties (Clarke, 1982). Most of these people have no other impairments and are less likely than people with more severe learning difficulties to be seen by therapists working in specialist teams for people with learning difficulties. They are, however, just as likely as any other person to become ill or have an accident and may be treated by therapists in general settings.

Learning difficulties have, to some degree, been 'created' as society has become more complex. It has, for example, become necessary to be able to read and write and communicate in a complex way with others. There is now less employment for people who find these particular skills difficult. Mild learning difficulties are often identified in childhood, where great emphasis is placed on skills such as reading and writing at school. The 'problem' may disappear or become less marked in adulthood when people have more control over their lives and roles.

Of the 15 per cent of people with more severe learning difficulties, a large proportion have physical and sensory impairments and epilepsy. According to Martin *et al.* (1988), 48 per cent have a sensory impairment and 1 in 3 has epilepsy which is not always completely controlled. Most of these people have a definite medical diagnosis. Almost one-third have chromosomal disorders which give rise to various syndromes. It is important to realize that not all features of a syndrome are present in any one individual and that they vary in degree (Petrie, 1993).

The most common syndrome associated with learning difficulties is Down's syndrome. This occurs once in every 700 live births and is linked to maternal age, being most common in women over 40 years (Watson, 1997). Down's syndrome is characterized by learning difficulties of varying degrees and a range of medical conditions and impairments including congenital heart disease, sensory impairments, hypothyroidism, diabetes, bone and joint disease, leukaemia and the early onset of dementia.

Most syndromes associated with learning difficulties are rare. Tuberous sclerosis, for example, occurs once in every 30 000 live births and Rett's syndrome, which is associated with scoliosis and epilepsy, has an incidence of 1 in 10 000 live female births. Fragile X syndrome is more common, occurring once in every 2000 live births and being more common in males. It is associated with epilepsy, joint laxity, autism and an increased vulnerability to cancer.

It is outside the scope of this chapter to describe all of these syndromes and for further information the reader is referred to O'Hara and Sperlinger (1997) and Gates (1997). Auty believes, however, that:

A diagnosis is not necessary, since the careful assessment of the client's referred needs provides all the information required to plan a programme for that client . . . we are not, nor should we be, in a medical model attitude of care. (1991:15)

Therapists, through their medical education, will be familiar with most of the individual medical conditions and impairments which may arise within these syndromes. They may, however, require a more detailed understanding of visual and hearing disability, as well as multiple disability, to work effectively within this field.

The aetiology of learning difficulties

In 75 per cent of people with learning difficulties the cause is unknown. The more severe the learning difficulty, the more likely it is to be linked with a specific medical diagnosis where there is evidence of damage to the brain (Watson, 1997). One way of classifying the biological causes of learning difficulties is to identify the stage of development at which they occur:

- *Pre-fertilization*. This includes genetic disorders such as tuberous sclerosis, and chromosonal syndromes such as Down's syndrome.
- Inter-uterine. This includes maternal infection (e.g. maternal rubella), radiation, drugs, rhesus incompatibility, poor maternal diet, maternal disease and trauma (e.g. falls and road traffic accidents).
- *Perinatal*. This includes birth trauma (e.g. a difficult forceps delivery), prematurity, hydrocephalus and asphyxia. If the brain is deprived of oxygen for 4–5 minutes, irreversible changes occur. This situation can arise if the second stage of labour is very prolonged or if the umbilical cord is wrapped around the baby's neck during delivery.
- *Postnatal*. This includes infections (e.g. meningitis), head injuries (e.g. falls, road traffic accidents and non-accidental injury), toxins (e.g. ingestion of household cleaning substances and lead poisoning), asphyxia, brain tumours, adverse effects from vaccines and malnutrition in infancy.

Learning difficulties are often associated with cerebral palsy – a condition with which all therapists will have some knowledge. It is caused by damage to the brain and has a similar list of aetiological factors to those described above. Cerebral palsy occurs once in every 500 live births and approximately 50 per cent of people with cerebral palsy have some degree of learning difficulty.

Most of these causal factors are, to some extent, 'socially created'. Disease and impairment are not randomly distributed throughout the population. Apart from genetic and chromosomal disorders, they are more likely to occur in people from social class 5 (the most deprived social class) and are thought to relate to poverty, poor diet, poor housing, high stress, poor child care facilities and social and educational deprivation (Jacobson *et al.*, 1991; Petrie, 1993). Mental distress, physical illness, impairment and accidents are all strongly associated with social status with those people in social class 5 being particularly disadvantaged.

The effect of the environment cannot be overemphasized as a causal factor in learning difficulties. The environment plays a major role in the development of the brain, particularly in infancy, where it influences the number of brain cells and the connections and arrangements among them (Lerner, 1997). An environment which is severely lacking in sensory and social stimulation can create learning difficulties in the absence of any other causal factor.

Mild learning difficulties are strongly associated with low socio-economic status where, through poverty and limited resources, social and cognitive stimulation may be inadequate. Although learning difficulties are sometimes associated with a dysfunction of the brain, this can be greatly modified by environmental factors. Most people need a satisfying and stimulating environment to develop emotionally and to gain confidence socially. People with learning difficulties have often lived in impoverished environments which are severely lacking in both sensory and social stimulation. Their learning difficulties may relate more to these environmental factors than to biological factors. Conversely, it is possible for people with learning difficulties to improve their skills if the environment is favourable.

Illness and impairment in people with learning difficulties

People with learning difficulties have a greater number and variety of health care needs compared with their peers in the general population (Rodgers and Russell, 1995). The demand on GPs is, however, less than would be expected, indicating that the health needs of people with learning difficulties are not being met (Howells, 1997; Vernon, 1997). People with learning difficulties have as much right to high-quality health care as other citizens, but the Health Service is not geared to their needs and they are, therefore, particularly disadvantaged as consumers of health care (Walmsley, 1997). For example, people with learning difficulties receive far less preventative medicine, such as breast screening and cervical cytology, than other members of the community (Rodgers and Russell, 1995; Vernon, 1997).

People with learning difficulties may have difficulty in recognizing signs and symptoms of illness and disease or have problems in communicating information to health professionals (Rodgers and Russell, 1995). Health professionals, in turn, may be ill-equipped to communicate with people who have learning difficulties, may interpret a physical sign of disease as a psychological problem and be reluctant to undertake full investigations because of issues of consent (Downie and Calman, 1987; Howells, 1997). They may believe that the person's life is of limited value and does not warrant costly medical investigations and treatments (Morris, 1991), or pessimistic about the extent to which the person can cooperate with treatment (Howells, 1997).

It is often very difficult to assess the cognitive ability of people who, in addition to learning difficulties, have physical and sensory impairments. Sensory impairments, in particular, are often overlooked, as the problems to which they give rise are thought to be part of the learning difficulty; for example, an inability to hear or see may be mistaken for an inability to comprehend information. There is also a tendency to regard minor health problems as trivial in the context of multiple impairment (Vernon, 1997).

Therapists with a sound knowledge of illness and disease, and the particular syndromes which may be associated with learning difficulties, are in a key position to identify the manifestations of disease in their clients and to ensure that they receive the health care which is their right. Physical illness may also be a causal factor in 'challenging behaviour', depression and anxiety, so its correct identification has the potential to improve the person's quality of life. If medical treatments and therapeutic interventions are imposed upon people against their wishes, however, or if the needs and lifestyle of the particular disabled person are not taken fully into account, they can become oppressive and abusive in themselves.

Therapists are likely to encounter particularly difficult ethical dilemmas with people who are unable fully to understand the situation or to give their informed consent. Someone may be distressed by treatment to reduce contractures of the hip, for example, even though the contractures are interfering with a valued leisure pursuit such as horse-riding. Such everyday ethical issues faced by therapists are explored in detail by Sim (1997). (For further information on ethical issues the reader is referred to Chapter 22A).

Therapists may need to understand the medical conditions that people with learning difficulties have in order to undertake effective interventions. An understanding of spasticity, for example, is essential when attempting to assist movement in people with cerebral palsy or when advising upon footwear or mobility aids. Attending to the person's physical needs, in the context of their own desired lifestyle and goals, can improve their quality of life; for example, achieving a comfortable sitting position may open up all kinds of opportunities for interaction and play. Similarly, joint deformity may be prevented or minimized by careful positioning, and various aids and equipment suitable to the person's impairment can be installed. 'Opening up opportunities' can, however, be used to justify all kinds of interventions which may not be welcomed. Activities such as these should not be used as 'ends in themselves' but in the context of a supportive relationship where the client is in control and where the client's interests are central.

The alleviation of symptoms can be a prerequisite of many valued activities. There may, in addition, be aspects of various syndromes which require the therapist to take extra care, for example epilepsy associated with Rett's syndrome, joint laxity associated with Fragile X syndrome and an insensitivity to pain associated with Prader–Willi syndrome.

People with learning difficulties, particularly when their learning difficulties are associated with physical and sensory impairments, need extra assistance in creating a stimulating environment for themselves (Clements, 1997). Therapists, with their knowledge of the effects of various impairments upon the person with learning difficulties, will be in a position to suggest ways of creating interesting and stimulating environments for clients according to their interests and whatever their level or type of impairment.

An overall knowledge of the biological factors associated with learning difficulties may also help the clients themselves, as well as their families and assistants, to make important lifestyle and financial decisions. People with learning difficulties have the right to health education and to knowledge concerning their own medical condition. As medically educated professionals, therapists may be expected to give information and advice on these issues. The medical condition may, for example, be progressive and some syndromes, for example Down's syndrome, are associated with a shortened life-span. Therapists may be able to predict how the ordinary ageing process will affect impairments and suggest ways in which valued activities may be preserved for as long as possible.

The incidence of depression, anxiety and schizophrenia is also higher in people with learning difficulties and is particularly difficult to diagnose if people are unable to describe their feelings (Vernon, 1997). Symptoms of depression tend to mirror those seen in other people involving sleep disturbances, weight loss, irritability, social withdrawal, somatic symptoms, tearfulness and a decrease in skills, but these symptoms are frequently misinterpreted as being part of the learning difficulty rather than an expression of distress which needs to be taken seriously and investigated.

Although people with learning difficulties are more prone to emotional disorders and 'challenging behaviour', this may not be directly or exclusively related to biological factors, although there is some evidence that biochemical imbalances may play a part in some people (Lerner, 1997, Birchenall et al., 1997). It could be related, wholly or partially, to one or more of the following interrelating factors:

- Under-stimulation.
- Other people's hostile attitudes and behaviour.
- Lack of social contact and reduced social networks.
- Deprivation and abuse.
- Inability to communicate or to be understood by others.
- Numerous environmental and social barriers.
- Lack of social skills. There may be a failure to grasp the complex rules of social interaction.
- Experiences of separation and loss. People with learning difficulties, particularly if they have lived in residential care, may have multiple experiences of separation and loss of people they value and trust. They may not have sufficient cognitive skills to comprehend these losses fully, nor sufficient language to express in words their feelings or to 'think their way through' the emotional upheaval. Birchenall et al. (1997) point out that learning difficulties may inhibit problem-solving abilities. Without help they may be denied the therapeutic expression of thoughts and feelings and the healing effect of bereavement itself. This may lead to the persistence of emotional disturbances such as depression and self-injurious behaviour.
- Lack of information and uncertainty, with regard to important issues in the person's life, may give rise to feelings of anxiety, stress and vulnerability. People with learning difficulties may not always

understand the information they are given or other people may not take the time or trouble to explain, or know how to explain, to somebody who cannot readily comprehend. This may lead to emotional disturbance and difficult behaviour such as aggression.

All of these factors may be intensified by the presence of other impairments.

Conclusion

For many years the lives of people with learning difficulties have been defined in biological and medical terms. This orientation has been partly responsible for the dehumanization and abuse of people with learning difficulties. There is a growing rejection of the biological and medical perspective among people with learning difficulties, as well as other disabled people and their allies (Oliver, 1996; Walmsley, 1997). It can be argued that therapists need knowledge of medical and biological factors in order to work effectively and safely, but these factors should be placed within a wide social context and should never be allowed to dominate the lives of people with learning difficulties nor the help that they receive.

References

Auty, P.O. (1991) *Physiotherapy for People with Learning Difficulties*, Woodhead-Faulkner, London

Bailey, R. (1996) Prenatal testing and the prevention of impairment: a woman's right to choose. In Morris, J. (ed.), *Encounters with Strangers: Feminism and Disability*, The Women's Press, London

Birchenall, M., Baldwin, S. and Morris, J. (1997) *Learning Disability and the Social Context of Caring*, The Open Learning Foundation/Churchill Livingstone, Edinburgh

Clarke, D. (1982) *Mentally Handicapped People: Living and Learning*, Baillière Tindall, London

Clements, J. (1997) Challenging needs and problematic behaviour. In O'Hara, J. and Sperlinger, A. (eds), *Adults with Learning Disabilities: A Practical Approach*, John Wiley, Chichester

Downie, R.S. and Calman, K.C. (1987) *Healthy Respect: Ethics in Health Care*, Faber and Faber, London

French, S. (1997) The psychology and sociology of pain. In French, S. (ed.), *Physiotherapy: A Psychosocial Approach*, 2nd edn, Butterworth-Heinemann, Oxford

Gates, B. (ed.) (1997) *Learning Disabilities*, 3rd edn, Churchill Livingstone, Edinburgh

Howells, G. (1997) A general practice perspective. In O'Hara, J. and Sperlinger, A. (eds), *Adults with Learning Disabilities: A Practical Approach*, John Wiley, Chichester

Jacobson, B., Smith, A. and Whitehead, M. (1991) *The Nation's Health: A Strategy for the 90s*, King Edward's Hospital Fund for London, London

Lerner, J.W. (1997) *Learning Disabilities: Theories, Diagnoses and Teaching Strategies*, 7th edn, Houghton Mifflin, Boston

Martin, J., Meltzer, H. and Elliot, D. (1988) *The Prevalence of Disability Among Adults*, OPCS Surveys of Disability in Great Britain, Report 1, OPCS, London

Melzack, R. and Wall, P. (1988) *The Challenge of Pain*, Penguin Books, Harmondsworth

Morris, J. (1991) *Pride Against Prejudice: Transforming Attitudes Towards Disability*, The Women's Press, London

O'Hara, J. and Sperlinger, A. (eds) (1997) *Adults with Learning Disabilities: A Practical Approach*, John Wiley, Chichester

Oliver, M. (1996) *Understanding Disability: From Theory to Practice*, Macmillan, London

Petrie, G. (1993) Physical causes and conditions. In Shanley, E. and Starrs, T.A. (eds), *Learning Disabilities: A Handbook of Care*, 2nd edn, Churchill Livingstone, Edinburgh

Potts, M. and Fido, R. (1991) *A Fit Person to be Removed: Personal Accounts of Life in a Mental Deficiency Institution*, Northcote House Publishers, Plymouth

Rodgers, J. and Russell, O. (1995) Health Lives: the health needs of people with learning difficulties. In Philpot, T. and Ward, L. (eds), *Values and Visions: Changing Ideas in Services for People with Learning Difficulties*, Butterworth-Heinemann, Oxford

Ryan, J. and Thomas, F. (1990) *The Politics of Mental Handicap*, revised edn, Free Association Books, London

Sim, J. (1997) *Ethical Decision Making in Therapy Practice*, Butterworth-Heinemann, Oxford

Sperlinger, A. (1997) Introduction. In O'Hara, J. and Sperlinger, A. (eds), *Adults with Learning Disabilities: A Practical Approach*, John Wiley, Chichester

Swain, J. and French, S. (1997) Whose tragedy? *Therapy Weekly*, **24**(13), 7

Toates, F. (1996) The embodied self: a biological perspective. In Stevens, R. (ed.), *Understanding the Self*, Sage Publications, London.

Vernon, D. (1997) Health. In Gates, B. (ed.), *Learning Disabilities*, 3rd edn, Churchill Livingstone, Edinburgh

Walker, A. and Walker, C. (1998) Normalisation and 'normal' ageing: the social construction of dependency among older people with learning difficulties. *Disability and Society*, **13**(1), 125–142

Walmsley, J. (1997) Learning difficulties: changing roles for physiotherapists. In French, S. (ed.), *Physiotherapy: A Psychosocial Approach*, 2nd edn, Butterworth-Heinemann, Oxford

Watson, D. (1997) Causes and manifestations. In Gates, B. (ed.), *Learning Disabilities*, 3rd edn, Churchill Livingstone, Edinburgh

8

Controversial issues: critical perspectives

Sally French

The area of learning difficulties is fraught with numerous conflicts and critical debates. These have emerged as people with learning difficulties have struggled to assert their rights as equal citizens and have moved from institutions to community living. In this chapter, three interrelating, controversial areas will be examined: labelling, the principle of normalization, and the 'disabled role'. These issues have given, and continue to give, rise to heated debate both among professionals and between professionals and disabled people themselves.

Labelling

Labelling refers to a process whereby people are categorized into groups and defined in a particular way, usually by more powerful people. Once labelled, people tend to be perceived and treated in a way which corresponds with the label. Until 1970, for example, some children with learning difficulties were labelled 'ineducable' which resulted in them receiving no formal education. Other children were labelled 'educationally subnormal' which led not only to low expectations of their abilities, but segregation in special schools. People with learning difficulties have, until recent times, been incarcerated in inhumane institutions on the basis of this labelling process.

Not all labels are negative; some are neutral, for example 'father' and 'child', and some are positive, for example 'talented' and 'diligent'. Some labels applied to disabled people, which appear positive, are regarded by disabled people themselves as negative. This is because they give a distorted or 'superhuman' image; examples of such labels are 'extraordinary' and 'brave'. It is sometimes the case that neutral labels become negative because of their association with the devalued group. The medical term 'geriatrics' is essentially neutral but has taken on a negative meaning because of the attitudes within society towards old people. The labels applied to people with learning difficulties are constantly changing and this is likely to continue.

Although the discourse is usually about the labelling of disabled people by others, disabled people have also labelled themselves both individually and collectively. They may, for example, turn negative labels into proud labels. People in the deaf community write 'Deaf' with a capital 'D' as a symbol of pride and strength and labels such as 'crip' are used by disabled people in a similar way. Labelling by disabled people themselves helps to provide a valid social identity which may foster a collective identity and celebration of difference.

Labelling theory was first applied to criminal behaviour, where it was noted that the application of labels such as 'criminal' and 'addict' tended to increase the deviant behaviour. One of the reasons for this is that we tend to live up to other people's expectations of us. Interacting with other people, and experiencing the way they treat us, influences how we define ourselves. Labelling somebody negatively may also lead to increased surveillance or segregation from the community which further increases (and even creates) the predicted behaviour. These processes, whereby people tend to live up to the expectations of others, have been termed the 'self-fulfilling prophecy'.

If disabled people view themselves in the same way as non-disabled people, and behave in a way expected of them, they may be experiencing a state of internal oppression. Such oppression can be very difficult to defeat. Woolley states:

> We are oppressed from without by a society which does not value us and therefore does not give priority to our needs, and we are oppressed from within because we have internalised these same attitudes towards ourselves. (1993: 81)

It is not at all surprising that disabled people internalize the views of the wider society as, with the exception of Deaf culture, there has been very little sense of cultural identity among them until recent times. This makes it difficult for disabled people to reject the expectations and beliefs, about how they should think and behave, which non-disabled people hold.

It is easy to see the labelling process at work with people with learning difficulties. The label 'learning difficulties' may lead us to segregate people from the mainstream of life, to reduce their opportunities, to neglect their rights as human beings and to expect very little of them. This, in turn, may lead to the 'self-fulfilling prophecy' and a state of internal oppression as people come to define themselves in a similar way and live out their lives in ways which are predicted by others. The self-fulfilling prophecy can, in turn, lead to 'proof' that the erroneous attitudes and beliefs are correct which can serve to justify the treatment people are receiving, creating a vicious circle. People with learning difficulties tend to dislike all labels which categorize them into a group. The slogan of People First, an organization run and controlled by people with learning difficulties, is 'Label jars not people'.

It can be seen that labels applied to people with learning difficulties, and disabled people generally, can be very harmful. There are, however, some positive advantages to being labelled. Labelling may entitle people to certain benefits and services and lead to positive discrimination (Eayrs et al., 1993), though this is rare. Labels can also give explanations of cause to self or others; it can be a great relief, for example, to receive a diagnostic label after a period of uncertainty. Labels can, as we have seen, also be used as symbols of pride and solidarity.

Normalization

The principle of normalization was articulated and developed by Nirje in Scandinavia in the late 1960s. It is a principle which has played a major role in the move from institutional to community living. Nirje defines normalization as:

> ... Making available to mentally retarded people patterns of life and conditions of everyday living which are as close as possible to the regular circumstances and ways of life of society. (1980:8)

This implies that people with learning difficulties should be permitted and assisted to live socially valued lives of their own choosing within the community.

The principle of normalization was further developed by Wolfensberger in North America where it was specifically applied to standards of behaviour. He believes, for example, that if the right to choose is in conflict with 'appropriate' behaviour, then the latter should take priority (Perrin and Nirje, 1989). Chisholm (1993), for example, speaks of the dilemma of image versus efficiency. An example is given of whether or not a disabled person should use a walking stick which, on the one hand is likely to improve his or her competency in walking, but on the other is likely to decrease his or her image in the eyes of others. Robinson (1989) believes that normalization as a human rights issue, as formulated by Nirje, was eroded by Wolfensberger because, in trying to rid people with learning difficulties of negative labels, they are forced to deny their own identity.

Despite the influence of the principle of normalization in the transfer of people with learning difficulties from institutions into the community, it has been subject to much criticism. The main critique has been that normalization attempts to 'normalize' people with learning difficulties and to impose traditional standards of behaviour upon them with which only a proportion of the non-disabled population adhere (Ryan and Thomas, 1993). Although the principle of normalization has not been applied to other disabled people, similar criticisms regarding pressures to be 'normal' abound (Sutherland, 1981; Morris, 1991; French, 1994).

The principle of normalization aims to disperse people with learning difficulties into the community and to minimize any differences between them and other people. Chappell believes that this does little to enhance the identity of people with learning difficulties and denies them valuable friendships. She states:

> Normalization encourages people with learning difficulties to mix with socially valued people, while distancing themselves from those who have stigmatised identities. Such an argument misunderstands fundamentally the nature of friendship as a voluntary relationship based on mutual respect and affection, which has at its centre shared experiences and interests. (1997:49)

Chappell believes too that the principle of normalization fails to take account of the material constraints in the lives of people with learning difficulties, that poverty is rarely questioned, and that the principle of normalization lacks a political context. She points out that notions of stigma and deviance are 'taken as given' rather than explained and that broad political analyses of disability, where it is found to be socially constructed, have been ignored. Chappell also refutes the idea that attitudes can be changed with training without taking into consideration the material context in which those attitudes are formed and maintained. She states:

> Normalization works through existing structures and strives to change them. It does not examine the material underpinnings of service provision. (1992: 40)

A further criticism of normalization, given by Chappell (1992), is that it is service orientated and lacks the voice of people with learning difficulties themselves. It is a model which has never been adopted by disabled people (Chappell, 1997), who instead have advocated the social model of disability which addresses the very issues that the normalization principle ignores.

Normalization can be regarded as a theory for professionals which serves their vested interests by enabling them to maintain an authoritative role in the lives of people with learning difficulties; indeed, Wolfensberger and Glen (1973) developed a tool, Program Analysis of Service Systems, to measure the efficacy of the normalization principle within human services. Similarly, Auty (1991) regards normalization as a tool for changing and improving services. Conversely, the principle of normalization can lead to a reduction in assistance on the grounds that people with learning difficulties are 'the same as everyone else' and that other people should not interfere (Walmsley, 1997). The principle of normalization fails to recognize the power imbalances between professionals and clients and assumes that they work in partnership with similar goals. Normalization has also been criticized for ignoring gender, class and race (Walker and Walker, 1998).

The principle of normalization is also underpinned by the assumption that the values, norms and behaviour of mainstream society are worth striving for. Walker and Walker (1998) make the point, in relation to older people with learning difficulties, that many of their non-disabled peers belong to an oppressed group where ageism is rife.

A more specific critique has been mounted by Brown (1994) with regard to sexuality which, she contends, the principle of normalization ignores. Although some people with learning difficulties are now supported in marriages and heterosexual partnerships, the support received and the living arrangements do not usually encourage this. People tend, for example, to live in small groups with people who are not necessarily their friends and where to change accommodation is administratively cumbersome.

Rather than encouraging satisfying sexual relationships, services may, instead, regulate sexual behaviour often in collusion with, or as a result of pressure from, parents and carers. Professional training in the area of sexuality is largely concerned with sex education and the prevention of sexual abuse. Sexual behaviour of people with learning difficulties is often denied by over-romanticizing their behaviour or giving it a child-like interpretation. In addition, sexual expression is seldom legitimated or supported outside heterosexual relationships.

Brown (1994) makes the important point that sexual expression is learned and, rather than being 'natural', it is determined in large part by the social environment. It follows from this that, in order to give people with learning difficulties maximum opportunity and support in this area of life, those who work with them need to provide suitable living arrangements and support.

The social model of disability has done much to undermine the principle of normalization. An important tenet of the social model is that disability resides within society, not within individuals, and that, rather than something to be hidden and denied, difference is a cause for celebration (Morris, 1991). In recent years people with learning difficulties have been embracing these ideas, in organizations such as People First and the Self-advocacy Movement, and demanding a lifestyle of their own choosing rather than one which is imposed by others. (For further information on normalization the reader is referred to Chapters 6 and 10).

The disabled role

Disabled people have articulated a set of disabling expectations that non-disabled people have of them which, taken together, have been termed the 'disabled role' (Sutherland, 1981; French, 1994). These role expectations, which apply to people with learning difficulties and have been challenged by them, demand that disabled people be 'independent' and 'normal' and that they 'adjust' to disability and 'accept' it. Such expectations encourage a denial of disability which is politically convenient as it maintains the status quo.

Independence

Physical independence is generally considered to be something disabled people desire above all else. In many ways this is so, for if a person is excessively dependent on others, then he or she must fit in with their schedules and plans with a subsequent loss of freedom and autonomy. In addition, it is all too easy for the relationship to develop into an unequal one, with the helper having undue power and the disabled person being compelled constantly to express gratitude, or at best never to complain. This oppression is difficult to challenge because many disabled people need some assistance and its continuance may depend on expressing a sufficient degree of appreciation (Sutherland, 1981).

Health professionals usually regard physical independence as a central aim in the rehabilitation process. But is it always in the best interests of disabled people to strive for physical independence? A disabled woman featured in Campling's book, thinks not: she explains, 'I can sew but so slowly that it bores me to do it'. (1981:1) Similarly, a person with a physical impairment may ask for assistance in cleaning and cooking, as so many non-disabled people do, in order to save time and energy to lead a full and satisfying life. Disabled people define independence, not in physical terms, but in terms of control. People who are almost totally dependent on others, in a physical sense, can still have independence of thought and action, enabling them to take full and active charge of their lives.

The pressures placed upon disabled people to achieve physical independence is regarded by Sutherland (1981) as a form of oppression. Corbett (1989) agrees, believing that self-help skills can be an intolerable chore for some disabled people, impeding their quality of life and inhibiting self-expression. She describes how people with severe learning difficulties can actually regress if independence is forced upon them indiscriminately.

We are, of course, all dependent on each other to a large extent, and we all use aids, such as washing machines, motor cars, eating utensils and aeroplanes, to save time and to overcome physical limitations such as our inability to move fast or to fly. We are also dependent on other people to produce and repair these aids. Despite the interdependency of us all, the dependency of disabled people tends to be regarded as 'special', as qualitatively different.

The problems disabled people face and the equipment they need, such as wheelchairs and hoists, are also regarded as exceptional. This creates beliefs among health professionals and others that disabled people should 'manage' in as 'normal' a way as possible and that 'unnecessary' aids may harm them by reducing the amount of exercise they take or by making them lazy and dependent. These beliefs, and the control of professionals over resources, exacerbate the considerable practical difficulties disabled people face in acquiring the aids and equipment they need.

The physical and psychological stress involved in gaining independence in basic tasks, as well as the wasted time and reduced social opportunities incurred, are rarely given much attention by anyone other than disabled people themselves. Yet we do not insist that people walk six miles (or even one) rather than using their motor cars, or that they dispense with labour-saving devices in case they become lazy, or dependent on the people who produced them. Indeed, to attempt to enforce such a plan would be considered extremely patronizing and a serious breach of human rights, even if it were motivated in terms of the person's 'own good'.

It is frequently the case that non-disabled people are dependent on disabled people in some way. There is, for example, a huge commercial industry around disability providing lucrative work for many people. Disabled people may also serve the needs, often incidentally, of those who want to care, be useful, or to help. There is often an erroneous assumption that disabled people are unable to reciprocate the help which they receive, whereas in reality people who require assistance are often carers themselves (Walmsley, 1993).

Normality

Closely associated with the concept of independence is that of normality. The pressures placed upon disabled people to appear 'normal' can give rise to enormous inefficiency and stress, yet many disabled people are well into adulthood before they realize what is happening or before they find the courage to abandon such attempts (Campling, 1981).

The pressure to be 'normal' is often at the expense of the disabled person's needs and rights. For example, if a person with a motor impairment who can walk short distances is denied a wheelchair, he or she may become isolated or unable to pursue certain types of education, employment or leisure. Mason believes that, 'Almost every activity of daily living can take on the dimension of trying to make you less like yourself and more like the able-bodied' (1992:27), and Ryan and Thomas (1987) contend that the conventional and conformist life-styles forced upon people with learning difficulties can be an exaggeration of normality.

The goal of 'normality' can also be physically dangerous, as when the person with a severe visual impairment avoids using a white stick. In addition, rendering an impairment less visible can create social problems which are equally or more difficult to manage than when the impairment is exposed. As a disabled woman in Sutherland's book explains, 'I'm happier with something that isn't a deception than with something that is'. (1981:75)

Because of the negative attitudes towards disability which prevail in society, disabled people and those who live and work with them may come to the conclusion that attempting to be 'normal' is the only way to succeed; the goal of normality is thus justified in terms of social acceptance. For example, it can be argued that one of the objectives of deaf people learning to talk, blind people learning to use facial expression and people with Down's syndrome having plastic surgery, is that they will be more socially acceptable, less isolated and better able to compete with non-disabled people. People with Down's syndrome have, however, shown opposition to this view:

> Usually it is other people who make decisions to have plastic surgery, not us. We feel that if you need plastic surgery for medical reasons that's OK. But it should not happen just to make us look like other people. Our faces are not just painted on. We can't just take them on and off. They are ours and we should be proud of them. (People First, 1995)

Morris (1991) believes that the assumption that disabled people want to be normal, rather than just as they are, is one of the most oppressive experiences to which they are subjected. She rejects the view that it is progressive and liberating to ignore difference, believing that disabled people have a right to be both equal and different. She states, '. . . I do not want to have to try to emulate what a non-disabled woman looks like in order to assert positive things about myself. I want to be able to celebrate my difference, not hide from it.' (1991:184)

Acceptance and adjustment

Therapists, nurses and others have viewed their role as one of helping disabled people 'accept' their disabilities and 'adjust' to them. Disabled people have been urged to 'overcome' what are viewed as 'their' problems, to learn to live with them and never to complain. Any anger or depression concerning lack of access, negative attitudes, inappropriate rehabilitation, poor housing, or non-existent educational or job prospects, have been viewed as evidence of maladjustment, denial, and 'chips on their shoulders'.

As well as making a physical adjustment, it is assumed that the disabled person must also make a psychological adjustment. It is thought that becoming disabled is inevitably psychologically devastating, a personal tragedy. For example, Weller and Miller (1977) believe that the adjustment to disability requires a process of mourning. Oliver (1983), however, rejects such ideas on the grounds that non-disabled people view disability and adjustment in terms of the individual, thus neglecting wider social influences. He has also found that these explanations fail to tally with the experiences of many disabled people who neither grieve nor mourn and who may indeed find the experience of disability enriching. Even people who do mourn may be mourning the loss of their autonomy rather than the loss of bodily function or appearance, a situation which could to a large extent be eliminated by social and environmental change.

It is very convenient for society that disabled people should accept what are viewed as their problems and adjust to them, for in that way the status quo is maintained.

Conclusion

This chapter has explored some key and controversial issues which are of relevance to all therapists working with people with learning difficulties. The closure of the large institutions and the move towards inclusion of people with learning difficulties into mainstream life are very recent occurrences which are still evolving. Although discrimination towards disabled people is embedded within our culture, institutions and organizations, therapists are in a position to influence practice and policy and to bring about changes in accordance with the wishes of people with learning difficulties themselves.

References

Auty, P.O. (1991) *Physiotherapy for People with Learning Difficulties*, Woodhead-Faulkner, London

Brown, H. (1994) An ordinary sexual life?: a review of the normalisation principle as it applies to the sexual options of people with learning disabilities. *Disability and Society*, 9(2), 123–144

Campling, J. (1981) (ed.) *Images of Ourselves: Women with Disabilities talking*, Routledge and Kegan Paul, London

Chappell, A.L. (1992) Towards a sociological critique of the normalisation principle. *Disability, Handicap and Society*, 7(1), 35–51

Chappell, A.L. (1997) From normalisation to where? In Barton, L. and Oliver, M. (eds.), *Disability Studies: Past, Present and Future*, The Disability Press, Leeds

Chisholm, A. (1993) Quality of care. In Shanley, E and Starrs, T.A. (eds), *Learning Disabilities: A Handbook of Care*, 2nd edn, Churchill Livingstone, Edinburgh

Corbett, J. (1989) The quality of life in the 'independence' curriculum. *Disability, Handicap and Society*, 4(2), 145–163

Eayrs, C. B., Ellis, N. and Jones, R. S. P. (1993) What label? An investigation into the effects of terminology on public perceptions of and attitudes towards people with learning difficulties. *Disability, Handicap and Society*, 8(2), 111–127

French, S. (ed.) (1994) *On Equal Terms: Working with Disabled People*, Butterworth-Heinemann, Oxford

Mason, M. (1992) Internalised oppression. In Rieser, R. and Mason, M. (eds), *Disability Equality in the Classroom: A Human Rights Issue'*, 2nd edn, Disability Equality in Education, London

Morris, J. (1991) *Pride Against Prejudice: Transforming Attitudes to Disability*, The Women's Press, London

Nirje, R. (1980) The normalisation principle. In Flynn, R.J. and Nitsch, K.E. (eds), *Normalisation, Social Integration and Community Services*, University Park Press, Baltimore

Oliver, M. (1983) *Social Work and Disabled People*, Macmillan, London

People First (1995) *Not Just Painted On*, A report of the first ever conference run by and for people with Down's syndrome. People First, London

Perrin, B. and Nirje, B. (1989) Setting the record straight: a critique of some frequent misconceptions of the normalisation principle. In Brechin, A. and Walmsley, J. (eds), *Making Connections: Reflecting on the Lives and Experiences of People with Learning Difficulties*, Hodder and Stoughton, London

Robinson, T. (1989) Normalisation: the whole answer? In Brechin, A. and Walmsley, J. (eds), *Making Connections: Reflecting on the Lives and Experiences of People with Learning Difficulties*, Hodder and Stoughton, London

Ryan, J. and Thomas, F. (1987) *The Politics of Mental Handicap*, Free Association Books, London

Ryan, J. and Thomas, F. (1993) Concepts of normalisation. In Bornat, J. *et al.* (eds), *Community Care: A Reader*, Macmillan, London

Sutherland, A.T. (1981) *Disabled We Stand*, Souvenir Press, London

Walker, A. and Walker, C. (1998) Normalization and 'Normal' Ageing: the social construction of dependency among older people with learning difficulties. *Disability and Society*, 13(1), 125–142

Walmsley, J. (1993) Contradictions in caring: reciprocity and interdependence. *Disability, Handicap and Society*, 8(2), 129–141

Walmsley, J. (1997) Including people with learning difficulties: theory and practice. In Barton, L. and Oliver, M. (eds), *Disability Studies: Past, Present and Future*, The Disability Press, Leeds

Weller, D.J. and Miller, P.M. (1977) Emotional reactions of patient, family and staff in the acute care period of spinal cord injury. Cited in Oliver, M. (1983) *Social Work and Disabled People*, Macmillan, London

Wolfensberger, W. and Glen, L. (1973) Program Analysis of Service Systems (PASS): a method for the quantitative evaluation of human services. Cited in Auty, P.O. (1991) *Physiotherapy for People with Learning Difficulties*, Woodhead-Faulkner, London

Woolley, M. (1993) Acquired hearing loss: acquired oppression. In Swain, J. *et al.* (eds), *Disabling Barriers – Enabling Environments*, Sage, London

9

Women speaking: personal experience in perspective

Lindsay Brigham

Introduction

This chapter is based upon a small-scale project, carried out in 1995 in North Tyneside Further Education College, with a group of five young women with learning difficulties, between the ages of 18 and 20 years. The original aim of the project was to create a women-only 'space' within the college context, and to use a combination of strategies to enable these young women to relate their personal life stories, present concerns and aspirations for the future. The outcome of the project was the collective production of a booklet: a record of the conversations, discussions and artwork produced over a six-week period. The intention behind this chapter is, first, to provide a forum for the voices of these young women to be heard; secondly, to draw upon debates within feminist thinking to explore the relationship between personal experience and theory; and thirdly, to tease out the implications for therapists.

The project was carried out within a broadly feminist framework in that it was 'by women, about women and for women' (Harding, 1987: 1–14). The discussions and conversations were about the lives of the five young women and the final outcome, i.e. the booklet produced, was for the participants and anyone they chose to share this with. The main concern was not about methodological rigour, the production of knowledge for external approval, or even claiming that the work had the status of 'research', but rather the intrinsic value of the activity for both the participants and myself.

However, on reflecting upon the process of enabling these young women to tell their stories several issues came to the fore. Although the meetings were of value in themselves and gave the young women time and space to talk about their personal life experiences, this was essentially a 'private' activity and the voices were not heard by a wider audience. Debates within feminism have focused attention on the idea that the personal is political and hence there has been value placed upon the importance of women's past and present experiences (Robinson, 1993:3). However, as Mary Eagleton has argued:

> Though the personal is political, the political isn't only the personal; an untheorised politics of personal experience may never get beyond the subjective. (1991:6)

The focus of this chapter is therefore upon the complex dialogue between personal experience and theory and the ethical and political dilemmas inherent in transforming the rich, diverse and detailed stories of private lives into public academic theories and perspectives. Recognizing the importance of this dialogue is important for therapists who draw upon theoretical models which have implications for policy and practice.

Women speaking

Before listening to the voices of the young women it is useful to describe the techniques and strategies used to encourage them to talk about their lives. The project itself was small scale and involved weekly meetings with the group over a six-week period. The agenda was open ended; by providing a women-only 'space' within the college context it was assumed that this would give the opportunity for issues of concern to the young women to be aired and discussed. To give some structure to these meetings, they were organized around the themes of memories of the past; present concerns and interests – hobbies, relationships/sexuality, college, families; hopes and aspirations for the future – work, relationships and independence.

The methodology evolved over the six-week period rather than being fixed at the beginning and a tape recorder was an essential part of the proceedings. The original intention had been to make each session a focus group for discussion but this became more varied as the young women gained confidence and decided what they wanted out of our meetings. They initiated the idea of producing creative artwork to illustrate their lives and this in turn meant there was time to conduct interviews with individuals or pairs and to ensure that everyone had the opportunity to tell their stories rather than one or two voices dominating the proceedings. There were still full group discussions but they formed a smaller part of the agenda.

Discussion of the past was characterized by memories of domestic life and family relationships. The following incident was described by one of the young women whose twin sister was also a participant in the group:

> I used to paint the fence when we lived in Howden – painted it white. And when we were little, me and De. used to jump on the beds you know, jump on them and mam says will you stop it or else you'll make a hole in the floor. We never bothered we kept on doing it then one day me and De. used to go out with no tops on. We used to go outside with no tops on you know and we used to get wrong for doing that'.

Working together as a group also enabled participants to describe traumatic events from the past as the following dialogue between a young woman with learning difficulties and her support worker illustrates. This interaction took place in the first session. The young woman, who was also autistic, had been quiet and withdrawn but suddenly became animated when one of the others remembered falling off a bike when she was little:

Su. I scratched my head. I just went sick all the time.

L. How did you scratch it?

Su. It was absolutely terrible.

K. How did you hurt your head Su., was this when you were a little girl?

Su. Fell off a bike . . . split my head. Dad was covered in blood . . . all over his shirt. I had to take her home.

K. Who took you home?

Su. C. took her home.

K. Is that your sister, is that your older sister?

Su. Yeah.

K. Was C. on a bike?

Su. No . . . dear me, absolutely terrible . . . the house was thick with blood . . . daddy's shirt covered in blood too.

K. Did you go back on your bike afterwards or did you not bother?

Su. I took her home . . . bandage on my head . . . I was alright. I thought eeh my god. I took her home, in the house. She was alright.

The telling of this story provided quite a dramatic moment in the first session. Because of her autistic tendencies the young woman concerned had interacted very little with the others in the group up until this point. The dialogue is interesting in that it switches from first to third person, firstly identifying herself as the person who was injured, then distancing herself from the situation to the role of bystander and helper, then back again. The support worker confirmed later that it was in fact the young woman talking who had been injured and expressed surprise that she had spoken for so long (this is a shortened extract). This was not usual in one-to-one conversation and it seemed that there was something about the group process itself which triggered this disclosure.

Memories of schooling were also a strong theme in discussions of the past, possibly accentuated by the fact of limited availability of 'special schools' and facilities for people with learning difficulties. This meant that there were networks of shared memories:

L. Did you have a special friend [at that school]?

Da. I used to go and Sa. used to meet us two didn't you?

L. When you were little?

Sa. Yeah.

Da. Yeah, I think we used to go to school together and we used to see each other.

L. And what did you used to like about school . . . or did you not like it?

Da. I know something I didn't like.

Sa. I didn't like doing maths.

Da. Why didn't you like doing maths?

Sa. 'Cos they were too hard and that.

L. What did it make you feel like when you couldn't do them?

Da. It made me cross when I couldn't do any maths. I couldn't do any maths, they were hard as well.

L.   What did you like doing at school?
Sa. English and that.
Da. I enjoyed cooking.
[ ]
Da. I remember something I didn't like at Southlands.
L.   What was that?
Da. You should know, you should know, you should know this.
     Injections, they used to give us them. We didn't quite enjoy it.
L.   Injections aren't very nice.
[ ]
Da. One day me and S. were having our dinner and we were going to
     have a pudding, right . . . the first one to say who wants the skin of
     the custard . . . we shouted but all the lads got them every day.
Sa. And you were cross.
Da. I didn't like that school. I did remember the first day, I was nervous.
     We used to wear dresses and I didn't like it.

Discussions about the present centred on various themes and topics.
The domestic setting and family relationships were a continuing theme:

C. has a baby called D. who is a lovely little boy and I do just love him
to bits and I do just love him all the time. And he comes on a Friday night
till a Saturday afternoon and he gets fed and I look after him if mam is
making the beds.

However, the present also encompassed an increasing focus on
relationships outside the family and particularly relationships with boys,
romance and sexuality. There were clearly some tensions around issues of
sexuality, with the young women preferring an idealized romantic
approach rather than a very overtly sexual one. Discussion about feelings
brought this to the fore, as the contrast between the following two
extracts illustrates:

L.   What makes you feel sad?
C.   Aww boyfriends and girlfriends.
L.   Boyfriends and girlfriends?
C.   Yeah.
L.   Other people make you feel sad?
C.   Yes.
L.   What makes you feel sad about boyfriends and girlfriends?
C.   Touching, touch me.
L.   When they touch you, who touches you?
C.   M., my boyfriend.
L.   That makes you feel sad?
C.   Yeah, touching.
L.   Why does it make you feel sad?
C.   Touch here and touch here (gestures to breasts and vagina), I no
     like it . . . I hate it, touching there.
L.   Right, so what do you say if he touches there.
C.   Mum said, no touching.

This dialogue was with a young woman in the group with Down's syndrome who had difficulty in articulating what she wanted to say. It was clear from the discussion that touching was something which had been discussed in the family context and that she was uncomfortable with behaviour which she had been told was wrong. The young woman speaking in the following extract also has Down's syndrome and expresses relationships in a much more romantically idealized way:

L.   What makes you feel happy S.?
S.   Boyfriends.
L.   Why do boyfriends make you happy?
S.   I like them.
L.   What do you like about them?
S.   I like passion.
L.   You like passion?
S.   A kiss . . . to hold me, hold me, kiss me.
L.   Hold you and kiss you, right?
S.   I'll be, I'll be his wife soon.
L.   You're getting married.
S.   Yeah.
L.   You hope to marry him.
S.   I want to marry him . . . he'll be a perfect man to go out with me . . . it'll be nice.

Popular music, fashion, friends and food were also topics which dominated the conversations based on the present time:

I used to do hospitality, right, and I went to C's house and me and C. were singing in her bedroom – 'Take That' – on her karaoke and we had like loads of things to eat – cakes, biscuits, crisps, tea. Then C. came to my house one day and we still had the tapes on.

I like dresses – my favourite colour dress is black and white – I like black first, white second, I like boyfriends, I like make-up – lipstick, a little bit of cream on my face and a little bit of talc on my face, deodorant to keep me fresh and clean.

The future was characterized by talk about independence, relationships, marriage and children, with paid work also featuring in the young women's aspirations:

I want to get a wedding dress and have a ceremony with flowers. I'd like a decent boyfriend to get married to. He'd be handsome and talented with personality. I'd like a honeymoon after I got married in San Francisco. We would go in an aeroplane from Newcastle.

I want a son, a boy . . . my best names Adam and Robin . . . I want to win the lottery.

. . . getting married . . . tidying up . . . I'd like having a child . . . take the kids out and have a ride in the car. . .

I'll have a dog and a cat, they'll be always fighting each other. I'll go shopping and that. You can do anything you want when you're by yourself. I'd cook. I'd ask my friends round – I'd make them a cup of coffee or tea.

I would like to be a nurse 'cos the way they dress, more grown up . . . and wear a hat . . . operations, gloves.

Personal experience in perspective

The accounts described in the previous section provide a detailed insight into the lives of the young women with learning difficulties. On their own terms they are powerful expressions of personal experience. So, is it necessary to attempt to transform the richness and detail of these private conversations into public academic discourse; to link these individual stories to feminist theory? If we are to make the personal political and to transform talk into action, or as Angela McRobbie puts it to 'make talk walk' (1991a:79), then it would seem that the answer to this question has to be yes.

In organizing and making sense of the detailed narratives, I start with my first impressions. I had gone into the group expecting to find differences, yet I found many commonalities with any group of young women who had not been labelled as having learning difficulties (Atkinson, 1997). To organize and interpret the findings it therefore made sense to draw upon frameworks of analysis which have been utilized by feminist researchers of youth culture (McRobbie, 1991b; Griffin, 1993).

A large percentage of the group discussions, one-to-one interviews and the artwork hinged round the way the young women interacted with texts of popular culture: music, comics, magazines, television programmes. These media carry powerful ideological messages relating to gender. McRobbie carried out a detailed analysis of one text, i.e. *Jackie* magazine, and identified a 'culture of femininity' related to an over-arching ideology of romantic individualism. She argued that the messages conveyed are constructed round sets of codes: the code of romance, code of personal/domestic life, code of fashion and code of pop music. In her study of working class girls in Birmingham she illustrates how the meanings embedded in these codes are lived out in the daily lives of the girls:

. . . they replaced the official ideology of the school with their informal feminine culture, one which was organized round romance, pop fashion, beauty and boys. (McRobbie, A., 1991c:51)

The extracts in the previous section mirror the concerns of the Birmingham schoolgirls in the study, illustrating that the 'culture of femininity' held a similar appeal for both groups of young women.

If making comparisons about 'femininity' from a discourse perspective can give insights, it is also useful to examine discourses of adolescence. Christine Griffin argues that 'both family life and sexuality have been crucial elements in discourses around adolescence' (1993:158). I would like to explore how one of the key discourses she identifies links to the personal aspirations of the group of young women with learning difficulties – the discourse of development.

Griffin describes the discourse of development as laying out the 'normal' path between childhood through adolescence to mature adulthood, heterosexuality, marriage, parenthood and full-time job. Adolescent sexuality is constructed as somewhat problematic, a 'natural' but rather disruptive force which must be channelled into the appropriate pathway. The extracts in the previous section illustrate how the young women with learning difficulties positioned themselves within this discourse of development. The emphasis on marriage and motherhood is particularly interesting, as work with older women has shown that this type of aspiration was outside their expectations (Atkinson, 1993)

If the 'discourse of development' constructs adolescent sexuality as somewhat problematic, with young people who stray from normative expectations being defined as 'deviant', it could be argued that sexuality for young women with learning difficulties is even more problematic. This has been touched upon in extracts from the previous section and Hilary Brown argues that, despite the rhetoric of 'normalization' (Wolfensberger, 1972), the implicit role of services for people with learning difficulties is to regulate sexuality and create sexual boundaries. This could also be compounded by protective parental attitudes. Service workers often fall short of enabling sexual relationships to take place and this lack of enabling practice can be linked to latent discourses of learning disability which are still prevalent in society, for example eugenic discourses which define people with learning difficulties as 'unfit' to reproduce (1994:114). Brown argues that,

> People with learning difficulties who do assert their right to what is perceived as an ordinary sexual life are actually breaking the rules for their 'kind' and should be supported in what is an act of rebellion rather than conformity. (1994:141)

Therefore, in actively positioning themselves as 'subjects' within the 'discourse of development' the young women who took part in the project were refusing to be subjected to discourses of learning disability which denied their rights to (hetero)sexuality, marriage and motherhood.

The dialogue between personal experience and theory

The previous section has illustrated how personal experiences can be potentially politicized by integrating them with broader perspectives. However, there is a long-standing debate within feminism concerning the personal experience/theory dichotomy and the value of different forms of knowledge constituted by each. The idea of the personal as political takes as its starting point the everyday lives of women and their experience of this reality. In terms of understanding gender and power relations, this approach sees knowledge as empirically and experientially based. The women's movement of the 1960s and 1970s stressed the importance of women sharing experiences in a group context to raise awareness that there was a commonality in their situation. This commonality was linked to the broader patriarchal structure of society, i.e. the personal became political and was theorized to an extent, but the starting point was always with personal experience.

This was a radical break from traditional social sciences which had focused upon the public sphere and been characterized by more abstract theorizing in an attempt to distance itself from what was perceived as the specific and subjective. Radical feminists tend to take a polemical stance within the experience/theory debate and see theory as essentially masculinist. For example, Mary Daly argued that,

> Under patriarchy, Method has wiped out women's questions so totally that even women have not been able to hear and formulate our own questions to meet our own experiences. Women have been unable even to experience our own experiences. (1973:11–12)

From this perspective, far from being disinterested, 'male-stream' theorizing presents a partial view of the world and represents this partiality as objectivity. In the process, women have been either misrepresented or excluded (Gunew, 1990). Some contemporary feminists have reiterated Daly's stance and classified theory as impersonal, public, objective and male, in contrast to experience which is seen as personal, private, subjective and female (Cixous, 1986). Other feminists have been much more sympathetic to the need to engage with theory in order to challenge patriarchal knowledge and associated policy and practice. However, this has not been without difficulties and feminist theorizing has often been accused of falling into a similar trap to 'male-stream' theorizing; being written from a white, middle class, heterosexual perspective which misrepresents or excludes the wide diversity of women's experiences (Hooks, 1984:1–15). In recent years disabled women have added their voices to the chorus of those excluded. For example, Jenny Morris has developed a critique of '... research and theorizing about "care" and "caring", dominated by a feminist agenda of challenging the economic dependence of women created by their role as unpaid carers within the family' (1998: 163–170). She argues that the focus on the 'burden of care' and the 'dependency' of older and disabled people excludes their subjective experience which is often more in tune with reciprocity of care and interdependence.

However, if dominant voices within feminism can be accused of failing to listen to the subjective experiences of others, even the disability movement, which initially placed a high value on the experiential validity of disabled people, can be charged with a tendency towards the abstract. To explore this assertion it is useful to look at the complex dialogue between theory and experience in this context.

Until recent years disability research was dominated by a 'medical model' which defined disability as synonymous with physical, sensory or mental impairment. This way of approaching disability has constructed it as something which is located in the individual and which can be objectively assessed by an 'expert' who is able to quantify the extent of the impairment. This model has come under strong criticism and it has been argued that constructing disability in this way contributes to the social oppression of disabled people by focusing upon the limitations of the individual rather than upon obstacles in the physical and social environment (Oliver, 1990:6–9). When disabled people have discussed their experiences, what has emerged from this more qualitative understanding is a 'social model' of disability which defines it as something which society imposes upon the individual by inappropriate structural, attitudinal and organizational barriers (Finklestein, 1993). The social model therefore developed out of a recognition of the experiential validity of disabled people and claims for this type of knowledge a status which can challenge accounts and practices imposed by 'experts'. In recent years the social model has also been seen as appropriate for people with learning difficulties (Williams, 1992) and the dominance of the medical model in this context is similarly being challenged.

This discussion can be seen as an example of how personal experience can be used to challenge disempowering models and produce new empowering models. The social model has provided a powerful tool for challenging disablist policies and practices. However, unless an ongoing dialogue is maintained with the experiential there is a danger that theory can stagnate and become limited in its application. As Sally French points out:

> In recent years a number of disabled people, particularly women, have sought to extend the social model of disability to include impairment. (1997a:341–342)

In currently ignoring impairment, the social model neglects to acknowledge that as human beings we are embodied subjects and our experiences of the world are mediated through our bodies. As Chris Schilling argues:

> ... we need to regard the body as a material and a physical phenomenon which is irreducible to immediate social processes or classifications. Furthermore, our sense, knowledgeability and capability to act are integrally related to the fact that we are embodied beings. Social relations may profoundly affect the development of our bodies [ ] but bodies can't be 'explained away' by these relations. (1997:81)

The benefits of the social model are that it has been inextricably linked with the development of a politics of disablement and has been used to explore the role of social causation and social construction in the oppression of disabled people (Oliver, 1990:12–14; 78–94). However, to deny embodiment is also to devalue the subjective experiential validity of pain, discomfort, limited mobility or sensory loss. Conversations with the young women with learning difficulties involved in the project often centred around bodily discomfort such as painful and irregular periods, headaches, and feeling sick and generally under the weather. The following conversation illustrates my attempts to move the conversation away from the physical body to place emotional feelings in a broader context. In attempting to do so I was working to my own agenda, influenced by the social model, rather than being sensitive to the importance of negative feelings associated with the physical body for these young women:

L.   What do we mean by feelings, what are the different sorts of feelings you can have?

De.   Awful, aw hey.

L.   Awful, when you feel at your worst?

De.   When you've got a lot of pain and you feel sick.

L.   If you're feeling ill that makes you feel awful, does anything make you feel awful other than being ill?

De.   Na.

L.   What other feelings?

Da.   Feeling awful if you get like your periods.

De.   Feeling awful if you're not well.

L.   What other sorts of feelings?

De.   When you've got a bad head.

L.   Well that's feeling ill, feeling poorly.

De.   If you've been sick.

L.   Yeah, that's feeling ill . . . other sorts of feelings.

These symptoms are not only associated with learning difficulties, of course, but there is growing evidence that people with learning difficulties have a greater than average amount of ill health (Walmsley, 1997). In privileging abstract theory over experience the politics of disablement are highlighted within the framework of the social model, but at the expense of devaluing the personal experience of physical impairment.

Ethical dilemmas

In carrying out the project an ethical framework was set which centred round issues of informed consent, confidentiality and honesty in explaining the purpose of the research. Plummer also includes issues of exploitation and betrayal in his overview of potential ethical dilemmas in life history research (1983:140–146). Others have highlighted particular issues in the research process when people with learning difficulties are involved (Walmsley, 1995; Goodley, 1996). As these concerns are well documented, what I would like to concentrate on here is the ethical and political dilemma highlighted at the end of the last section.

As argued previously, the social model of disability has been essential to the development of a political analysis of the situation of disabled people. This analysis has been central to challenging individualizing accounts of disability perpetuated by the medical model. It has taken as its starting point the social oppression of disabled people, and researchers working within this framework have taken the ethical stance that research should be emancipatory; it needs to actually change the situation of disabled people before it can be recognized as successful. The researcher is considered to be part of the struggle against the oppression of disabled people rather than a neutral and disinterested searcher after the 'facts'. The ethical dilemma occurs when the shift towards the abstract goes too far and whole groups of people are defined by a generalized model which does not recognize diversity and individual experience. Opie (1992) suggests that for research to remain empowering it must:

- incorporate a reflexive dimension;
- recognize differences between the voices of participants and the contradictoriness of individual voices;
- employ a deconstructive textual analysis which does not aim to be definitive;
- incorporate the diverse voices of participants in published research;
- encourage individual and collective challenging of the system.

In other words, to remain empowering, research must create a more extensive dialogue between personal experiences and theory.

Conclusion

The discussion in this chapter has placed an emphasis on the value of personal experience and explored the benefits as well as the pitfalls of theorizing experience. In doing so there have been several implicit messages for therapists.

First, it is necessary to use an appropriate method to elicit information and enable people to talk about their experiences. In a clinical context, the usual method is the one-to-one interview which ranges from a structured interview, which is relatively easy to code and analyse, to a semi-structured or unstructured interview which gives access to a more rich, detailed and qualitative account (French, 1997b). If the interviewer is to avoid imposing their framework of meaning on the interview process, the latter is a more useful tool. When working with people with learning difficulties it is important to use appropriate strategies to facilitate communication and it may be necessary to explore other possibilities than the one-to-one interview. For example, the creative artwork produced over the duration of the project provided insight into the experiences, interests and concerns of the young women, as well as forming a stimulus for further discussion.

Secondly, there must be an awareness of the imbalance in the power relationship between the therapist and client. The therapist has at his or her disposal a body of knowledge gained from abstraction and theorizing which has a greater status as knowledge than the personal experience of the client. This can lead to professionals ignoring or overlooking information which might be of value because it does not fit within their framework of reference.

Thirdly, a more general point can be made relating to the balance between theory and experience. Personal experience has tended to be devalued and associated with the feminine and subjective, whereas theory has been associated with the masculine and objective. This bias towards the abstract rather than the specific creates an imbalance which, if unchecked, leads to a one-sided monologue instead of a dialogue between theory and experience, and those with power can impose their definitions and realities on those who have less power. Daly's argument that we have a situation whereby 'women have been unable even to experience our own experiences' further highlights that experience itself is not untainted by theory and discourse. The experiences of the young women with learning difficulties were not just features of their individual life stories but were structured by gender, age and the fact that they had been labelled as having learning difficulties and, prior to that, mental handicap; discourses which are historically specific and have particular consequences in terms of policies and practices which affected their lives. Rather than thinking about personal experience/theory as binary opposites a new form of theorizing is required, a dynamic theory in process, which recognizes the blurred boundaries and the mutually constitutive relationship between personal experience and theory.

References

Atkinson, D. (1993) *Past Times. Older People with Learning Difficulties Look Back on their Lives*, private publication, Milton Keynes

Atkinson, D. (1997) *An Auto/Biographical Approach to Learning Disability Research*, Ashgate Publishing, Aldershot

Brown, H. (1994) An ordinary sexual life?: a review of the normalisation principle as it applies to the sexual options of people with learning difficulties. *Disability and Society*, **19**(2), 123–143

Cixous, H. (1986) 'Sorties: out and out: attacks/ways out/forays. In Cixous, H. and Clément, C. (eds) *The Newly Born Woman*, University of Manchester Press, Manchester

Daly, M. (1973) *Beyond God the Father: Towards a Philosophy of Women's Liberation*, Beacon, Boston

Eagleton, M. (1991) *Feminist Literary Criticism*, Longman, London and New York

Finklestein, V. (1993) *K665: The Disabling Society*, Workbook 1, The Open University, Milton Keynes

French, S. (1997a) Defining disability: its implications for physiotherapy practice. In French, S. (ed.), *Physiotherapy: A Psychosocial Approach*, 2nd edn, Butterworth-Heinemann, Oxford

French, S. (1997b) Clinical Interviewing. In French, S. (ed.), *Physiotherapy: A Psychosocial Approach*, 2nd edn, Butterworth-Heinemann, Oxford

Goodley, D. (1996) Tales of hidden lives: a critical examination of life history research with people who have learning difficulties. *Disability and Society*, **11**(3), 333–348.

Griffin, C. (1993) *Representations of Youth: The Study of Youth and Adolescence in Britain and America*, Polity Press, Cambridge

Gunew, S. (1990) *Feminist Knowledge: Critique and Construct*, Routledge, London and New York

Harding, S. (1987) Introduction: is there a feminist method. In *Feminism and Methodology*, Indiana University Press, Bloomington, Ind.

Hooks, B. (1984) *Feminist Theory: From Margin to Centre*, South End Books, Boston

McRobbie, A. (1991a) The politics of feminist research: between talk, text and action. In *Feminism and Youth Culture: From Jackie to Just Seventeen*, Macmillan Press, London

McRobbie, A. (1991b) *Feminism and Youth Culture: From Jackie to Just Seventeen*, Macmillan, London

McRobbie, A. (1991c) The culture of working class girls. In McRobbie, A. (ed) *Feminism and Youth Culture: From Jackie to Just Seventeen*, Macmillan, London

Morris, J. (1998) Creating a space for absent voices: disabled women's experience of receiving assistance with daily living activities. In Allott, M. and Robb, M. (eds) *Understanding Health and Social Care: An Introductory Reader*, Sage, London

Oliver, M (1990) *The Politics of Disablement*, Macmillan, London

Opie, A. (1992) Qualitative research, appropriation of the 'Other' and Empowerment. *Feminist Review*, **40**, 52–69

Plummer, K. (1983) *Documents of Life: An Introduction to the Problems and Literature of a Humanistic Method*. George Allen and Unwin, London

Robinson, V. (1993) Introducing Women's Studies. In Richardson, D. and Robinson, V. (eds), *Introducing women's studies* Macmillan, London

Schilling, C. (1997) The body and difference. In Woodward, K. (ed.), *Culture, Media and Identities: Identity and Difference* Sage/The Open University, London

Stacey, J. (1993) Untangling feminist theory. In Richardson, D. and Robinson, V. (eds), *Introducing Women's Studies*, Macmillan, London

Walmsley, J. (1995) Life history interviews with people with learning disabilities. *Oral History*, Spring, 71–77

Walmsley, J. (1997) Learning difficulties: changing roles for physiotherapists. In French, S. (ed.), *Physiotherapy: A Psychosocial Approach*, 2nd edn, Butterworth-Heinemann, Oxford

Williams, F. (1992) Women with learning difficulties are women too. In Langan, M. and Day, L. (eds), *Women, Oppression and Social Work: Issues in Anti-Discriminatory Practice*, Unwin Hyam, London

Wolfensberger, W. (1972) *The Principle of Normalisation in Human Services*, National Institute on Mental Retardation, Toronto

10	# Research and people with learning difficulties
	Anne Chappell

Introduction

This chapter will examine the development of methodology in qualitative research into the lives of people with learning difficulties. Given the breadth of this topic, I do not claim to provide a comprehensive review of research in this field, but I will endeavour to explore the principal strands of this body of research. The aim of the chapter is to enable therapists to think critically about the development of methodology in learning difficulty research, so that they may reflect on methodological issues when undertaking their own research and in their reading of other people's research.

The chapter will be divided into three sections. First, a brief definition of qualitative research is given. Secondly, the development of methodology in research into services for people with learning difficulties is discussed. The final section explores methodologies used in research which investigates the lives of people with learning difficulties, particularly research which seeks to elicit their views.

What is qualitative research?

Mason emphasizes the diversity of methodological approaches which can be put under the heading of qualitative research. However, she suggests a working definition as research which explores the production and interpretation of the social world; uses methods of data collection which are flexible and sensitive to the social context of the research; and analyses rich, complex and detailed data (1996:4).

Barnes, discussing disability research, explains why qualitative methods may be attractive to researchers. First, they recognize the impossibility of achieving objectivity in their research. Secondly, survey and statistical methods do not assist understanding of the everyday world and, thirdly, striving for objective understanding of the world is both analytically and politically contentious (1992:116). Qualitative research encourages the recognition of researcher subjectivity, as well as the subjectivity of respondents' accounts, and these have been key themes in social policy and sociological research into learning difficulty.

Research into services for people with learning difficulties

One very important tradition in learning difficulty research has been the wealth of prescriptive and evaluative research which has focused on the quality of services. In the 1970s and 1980s, the emergence of the principle of normalization had a great influence over the development of services, to the extent that the goals of normalization became synonymous with the goals of community care. Research in this field was intended to disseminate good advice and practical experience to service planners and providers on how they could operationalize normalization in their own services.

In order to explain the way that normalization gained so great an influence, it is necessary to refer briefly to its history. A simple definition of normalization by the campaign for People with a Mental Handicap (CMH) is:

> The use of means which are valued in our society in order to develop and support personal behaviour experiences and characteristics which are likewise valued. (1981:1)

The normalization principle developed in Scandinavia in the 1960s. In these early stages it took a pragmatic approach to improving services. However, the transfer of normalization from Scandinavia to the USA shifted its emphasis and it became theorized and radicalized. This new and elaborate American version is most closely associated with Wolf Wolfensberger. His reformulation of normalization was influenced heavily by interpretive sociology, which itself appeared to be a radical and exciting departure from an essentially conservative sociology dominated by functionalism.

Interpretive sociology is concerned traditionally with those marginalized within society. It is interested in how such 'outsiders' perceive the world and interpret their experiences. The emphasis of interpretive sociology on deviance, labelling and stigma was very significant for the development of normalization (Chappell, 1992; Emerson, 1992). The work of Goffman (e.g. *Asylums*, 1961) was of particular relevance. Furthermore, the scope within interpretive sociology for researchers to sympathize with the underdog and portray her/his view of the world also shaped the kind of research that was generated by normalization.

Wolfensberger's adaptation of normalization argues that people with learning difficulties are a devalued social group whose identities are stigmatized. The warehousing of people with stigmatized identities in poor quality services merely reinforces their deviance. This sets in motion a vicious circle. By putting the normalization principle into practice, the vicious circle can be transformed into a virtuous circle. If devalued people are integrated into the wider community, live in locally-based services of high quality and meet and mix with people with socially valued identities (such as non-disabled people), this will undo the stigma attached to people with learning difficulties and create a high-quality lifestyle for them.

The model of normalization developed by Wolfensberger was the one adopted by service planners and academics in the UK who were concerned at the poor standards of care in many long-stay hospitals.

Gradually, normalization became accepted as the foundation for good community care services. (For a more detailed account of this process see Chappell, 1992, and Emerson, 1992). Certain organizations and academics were enthusiastic supporters of normalization (e.g. the King's Fund, Campaign for People with a Mental Handicap) and produced a great deal of influential research. This research played a vital role in spreading the word of normalization and it emerged as the progressive model for those who wanted to improve services for people with learning difficulties.

This research tradition shared certain key features. First, it produced policy-based, evaluative and prescriptive research aimed at service planners and providers. The objective was a very practical one: to convince people that the provision of high-quality community care for people with learning difficulties (regardless of the severity of their impairments) was an achievable goal if normalization was used as the blueprint. The primary focus was how to improve services. This research was aimed at service planners and providers to enable them to learn from the experiences of successful community care projects which were founded on normalization (such as the NIMROD project, New Initiatives for the Mentally Retarded in Ordinary Dwellings project in South Wales and the Wells Road project in Bristol).

This body of research examines issues which are important to professionals, such as staff training (Ward, 1986, 1987; Williams and Tyne, 1988); user assessment (O'Brien, 1987) or the evaluation of a community care initiative (Evans et al., 1987; Blunden, 1988a; Alaszewski and Ong, 1990). In this way, normalization enabled service providers to develop new models of practice and retain a central role in the way that good community care is defined.

What it has not done is to challenge the authority that service providers have over disabled people. Whitehead notes that normalization has been adopted by:

> ... professionals and service providers, rather than disabled people themselves. So, whilst services have moved away from a treatment model, they have only moved to an advocacy model – others speaking up on behalf of disabled people. (1992: 57)

Furthermore, the clear focus of normalization is services. It neglects issues outside the narrow world of service provision which make up the wider context of the lives of disabled people, for example, poverty and the poverty trap, the isolation of disabled people from each other, the relationship between the social construction of disability and wider social, economic, political and historical forces.

Secondly, it was research based on an explicit set of values (i.e. the values of normalization). This is a common approach in qualitative research. Feminist research, for example, tends to reject the concept of researcher objectivity on the basis that it is impossible to be objective (see, for example, Oakley 1981; Graham, 1983; Stanley and Wise, 1983; Finch, 1984). What researchers should strive for is to be clear about their subjectivity.

One of the principal tenets of normalization is that we all have subconscious beliefs about devalued people. These beliefs shape the design and organization of services for people with learning difficulties and mark them out as being odd or dangerous. For example, hospital wards may be named after animals conveying, unconsciously, the message that people with learning difficulties are subhuman and bestial. This is known as 'symbolic marking' (Race, 1987: 68–69). Thus, services may claim to provide good quality of care, but in reality they may be oppressive and degrading. Normalization, drawing on the work of Goffman, refers to this as the difference between the manifest, publicly acknowledged function of services and their latent, but real, function (Wolfensberger, 1989). The subconscious and hidden objectives of services must be brought into the open. For this reason, much of the research in this tradition is founded on an explicit statement of values: a clear and passionate conviction that normalization represents the only way to transform services. In this kind of research, the researcher is an advocate of normalization and adopts it as a yardstick to measure the reality of the service against the criteria for quality set out within normalization (Ward, 1984; Blunden, 1988b).

The third feature of normalization that influenced this kind of research relates to the presumed nature of social values. Supporters of normalization see social values as homogeneous and easily identifiable (CMH, 1981; Williams and Tyne, 1988). This is not seen as problematic because normalization is essentially functionalist (Chappell, 1992). In this way, researchers are able to use the normalization principle as a proxy to define the aspirations of people with learning difficulties. They can then measure the extent to which services enabled people with learning difficulties to emulate these social values. This approach is problematic for a number of reasons. Do all members of society share the same social values? Society is unequal and some social groups, their beliefs and behaviours, are valued more highly than others. Social norms, therefore, are not neutral but products of the society that creates them. Brown and Smith (1989) and Baxter et al. (1990) argue that normalization's unquestioning acceptance of existing social mores is in danger of reproducing discriminatory social norms, such as sexism and racism. This worrying aspect of the notion of social norms is not recognized within normalization or the community care research it inspired.

Furthermore, the views of people with learning difficulties were assumed to be the same as the goals of normalization, without this ever being investigated empirically or researchers feeling compelled to evaluate services based on the views of the people who used them. For researchers, adopting normalization was insight enough into understanding the experiences and aspirations of people with learning difficulties (Chappell, 1992). It is significant that, as Oliver points out, no democratic or accountable organization of disabled people has adopted normalization as its founding philosophy (1994: 10).

This section has explored the development of the normalization principle and the way that it came to dominate much social research into learning difficulty. I have indicated the narrow focus of this research and some of the questionable assumptions that it makes. The enthusiasm, if not zeal, associated with normalization and its followers meant that it was very difficult to criticize openly. By the end of the 1980s, however, the consensus surrounding normalization began to crack (Chappell, 1997). The growing politicization of disabled people through the disability and self-advocacy movements means that social research which impacts on their lives, but fails to take account of their views, has become increasingly unacceptable. Alternative qualitative methodologies began to gain in popularity. (For further information on normalization the reader is reformed to Chapters 6 and 8.)

Research based on the views of people with learning difficulties

People with learning difficulties have been the subjects in countless pieces of social research. However, much of this research has either not attempted to elicit their views or has cast them as unreliable recorders of their experiences whose opinions must be treated with caution. In this section, I will discuss different approaches to including the views of people with learning difficulties in the research process: social-psychological research; ethnography, narrative and autobiographical research, and the critique of research developed by the disability movement and some of the research responses to this critique.

It is not uncommon for research which attempts to uncover the perspectives of people with learning difficulties to grapple with the question of the reliability of their accounts. To some extent, this is an issue of concern to all researchers – are respondents telling the 'truth'? Is the sample representative? Can the findings be generalized? When the respondents are people with learning difficulties, however, these issues have been of particular concern as researchers have wondered if the nature of intellectual impairment means that people are unreliable and inconsistent in the expression of their views. Social researchers have responded to this debate in different ways.

Social psychological research which seeks to elicit the views of people with learning difficulties has been very concerned over this issue of reliability. It is important to discuss these views in this chapter because this literature has influenced social research into learning difficulty. The work of social psychologists, such as Sigelman et al. (1981), Sigelman and Budd (1986) and Heal and Sigelman (1995) are cited frequently.

This social psychological approach has attempted to test out different interview techniques to highlight their influence on the reliability of responses. An issue of great concern is the wording of questions. Sigelman et al. (1981) claim, for example, that particular question formats increase the risk of respondents with learning difficulties displaying acquiescence (saying 'yes') to whatever the researcher asks or recency (opting for the latter option given in an either – or question). The authors argue that data should be cross-checked by the researcher asking questions to which the correct answer is 'no' or altering the order of options given in questions to test for recency.

However, other researchers have questioned the assumptions of writers such as Sigelman or have undertaken research in such a way that does not use as its starting point the assumption that people with intellectual impairments are unreliable witnesses. The work of Booth and colleagues, for example, attempted in a very explicit way to discover the views of people with learning difficulties regarding a move from a long-stay hospital to community-based housing. Although the researchers (1990: 121) note that it is important to be sensitive to the appropriateness of different question formats and use other means of data collection, such as pictures and photographs, they argue that issues concerning the validity of data must be treated with caution.

First, they question the connection made by Sigelman *et al.* (1981) between acquiescence, recency and intellectual limitation. Booth and colleagues suggest that the social context of people's lives and their limited control over their environments may lead to these phenomena. Secondly, cross-checking data by asking confusing and misleading questions is likely to make respondents uneasy and more likely to acquiesce. Thirdly, inconsistencies in the data may signal possible ambiguities or conflicting feelings that respondents may have about their circumstances. Such ambiguities might represent data in their own right and be worthy of follow-up, rather than simply representing a problem in interviewing technique or a sign of the inability of people with learning difficulties to be reliable respondents.

Other methodologies in social research have taken a different stance and have been more interested in allowing people with learning difficulties to tell their stories to an interested and sympathetic audience than with assumptions of reliability and inconsistency. In this section, the use of ethnographic, narrative and autobiographical methodologies in research into the lives of people with learning difficulties is discussed.

Ethnography is an extremely important methodology in qualitative research. While there is some disagreement over its distinctive features, a useful definition of ethnography is a methodology which relies:

> ... on a wide range of sources of information. The ethnographer participates, overtly or covertly, in people's daily lives for an extended period of time, watching what happens, listening to what is said, asking questions; in fact, collecting whatever data are available to throw light on the issues with which he or she is concerned. (Hammersley and Atkinson, 1983: 2)

The ethnographic tradition is well established in learning difficulty research. First, it takes a long-term approach. Ethnographers operate in their research setting and collect data for a protracted period of time. They also draw on a range of methods for collecting data (observation, conversation, interviewing, reading documents). This flexibility about data collection, particularly the use of naturalistic methods, means that they can develop a wider understanding of the social context of respondents' lives. Researchers take time to get to know their respondents and the circumstances of their lives. This can be very important in building up a rapport between researcher and respondent. It helps to avoid the problem of respondents being intimidated by the research process and giving the answers that they think the researcher wants to hear. Furthermore, ethnographers tend to be interested in social relationships in specific, clearly bounded locations. Settings such as hospitals or residential homes meet these criteria.

One of the classic pieces of social research into the lives of people with learning difficulties is Edgerton's *The Cloak of Competence* (1967). This is an ethnographic study of the experiences of people with mild learning difficulties discharged from long-stay hospitals in the USA. Edgerton followed up this research with further investigations of his original group of respondents (Edgerton and Bercovici, 1976; Edgerton *et al.*, 1984). As an interpretive sociologist, he was interested in the notion of stigma and the strategies that his respondents developed for coping with the stigma attached to them because of their time in an institution. Methodologically, therefore, Edgerton's research was significant: it was a longitudinal study and respondents were allowed to tell their stories.

Drawing on the tradition of sympathetic research into the lives of people with learning difficulties, research which uses narrative and autobiographical approaches appears to be undergoing a resurgence of popularity. There are a number of reasons for this. First, disadvantaged groups are seeking to reclaim their previously suppressed histories, at both an individual and collective level. As Atkinson and Williams point out:

> It has often been assumed not simply that the opinions of people with learning difficulties did not matter, but they did not exist. (1990: 8)

It is useful to mention the social psychological approach in this context. Their position was that these opinions did exist, but that they were inconsistent and unreliable for the purposes of research. The starting point of narrative and autobiographical research, by contrast, is that people with learning difficulties have interesting stories to tell, their accounts of their lives are reliable and that it is important that their stories reach a wider audience. The development of self-advocacy has been very significant as it has encouraged people with learning difficulties to 'speak out' to an interested and sympathetic audience of researchers. It has helped people with learning difficulties gain experience and confidence in telling their stories. It has also set these individual accounts in a political context as a collective experience begins to emerge.

Despite their methodological significance, however, what ethnographic, narrative and autobiographical research do not do is address the question of *control* over the research process. People with learning difficulties are still dependent on the goodwill of researchers for the ways that their stories are interpreted, edited and disseminated. Thus, for example, Edgerton's ethnographic work has been criticized in recent years for failing to recognize the validity of his respondents' accounts. Gerber argues that Edgerton and his colleagues interpret the accounts of people with learning difficulties merely as rationalizations as they struggle to maintain their self-esteem and deny their stigmatized identities (1990: 16). Gerber's critique highlights an extremely important point in research. Simply encouraging people with learning difficulties to speak about their experiences via research does not, in itself, guarantee people with learning difficulties any control over the research process.

This is an issue which Atkinson has considered in her autobiographical research with a group of people with learning difficulties. She argues that, although the research began as 'her' project, as the work progressed:

> . . . ownership passed from me to the group when I produced the first draft of the book. At that point I began to become the group's scribe, perhaps even its servant; my skills were at the group's disposal. (1997: p 131)

Atkinson's account of the research process is important because it conveys the experience of research as dynamic, negotiable between researcher and respondents and one where the balance of power may shift away from the researcher to the researched. What the researcher intends at the outset of the project may not be what emerges during the long process of work.

However, the willingness of Atkinson to permit the increased participation of people with learning difficulties in the research depends heavily on her skills and sensitivity as an experienced researcher. It was not built into the methodology from the start. As such, this methodological position does not meet the demands of the disabled people's movement regarding research methodology. The critique of research which the disabled people's movement has developed demands a far more systematic involvement of disabled people at all stages of the research process.

Critiques of Disability Research

The increasing political organization of disabled people over the last 10 years has set out numerous challenges for social researchers. In this section, critiques of the research process developed by the disabled people's movement and the methodological implications of these critiques are examined. In 1992, the journal *Disability, Handicap and Society* produced a special issue which explored methodological issues in disability research and proposed strategies for radical change. From these articles emerged what is termed the emancipatory model of research.

In brief, the emancipatory model comprises the following features: research into disability issues should be used as a tool for improving the lives of disabled people; there should be greater opportunities for disabled people to participate in disability research; non-disabled researchers must demonstrate reflexivity and allow disabled people to set the research agenda, and there should be far greater accountability to the organizations of disabled people who will act as commissioners of and consultants for research.

It must be pointed out, however, that not all academics who are committed to the political struggles of disabled people accept the premise of the emancipatory paradigm. Shakespeare, for example, draws a distinction between political commitment and political accountability. He describes himself as someone who is committed to supporting the struggles of disabled people for civil rights, but he argues there are serious dangers if researchers make themselves too beholden to the agendas of political organizations. Academics have a duty to be reflective, critical and to 'take an independent line' (1996: 117).

Methodological debates in learning difficulty research appear to be developing on a rather different track. In this field, the emerging paradigm is participatory research. This has some commonality with the emancipatory paradigm, but differs at certain key points.

Participatory research can be defined as the involvement of people with learning difficulties in the generation of knowledge about the research problem and analysis of data, and discussions on collective action to address the issues raised by the research findings (Cocks and Cockram 1995). In this model, however, Cocks and Cockram indicate that the identification of the research problem itself can be done by non-disabled researchers and then brought to the constituency of people with learning difficulties.

This is a significant difference to the emancipatory paradigm where it is disabled people who set the research agenda and researchers must put their:

> . . . knowledge and skills at the disposal of their research subjects, for them to use in whatever ways they choose. (Oliver, 1992: 111)

Thus, the key difference between emancipatory and participatory research is the relationship between researchers and disabled people. In the former, researchers are accountable to the organizations of disabled people; in the latter, the relationship is looser and is based on alliances.

It is possible to see the emergence of participatory research as a staging post on the way to the widespread use of emancipatory methodologies (Zarb, 1992). Another possibility is that the participatory model will emerge as a research methodology in its own right. It appears to be more pragmatic and achievable than emancipatory research. One reason for this is that funding agencies are unwilling to support 'political' research because this contravenes their charitable status (Ward and Flynn, 1994: 43). In this light, participatory research is more attractive to the research establishment because it permits some involvement of disabled people in the research process, while maintaining notions of researcher integrity and distance from an explicitly political agenda.

Furthermore, the inheritance of normalization and 'underdog' research influenced by interpretive sociology means that there is a long tradition of sympathetic non-disabled researchers engaging in learning difficulty research. Thus, participatory methodology has both strengths and weaknesses. Its strength is that it provides an achievable way for people with learning difficulties to participate in research, not just as respondents, but as co-researchers, consultants, members of a steering group or as researchers themselves (Whittaker et al., 1991; March et al., 1997). Its weakness is that although it permits a greater role than hitherto, it maintains the authority of non-disabled researchers and institutionalizes the relative power positions of researcher and researched.

Conclusion

This chapter has traced the development of qualitative research methodology into the lives of people with learning difficulties. A range of methodological issues in research into the quality of services for people with learning difficulties and research into the perceptions and experiences of people with learning difficulties themselves has been examined.

The rise of the normalization principle in the 1970s shaped the meaning of 'good' community care. It generated a particular style of research based on an explicit commitment to the tenets of normalization and the dissemination of information to service planners and providers. This body of research is problematic, however. For example, it tends not to ascertain the views of people with learning difficulties themselves. Neither does it think critically about the question of social norms and what it means for people with learning difficulties to emulate them.

In recent years, there has been a growing recognition that the views of people with learning difficulties must be at the centre of social research which seeks to investigate their lives. Ethnographic and, in particular, autobiographical methods are undergoing renewed popularity. Of even greater significance, is the emergence of participatory and emancipatory methodologies. These methodological approaches open up exciting possibilities for therapists involved in research, as well as providing important challenges, about the development of the whole process of research and the relationship between researcher, researched and the wider community of disabled people. (For further information on research the reader is referred to Chapters 2, 4, 5 and 20).

References

Alaszewski, A. and Ong, B.N. (eds) (1990) *Normalisation in Practice: Residential Care for Children with a Profound Mental Handicap*, Routledge, London

Atkinson, D. (1997) *An Auto/Biographical Approach to Learning Disability Research*, Ashgate, Aldershot

Atkinson, D. and Williams, F. (eds) (1990) *'Know Me As I Am': An Anthology of Prose, Poetry and Art by People with Learning Difficulties*, Hodder and Stoughton, London (in association with the Open University Press)

Barnes, C. (1992) Qualitative research: valuable or irrelevant? *Disability, Handicap and Society*, **7**(2), 115–124

Baxter, C., Ward, L., Poonia, K. and Nadirshaw, Z. (1990) *Double Discrimination: Issues and Services for People with Learning Difficulties from Black and Ethnic Minority Communities*, King's Fund/Commission for Racial Equality, London

Blunden, R. (1988a) Quality of life in persons with disabilities: issues in the development of services. In Brown, R. (ed.), *Quality of Life for Handicapped People*, Croom Helm, London

Blunden, R. (1988b) Safeguarding Quality. In Towell, D. (ed.), *An Ordinary Life in Practice: Developing Comprehensive Community-based Services for People with Learning Disabilities*, King's Fund, London

Booth, T., Simons, K. and Booth, W. (1990) *Outward Bound: Relocation and Community Care for People with Learning Difficulties*, Open University Press, Milton Keynes

Brown, H. and Smith, H. (1989) Whose 'ordinary life' is it anyway? *Disability, Handicap and Society*, **4**(2), 105–119

Campaign for People with a Mental Handicap (1981) *The Principle of Normalisation: A Foundation for Effective Services*, CMH, London

Chappell, A.L. (1992) Towards a sociological critique of the normalisation principle. *Disability, Handicap and Society*, **7**(1), 35–51

Chappell, A.L. (1997). From normalisation to where? in Baston, L. and Olives, M. (eds) *Disability Studies: Past, Present and Future*, The Disability Press, University of Leeds

Cocks, E. and Cockram, J. (1995) The participatory research paradigm and intellectual disability. *Mental Handicap Research*, **8**(1), 25–37

Edgerton, R.B. (1967) *The Cloak of Competence: Stigma in the Lives of the Mentally Retarded*, University of California Press, Berkeley

Edgerton, R.B. and Bercovici, S.M. (1976) The Cloak of Competence: years later. *American Journal of Mental Deficiency*, **80**, 485–497

Edgerton, R., Bollinge, M. and Herr, B. (1984) The Cloak of Competence after two decades. *American Journal of Mental Deficiency*, **88**, 345–351

Emerson, E. (1992) What is normalisation? In Brown, H. and Smith, H. (eds), *Normalisation: A Reader for the Nineties*, Tavistock/Routledge, London

Evans, G., Todd, S., Blunden, R., Porterfield, J. and Ager, A. (1987) Evaluating the impact of a move to ordinary housing. *British Journal of Mental Subnormality*, **33**(64), part 1, 10–18

Finch, J. (1984) 'It's great to have someone to talk to': the ethics and politics of interviewing women. In Bell, C. and Roberts, H. (eds) *Social Researching: Politics, Problems, Practice*, Routledge and Kegan Paul, London

Gerber, D.A. (1990) Listening to disabled people: the problem of voice and authority in Robert B. Edgerton's 'The Cloak of Competence'. *Disability, Handicap and Society*, **5**(1), 3–23

Goffman, E. (1961) *Asylums: Essays on the Social Situation of Mental Patients and Other Inmates*, Doubleday, New York

Graham, H. (1983) Do her answers fit his questions? Women and the survey method. In Gamarnikow, E. *et al.* (eds), *The Public and the Private*, Gower, Aldershot

Hammersley, M. and Atkinson, P. (1983) *Ethnography: Principles in Practice*, Tavistock, London

Heal, L.W. and Sigelman, C.K. (1995) Response biases in interviews of individuals with limited mental ability. *Journal of Intellectual Disability Research*, **39**, part 4, 331–340

March, J., Steingold, B. and Justice, S. with Mitchell, P. (1997) Follow the Yellow Brick Road! People with learning difficulties as co-researchers. *British Journal of Learning Disabilities*, **25**(2), 77–80

Mason, J. (1996) *Qualitative Researching*, Sage, London

Oakley, A. (1981) Interviewing women: a contradiction in terms. In Roberts, H. (ed.), *Doing Feminist Research*, Routledge and Kegan Paul, London

O'Brien, J. (1987) A guide to life-style planning using the *Activities Catalog* to integrate services and natural support systems. In Wilcox, B. and Bellamy, G.T. (eds), *A Comprehensive Guide to the Activities Catalogue: An Alternative Curriculum for Youth and Adults with Severe Disabilities*, Paul H. Brookes, Baltimore

Oliver, M. (1992) Changing the social relations of research production? *Disability, Handicap and Society,* **7**(2), 101–114

Oliver, M. (1994) Capitalism, disability and ideology: a materialist critique of the normalization principle. Paper presented to the conference *Twenty-five Years of Normalization, Social Valorization and Social Integration: A Retrospective and Prospective View,* University of Ottawa, Ontario, 10th–13th May

Race, D. (1987) Normalisation: theory and practice. In Malin, N. (ed.), *Reassessing Community Care (With Particular Reference to Provision for People with Mental Handicap and for People with Mental Illness),* Croom Helm, London

Shakespeare, T. (1996) Rules of engagement: doing disability research. *Disability and Society,* **11**(1), 115–119

Sigelman, C.K. and Budd, E.C. (1986) Pictures as an aid in questioning mentally retarded persons. *Rehabilitation Counselling Bulletin,* **29**, 173–181

Sigelman, C.K. Budd, E.C., Spanhel, C.L. and Shoenrock, C.J. (1981) When in doubt, say yes: acquiescence in interviews with mentally retarded persons. *Mental Retardation,* **19**, 53–58

Stanley, L. and Wise, S. (1983) *Breaking Out: Feminist Consciousness and Feminist Research,* Routledge and Kegan Paul, London

Ward, L. (1984) *Planning for People: Developing a Local Service for People with Mental Handicap, Recruiting and Training Staff,* Project Paper No. 47, King's Fund, London

Ward, L. (1986) Changing services for changing needs. *Community Care,* 22nd May, 21–23

Ward, L. (1987) After induction – then what? Providing on-going staff training for 'an ordinary life'. *British Journal of Mental Subnormality,* **33**(65), part 2, 131–142

Ward, L. and Flynn, M. (1994) What matters most: disability, research and empowerment. In Rioux, M.H. and Bach, M. (eds), *Disability is not Measles: New Research Paradigms in Disability,* Roeher Institute, North York, Ontario

Whitehead, S. (1992) The social origins of normalisation. In Brown, H. and Smith, H. (eds), *Normalisation: A Reader for the Nineties,* Tavistock/Routledge, London

Whittaker, A., Gardner, S. and Kershaw, J. (1991) *Service Evaluation by People with Learning Difficulties,* King's Fund, London

Williams, P. and Tyne, A. (1988) Exploring values as a basis for service development. In Towell, D. (ed.), *An Ordinary Life in Practice: Developing Comprehensive Community-based Services for People with Learning Disabilities,* King's Fund, London

Wolfensberger, W. (1989) Human service policies: the rhetoric versus the reality. In Banton, L. (ed.), *Disability and Dependency,* Falmer Press, London

Zarb, G. (1992) On the road to Damascus: first steps towards changing the relations of disability research production. *Disability, Handicap and Society,* **7**(2), 125–138

Part II

Towards Participation: Learning Disabilities in a Social World

11

Disabled transitions: negotiating identities in a prescriptive world

Mairian Corker

Introduction

The idea that life can be conceived as a process of physical, cognitive, emotional, moral and social maturation which results in some 'ideal', 'healthy' or 'desired' outcome where people are able to formulate some tentative answers to the questions 'Who am I?', 'Where do I come from?' and 'Where do I belong?' has preoccupied scholars and researchers for many years. These are questions which relate to *identity*, itself a complex term with many dimensions to which a single chapter could not do justice, and the significant *life transitions* people make on their different 'routes' to these answers. The term 'transitions' is also complex. It can, for example, refer to changing contexts such as the movement from education to work as well as to developmental transitions such as those between dependence and independence or between impairment and empowerment.

The aim of this chapter is to explore and critique different approaches to theorizing life transitions. It will ask whether these approaches can adequately explain the experience of people with learning difficulties for whom

> Much of the emphasis in the literature . . . has concentrated, importantly, on the process of stigmatization. Part of this process has meant, especially for those living in institutions, a stripping away of personal and social identity, and the imposition of a label, or a 'spoiled' identity – a lens through which the person's identity is given distorted and often unwanted meanings. (Atkinson and Williams, 1990: 13)

Because issues of identity and life transitions are intricately linked, the 'lens' that Atkinson and Williams mention above has particularly significant implications for the way in which we understand transitions. It emphasizes from the outset the importance of these issues for professionals working predominantly in medical settings and within medical or individual frameworks because identity and life transitions clearly have both structural and sociocultural dimensions. For example, occupational therapists may focus on therapy related to structural transitions from one physical environment to another but lack an understanding of how the latter will influence the person's ability to take advantage of the former. Similarly, physiotherapists, in their emphasis on bodily structures, functions and practices may fail to understand or may make assumptions about how the life histories of people with learning difficulties influence the relationship between mind and body. These comments may in themselves be diagnostic, stereotypical, inaccurate and full of assumptions about different kinds of therapy – in fact, they are deliberately so, because most of us have limited knowledge about what such professionals actually do. But this illustrates perfectly the importance of what knowledge we have, where it comes from and how we apply it in work with people with learning difficulties and in our understanding of these questions from the perspective of people with learning disabilities themselves.

The ideas in this chapter draw both upon my understanding of disability as a form of social oppression and institutionalized discrimination – a collective experience – and my own life story as one strand of that collective experience. As I child, I was variously described as having 'emotional and behavioural problems' or as being a 'slow learner' when I was in fact deaf. Then, later, as I struggled to resist these labels, I was variously and wrongly ascribed the terms 'psychotic' and 'bookish', the former because I was tested with psychometric instruments standardized on 'normal' hearing people. It is only now through my contacts with disabled academics that I have been able to reclaim the self-definitive description of a scholar who developed late and who has to run twice as fast to negotiate extra hurdles which symbolize a life of mislabelling. This brings me to the issue of terminology. Throughout this chapter, I use the term 'people with learning difficulites'. However, I do this in full awareness of the controversy surrounding such terminology, which is viewed differently depending on whether we use the gaze of the individual or social models of disability or that of organizations of people with learning difficulties such as People First. Using this term is particularly problematic in relation to the social model of disability with its claims that there are no people with disabilities, only 'people with impairments' and 'disabled people' (Darke, 1998). I nevertheless wish to emphasize that I see people with learning difficulties as disabled people.

Psychosocial perspectives on development

The process of early identity development has frequently been described in terms of *individuation* (Baumrind, 1991 Cooper *et al.*, 1983), which refers to striking the balance between dependency on and detachment from the family or other significant adults. Development is charted in relation to discrete, usually age-related stages demarcated by barriers or crises through which people have to go in order to make a successful transition from one stage to the next. *Stage theories* are epitomized by the work of Havighurst (1953, 1956, 1972), Erikson (1950, 1968) and Allport (1955, 1964). Erikson (1968), for example, describes the human life cycle in terms of eight different phases of ego development which he calls:

- basic trust vs. mistrust
- autonomy vs. shame/doubt
- initiative vs. guilt
- industry vs. inferiority
- identity vs. identity confusion
- intimacy vs. isolation
- generativity vs. stagnation
- ego integrity vs. despair.

He sees each of these diads as representing a conflict within the self which must be resolved in some way if development is to progress. These resolutions can be positive, negative or ambivalent; so, for example, individuals can learn to appreciate the difference between those people they can trust all of the time, some of the time or not at all by 'trying out' trusting in the social contacts they make. Stage theory is also implicit in the work of Piaget (1952), who sees children as developing more and more sophisticated cognitive structures with which to apprehend the world, and these are manifested in a series of intellectual stages through which the child passes *en route* to adult intelligence.

However, it is important to recognize that the developmental goals specified in different stage theories are strikingly similar and that their achievement seems to be underpinned by two key processes: a challenging but secure self-reflection, and finding a recognition within society. That is, development has both personal and social goals. Social identity is achieved as the result of a process of social differentiation, evaluation and identification. Most stage theories stress the importance of self-acceptance and a coherent identity which incorporates all the dimensions which are said to be necessary for the integration of the ego identity:

- gender
- mature physical capabilities
- sexuality
- ability to reason beyond the concrete operational level
- responses to social expectations to become more than a child

I will return to these dimensions in the section on disabled transitions. The *common* characteristics of psychosocial theories of development are summarized in Figure 11.1. As can be seen, all suggest progression in stages to something which is called identity, and I have suggested that 'identity' is itself a highly complex and contested term. But what is equally striking is that each and every one of these stages is under the influence of a large number of sociocultural variables, which in turn allows us to suggest that 'stages' are at best sterotypes and at worst 'norms' – benchmarks against which all development is compared. This realization underpins various critiques of stage theory.

Changing perspectives of development

As Honess (1992) has noted, there is very little in the way of direct empirical evidence for stage theories, though an important exception to this rule can be found in the research of Marcia, who explored *identity*

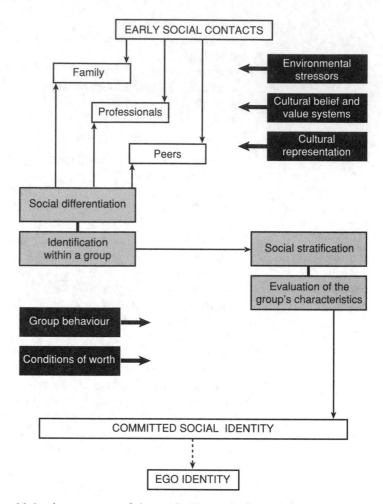

Figure 11.1 A summary of the main 'stages' of psychosocial development

statuses and Grotevant and colleagues who extended this into the interpersonal domain (see Bosma *et al.*, 1994 and Corker, 1996 for examples and an overview of this work). These authors attempt to break down the presumed homogeneity of developmental stages and this has formed the basis of a critique of stage theory on three main levels:

● There is an increasing understanding of our identities as *strategic* – multiply constructed across different, often converging and conflicting discourses, practices and positions. It is difficult, then, to see identities as developing in the orderly or predetermined manner suggested by many stage theories.
● In this context, such theories fail, as a whole, to take into account the structural and cultural inequality and discrimination which are institutionalized in Western society.

● Hence, stage theories often reflect culturally conditioned, socially acceptable views, of development, maturity, dependence, independence and *normalcy*. For example, the emphasis on the significance of achieving an 'appropriate' masculine or feminine role suggests a stereotyped perception of gender and sexuality.

Unsurprisingly, dominant critics of stage theory have tended to come from social groups who are designated as being outside the 'normal' self by the dominant culture – that is, they do not conform to the white, intelligent, non-disabled male 'norm' and so they become alien or what is described in sociological terms as *Other*. More recent research has uncovered deficiencies and inconsistencies in stage theory when it is analysed in terms of disability (Corker, 1996; Peters, 1996; Shakespeare *et al.* 1996). Indeed, at a fundamental level, Coupland *et al.* (1993: xi) suggest that

> . . . we need to think critically about taken-for-granted social categories such as 'child' and 'adult', 'youth', 'middle age' and 'old age'. Where do they come from, and what cultural assumptions sustain them as sense-making concepts in our lives and in our language? What social rituals endorse our accepted views of 'coming of age', 'turning 40' 'entering retirement', or generally 'acting our age'? What conventional forms of talk do we have for discussing life 'stages', life changes, and age itself?

For people with learning difficulties this has important implications for the distinction between theoretical ideas about 'age' and 'maturity' and society's tendency to view them as being in a state of perpetual childhood or as pre-sexual, asexual or immature, for example, as I will explore further in a later section. Added to this is the incommensurability of disability and childhood research which tends to compound stereoypes (Priestly, 1998). This raises further questions about the goal(s) of transition and development, for example 'transition to what?' and 'as determined by whom?' because within orderly predetermined and universal frameworks, alternative developmental 'routes' which are taken because of disabling barriers, for example, can be labelled as deviant. So too can a failure to resolve certain life conflicts because this failure is attributed to differences, for example differences in education or cognitive differences, which are not fully acknowledged outside of a pathologizing framework.

In this sense, stage theories risk being seen as parallels to medical and individual models of learning disability. In the example given about trust in the previous section it is not difficult to see that, as we develop, we are often impressed upon with the idea that there are some people who are unquestionably trustworthy – our parents and professional experts among them – and it is when we have experienced the damage of our trust in these people that we may develop conditional ideas about trust. This can only happen, however, if we are aware that our trust has been breached, aware of alternative meanings of trust and ways of trusting, and if we have, in consequence, developed an ability to resist cultural demands that we must place our trust in these people.

The professionals and parents in whom we invest our trust must also understand that they are capable of breaching that trust through denial that they harbour conditional love, for example. At the extreme end of the equation, this might mean that they will only love us if we strive to be 'normal'. For people with learning difficulties, awareness may depend on being told about alternatives, but clearly if parents and professionals are in denial, this cannot happen. Even when awareness is in evidence, there are other factors which determine how we use this awareness. We might consider, for example, why children who have been abused continue to believe that they are 'wrong', rather than acknowledging that their trust in an adult has been betrayed.

New perspectives on life transitions

Perspectives on development and life transitions, in an attempt to incorporate the 'turn to culture' (du Gay and Hall, 1997), have more recently acquired a different emphasis which is epitomized by the work of Rom Harré (1986). Harré avoids notions of finite or fixed states of mind and processes, suggesting instead that people learn their culture's rules as they grow up and gradually become adept in their use. The process of development implied by this is very different to those that psychologists are used to and which typify stage theory. For Harré, development consists not in the transformation of the way we think and feel, but in the gradual acquisition of accounting skills – itself dependent on the ability to learn, formal and informal opportunities for learning, and access to knowledge. 'Normal' development is therefore a process of becoming more and more sophisticated in one's ability to manufacture accounts *by using the linguistic and accounting rules of one's culture*. He sees this ability as developing, at least in part, through the social interactions that take place between infants and their caretakers. Adults interact with and talk to (some) babies as *if* they had desires, intentions, wishes and so on, so that infants, as they also develop language, gradually come to structure their own experience in these terms too. This puts the emphasis firmly on the social and linguistic practices embedded in a culture:

> The discursive positions on offer to us during social interaction may play a central role in the extent to which we are able to negotiate satisfactory identities for ourselves, and in our ability (physically and morally) to behave and to take action as we would like. To the extent that material conditions and social practices are inextricably bound up in discourses then our ability to, say earn a living, go out at night, tell people what to do or refuse to do what others say depends upon the positions in discourses that we can take up or resist. It follows therefore that an understanding of positioning and an ability to use it skilfully could be important tools in people's efforts to change themselves and their circumstances. (Burr, 1996; 150)

But it implies that if children's experience is fundamentally different in some way to that of their parents, such that they are *prevented* from structuring their experience in their parent's terms, the dynamics and the process of development will change. Put another way, such a child will be faced with additional and often more complex tasks in negotiating their route through life because they in some way disturb the relatively 'settled' path taken by the dominant self (their parents). A 'new' emphasis on language may, however, prove to be a mixed metaphor for people with learning difficulties, especially those who have spent most of their lives in institutions and/or who are disabled by environmental attitudes towards communication or language impairments. Some examples are given below.

People with learning difficulties – disabled transitions

The development of people with learning difficulties is often described as a series of transitions between dependence and independence or between impairment and empowerment. But the literature suggests that independence and empowerment are both defined differently in relation to people with learning difficulties. Independence may mean simply 'productive activity' rather than paid work because the goal of paid work may not be seen as 'realistic' for people with learning difficulties, and they do not, in outcome, have control over their own lives:

> It would appear that for many young disabled people, structural factors continue to outweigh individual agency. . . . Having a disability – and society's (re)action to this – seems to create a 'collective biographical pattern' (Evans and Furlong, 1997), particularly for those seen as having 'learning difficulties' or a range of disabilities. Rather than being faced with an array of confusing choices, young disabled people can find themselves on a 'conveyor belt' (Tisdall, 1996) with a limited number of options. (Tisdall, 1997 and references therein)

This may be why some people with learning difficulties criticize the dominant view of self-advocacy training for people with learning difficulties because

> Due to only having knowledge about rights within a moral context, self-advocates see themselves as only needing to negotiate with staff and managers to get changes to a given service. Service providers have ultimate control, their authority going unchallenged by people with learning difficulties and maintaining full control over services. . . . This leads to people with learning difficulties only being able to see what they want in terms of services and only receiving the benefits of change depending upon the manager or staff on duty in a given service. (Aspis, 1997: 652–653)

Riddell *et al.* (1997), in a preliminary report from their project *The Meaning of the Learning Society for Adults with Learning Difficulties*, funded by the Economic and Social Research Council, support this view in their findings that 'people with learning difficulties, who were likely to have problems understanding the system, were further penalized by lack of both guidance, choice and involvement in service planning and evaluation. They were thus deprived of opportunities for both exit and voice'.

Transitions must also be described in terms of changes in the physical setting or *changing contexts* such as the movement from education to work

– indeed much of the literature on transitions has emphasized this angle in relation to disabled people (see, e.g. Corbett, 1990) – but also that when context remains static, as often happens in institutional life, people can be significantly deprived of developmental stimulants and are consequently more prone to stereotyping. In these circumstances, people with learning difficulties can become trapped within language and attitudes which describe them as 'childlike', 'immature', 'simple', 'vulnerable' and 'incompetent' and deprived of access to alternative discourses which could be taken up or resisted in attempting to break out of this stranglehold. Recently, Capability Scotland (1998) has called for the censorship of language such as 'poor wee souls' as it is applied to disabled young people. Further, Gillman *et al.* (1997) note that case histories of people with learning difficulties tend to emphasize and give preference to information which is useful to professionals, such as IQ and medical diagnosis. In terms of stage theories, this may mean, for example, that there is a concentrated focus on the (in) ability to reason beyond the 'concrete operational level' and '(im)mature physical capabilities', a lack of 'social expectations to become more than a child', with the accompanying assumption that people with learning difficulties are asexual, genderless because this focus excludes other more 'human' ways of viewing the person. Life stories are thus replaced by 'objective' case histories with the result that

> A common theme that arose during the interviewing of key workers and care staff was the lack, loss or unavailability of background information and life history material relating to people with learning difficulties in their care. . . . For many people with learning difficulties who have been in long-term institutional care and who have lost contact with relatives, official files are the only record of their lived experiences. Yet such records are often inaccessible (both literally and conceptually) to those who are the subjects of their deliberations. (Gillman *et al.* 1997: 676)

As indicated earlier, objectification is frequently reinforced by strategies of denial employed by family members who are unable to face up to the idea that their child is different, as Example 1 shows.

Example 1

The family . . . was initially encountered in a large psychiatric institute to which they had turned in their search for a remedy for five and a half year old Mary's unusual behaviour. Family members stated that Mary was a verbal and intelligent child who malingered and refused to speak in public in order to embarrass the family. Extensive clinical examination revealed Mary to be severely retarded (sic) and unable to perform at anywhere near the level of confidence claimed by her parents and two older siblings. . . . Initial viewings of the videotapes suggested that family members' transactions were permeated by subtle, almost artful, practices that could function to create the image of Mary as an intelligent child. (Pollner and Wikler, 1985)

Even in situations where children with learning difficulties are educated in mainstream schools, their experience may be characterized by tense social relationships with their non-disabled peer group. For example, in Lewis's study, nearly two-thirds of children with moderate learning difficulties recalled playtime as a disliked aspect of mainstream schools and associated this with verbal or physical aggression from other children:

> Many children drew pictures of themselves as recipients of fighting and teasing in the playground. Some pictures showed the fighting or name-calling in progress; others depicted the aftermath. When showing the aftermath, children always drew themselves alone: 'I got jumped on by loads of kids. Got hurt. Crying.' (1995: 34)

This gives a different meaning to the processes of socialization which are integral to identity formation.

Armstrong (1997) builds on this picture of objectification and denial by pointing out that when people with learning difficulties say they 'have no memories' of their lives other than feelings of 'helplessness' and 'usefulness', they are implying that their human identity has been 'stripped away'. This is particularly important in the light of Okeley's (1996) view that life stories are one very important way of challenging the homogeneity of experience suggested by objectified case studies and, therefore, in challenging the power relations which create 'helplessness' and 'powerlessness'.

When we are able to access the life stories of people with learning difficulties (Atkinson and Williams, 1990) it is common for institutional life to be described in terms of monosyllabic negative evaluations, invasion of privacy and abuse of different kinds. We also find that even feelings and often involuntary transitions which most of us experience at some time in our lives can be manipulated to 'fit' the dominant view of people with learning difficulties by significant others. People with learning difficulties may have their feelings and experiences denied because it is felt that they (or their 'carers') need protection from the repercussions. However, this strategy can backfire, as Example 2 shows.

Example 2

After Mrs Z was widowed, the doctor advised: 'Don't tell your son.' She had enough problems. 'He might make more problems for you, and anyway he won't understand.' Acting on his advice Mrs Z kept the death of her husband secret for several months and merely told her mentally handicapped (sic) son that father had 'gone away'. It was a dreadful strain for her, grieving for her husband and at the same time having to keep the death secret from her adult son who was sharing the same house. When she finally did tell him, she discovered that he had known for some weeks, and felt very resentful that she had not talked about it to him before. He had somehow found out from things he had overheard at the day centre. (Oswin, 1990)

It is clear that change is perceived by people with learning difficulties in terms of feelings which reverse this negative trend, often associated with an abrupt change of physical environment, though not always by choice because institutional life for some people with learning difficulties who have no experience of other environments can feel 'safe' and 'familiar' and change is therefore frightening. Nevertheless change is frequently described as ' "growing up" and becoming "more independent" ' (Atkinson and Williams, 1990). However, this change can itself be narrowly defined in terms of learning basic life skills, for example cooking, or ongoing 'social training' – moving from one training course to another with little or no evaluation of progress – which cannot be equated with empowerment. 'Dependency' is well documented in the literature on disability (see, e.g., Barton, 1989 and Barnes, 1990), with some disabled people arguing that such an emphasis on *physical* independence confines understanding of independence to whether a person with learning difficulties can *enact* their own decisions and choices rather than on the ability to *make* the decisions and choices (Morris, 1993). This leaves us with the question of what needs to be done, and perhaps more importantly, by whom?

Invoking the social model of disability

A society which valued people with learning disabilities (sic) would have to question seriously the primacy it gives to cognitive skills at the expense of other attributes, such as emotional wisdom, insight and imagination. In turn, it would have to examine the institutions of education, paid work and financial rewards which sustain these priorities. This appears to strike at the very root of social and economic organization of most industrialized societies. . . . Whilst they may not be achievable in the here and now, they provide signposts to the goals which we might be aiming towards; they provide a framework within which more short-term achievable goals, like the representation of people with learning disabilities in these institutions can be placed. (Williams, 1989: 259–260)

Fiona Williams's interpretation of the social model, as it relates to people with learning difficulties, implies that the removal of barriers resides in social change rather than in the individual with learning difficulties. However, as the above discussion demonstrates, it is important to grasp that many people, including some people with learning difficulties, are not the passive recipients of nor do they have control over social change. People initiate, respond to and make use of change in different ways. Some people find change liberating whereas others find it terrifying and it must be understood that sometimes this response will be a product of power relations. This is particularly so for groups of people who are perceived by society as being 'incompetent' to make decisions or to negotiate outcomes, who are therefore labelled as 'vulnerable' and for whom society becomes the custodian of change in determining to do 'what is best' for them; it is also true for people who have not had access to a *variety* of alternative life experiences from which they can choose something which has meaning for them. The accent here is on variety, because life transitions are generally about how we sort out the wood from the trees in arriving at a clearing which becomes central to our sense of who we are in the forest of life. A clear or tangible sense of oneself in relation to the social world cannot be built from a single sapling, so there is as much here about providing opportunities, or what Mithaug (1996) refers to as 'optimal prospects', to encounter varied people and environments as there is about sustaining such encounters.

For some people with learning difficulties there will be substantial barriers to access to opportunities for learning and to 'remembering' what has been learnt. As an extreme example, legal case-work with some people with learning difficulties who have been abused is hampered by the need to constantly 'remind' them of the facts of their abuse, something that sheds an entirely different light on our definition of sustaining encounters. The irony is that such 'reminders' do not easily stand up in court within the current legal system because they can be construed as 'leading questions', which effectively reinforces society's view of learning disability and, in outcome, gives permission for the abuse to continue since there is no apparent way that the law can be used to resist it.

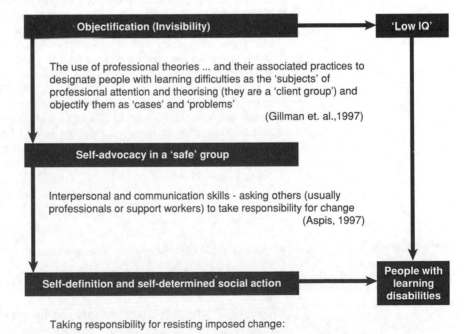

Figure 11.2 The transition from objectified labels to self-determination

Invoking the social model of disability suggests that 'stunted' development and dysfunctional life transitions are a result of the barriers imposed by those who restrict opportunities for people with learning difficulties to engage in a variety of social contacts through institutionalization, and limit opportunities for change by adopting stereotyped perspectives of ability, competence, independence and empowerment in relation to people with learning difficulties. If we take the view of development proposed by Harré, then removing these barriers means adopting a different world-view which acknowledges the way in which these perspectives are socially and culturally constructed to limit the goal of life transitions to one of continued dependency. A different world-view would give us a picture of development which looks something like Figure 11.2.

Demaresse, herself a person with a learning difficulty, sums this up in Example 3.

Example 3

I've never heard these professionals speak of 'true hope', but it seems to me that [false hope] might be the opposite. Must hope be either true or false? Doesn't hope imply something that has not yet come to pass? Isn't there really something wrong with telling a despairing young person who wants to live independently out in the community that such ideas are ludicrous? Should you let bright, vibrant, sensitive or just plain feeling people, worthy of dignity and love, lose all hope rather than give them 'false' hope, because you assume that if you've never seen it before, it's not a possibility? [. . .] In the end, I did move out of the institution and into the community; I am living with the kind of roommates I had hoped for, in the kind of quiet country setting I dreamed about; I do have the kind of assistance and help I had hoped for; and my time is spent writing the book I have always dreamed of, without the institution dictating where and when I could do all kinds of things I like best. I am glad that a group of us got together to share some 'false hope'. (1989: 9)

References

Allport, G. (1955) *Becoming: Basic Considerations for a Psychology of Personality*, Yale University Press, New Haven, CT

Allport, G. (1964) *Pattern and Growth in Personality*, Holt, Rinehart & Winston, New York

Armstrong, D. (1997) Special education and the construction on adult identities. Paper presented at the Disability Studies Seminar, Edinburgh, December

Aspis, S. (1997) Self-advocacy for people with learning difficulties: does it have a future? *Disability & Society*, **12**(4), 647–654

Atkinson, D. and Williams, F. (eds) (1990) *Know Me as I Am: An Anthology of Prose, Poetry and Art by People with Learning Difficulties*, Hodder and Stoughton, London (in association with the Open University Press)

Barnes, C. (1990) *Cabbage Syndrome: The Social Construction of Dependence*, Falmer Press, London

Barton, L. (ed) (1989) *Disability and Dependency*, Falmer Press, London

Baumrind, D. C. (1991) Parenting styles and adolescent development. In Brooks-Gunn, J., Lerner, R. and Peterson, A. C. (eds) *The Encyclopaedia of Adolescence*, Garland Press, New York

Bosma, H.A., Graafsma, T.L.G., Grotevant, H.D. and de Levita, D.J. (eds) (1994) *Identity and Development: An Interdisciplinary Approach*, Sage, Thousand Oaks, California

Burr, V. (1996) *An Introduction to Social Constructionism*, Routledge, London

Capability Scotland (1998) Plain Talking, Edinburgh

Cooper, C. R., Grotevant, H. D. and Condon, S. M. (1983) Individuality and correctedness in the family as a context for adolescent identity and role-taking skill. In Grotevant, H. D. and Cooper, C. R. (eds) *New Directives for Child Development No. 22. Adult Development in the Family*, Jossey-Bass, San Francisco

Corbett, J. (ed) (1990) *Uneasy Transitions: Disaffection in Post-compulsory Education and Training*, Falmer, London

Corker, M. (1996) *Deaf Transitions*, Jessica Kingsley, London

Coupland, N., Nussbaum, J.F. and Grossman, A. (1993) Discourse, selfhood and the lifespan. In Coupland, N. and Nussbaum, J.F. (eds), *Discourse and Lifespan Identity*, Sage, Newbury Park, California

Darke, P.A. (1998) Review of Rob Imrie's Disability and the City: international perspectives. *Sociology*, **32**(1), 223–224

Demaresse, R. (1989) On avoiding false hope. In Wetherow, D. (ed.), *Introduction to the Whole Community Catalog*, Communitas, Manchester, CT

Erikson, E.H. (1950) *Childhood and Society*, Norton, New York

Erikson, E.H. (1968) *Identity, Youth and Crisis*, Norton, New York

du Gay, P. and Hall, S. (1997) *Doing Cultural Studies*, Sage in association with The Open University, London

Gillman, M., Swain, J. and Heyman, R. (1997) Life history or 'case' history: the objectification of people with learning difficulties through the tyranny of professional discourses. *Disability and Society*, **12**(5), 675–694

Harré, R. (1986) The step to social constructionism. In Richards, M. and Light, P. (eds), *Children of Social Worlds*, Polity Press, Cambridge

Havighurst, R. (1953) *Human Development and Education*, Longman, New York

Havighurst, R. (1956) Research on the developmental task concept. *School Review*, **64**, 215–223

Havighurst, R. (1972) *Developmental Tasks and Education*, 3rd edn, David McKay, New York

Honess, T. (1992) The development of self. in Coleman, J.C. (ed.) *The School Years: Current Issues in the Socialisation of Young People*, Routledge, London

Lewis, A. (1995) *Children's Understanding of Disability*, Routledge, London

Mithaug, D.E. (1996) *Equal Opportunity Theory*, Sage, London

Morris, J. (1993) *Independent Lives: Community Care and Disabled People*, Macmillan, Basingstoke

Okeley, J. (1996) *Own or Other Culture*, Routledge, London

Oswin, M. (1990) The grief that does not speak. *Search*, **4**, 5–7

Peters, S. (1996) The politics of disability identity. In Barton, L. (ed.), *Disability and Society: Emerging Issues and Insights*, Longman, London

Piaget, J. (1952) *The Origins of Intelligence in Children*, W.W. Norton, New York

Pollner, M. and Wikler, L. (1985) The social construction of unreality *Family Process*, **24**(2), 241–259

Priestley, M. (1998) Childhood disability and disabled childhoods. *Childhood*, **5**(2), 207–223

Riddell, S., Baron, S. and Wilkinson, H. (1997) Cradle to grave training? Local enterprise companies, the marketisation of training and young people with learning difficulties. Paper presented to The Disability Studies Seminar, Edinburgh, December

Shakespeare, T., Gillespie-Sells, K. and Davies, D. (1996) *The Sexual Politics of Disability*, Cassell, London

Tisdall, K. (1997) Failing to make the transition? Theorisation of the 'transition to adulthood' for young disabled people. Paper presented to The Disability Studies Seminar, Edinburgh, December

Williams, F. (1989) Mental handicap and oppression. In Brechin, A. and Walmsley, J. (eds), *Making Connections: Reflecting on the Lives and Experiences of People with Learning Difficulties*, Hodder and Stoughton, London

12

Inclusive schools need an inclusive national curriculum

Chris Whittaker and Carol Potter

Introduction

The issue of inclusive schools for children with learning difficulties is of importance to physiotherapists and occupational therapists in various ways. Therapists working within the paediatric community service frequently work within educational settings and are considered to be full members of a multidisciplinary team. In addition, many special schools employ therapists on a full-time basis. There have been many criticisms of the ways in which medical treatment has taken priority over education for disabled children. However, if therapy were to be integrated into the National Curriculum, in a sensitive way which did not deprive disabled children of other aspects of their development, such criticisms may be unjustified. As we will argue later, the denial of therapy to children who may benefit from it is just as much an infringement of their rights as lack of formal education.

The history of disabled people is replete with externally imposed labelling, designed to distance them from others by classifying, emphasizing and devaluing their differences. This is particularly true of people with learning difficulties whose rights have been systematically denied by legislation perpetuating self-fulfilling prophecies of low achievement. We believe that the concept of 'Inclusion', manifest in an Inclusive National Curriculum and Inclusive Schools, is fundamental to the advancement of the rights of all disabled people, but that this is not best served by the current National Curriculum, nor by the way that inclusive education is often formulated. We will begin by examining curriculum issues.

Towards an empowerment curriculum

A research-based curriculum for children with Severe Learning Difficulties (SLD) developed rapidly following the Education Act 1971 which transferred responsibility for their education from Health to Education. A major debate surrounded the concept of development versus difference (Zigler, 1969) – whether the children followed a delayed pattern of development similar to typical children (Cunningham and Sloper, 1978;

McConkey and Martin, 1980) or were so damaged that the curriculum should be based on the task analysis of skills to be learnt (Kiernan *et al.*, 1978). As more developmental evidence emerged, some authorities appeared to alter their position (cf. Hogg, 1975 with Hogg, 1987). Although some adhered to an essentially behavioural paradigm (Gardner *et al.*, 1983), others favoured a more process-oriented approach where the child was seen as an active participant in the learning situation (McConkey, 1981; Whittaker, 1985; Wood and Shears, 1986).

Process-oriented approaches are important aspects of the concept of empowerment, which includes the aims of full community participation and personal autonomy. It has become a primary issue for people with learning difficulties, and is strongly reflected in the current literature (Coupe O'Cane and Smith, 1994; Brown and Cohen, 1996; Wehemeyer, 1997). We will now examine the impact of the Education Reform Act (ERA) 1988 on this empowerment agenda.

The ERA and empowerment

The ERA, described as 'one of the most significant UK educational reforms of this century' (Halpin and Lewis, 1996: 95), introduced a National Curriculum, imposing a statutory obligation upon Local Education Authorities to provide a 'broad, balanced and relevant curriculum' with entitlement for *all* pupils, primarily through its core and foundation subjects. From its inception, however, it gave cause for concern. The absence of reference to disabled children in the draft Bill exposed a serious lack of consideration of their needs. Kelly (1994) asserted that it represented a 'power-coercive' model in which curriculum change was imposed through legislation rather than derived from negotiation. Lloyd-Smith (1992) argued that the National Curriculum was driven more by political dogma than educational rationale, reflecting a government desire to introduce market forces, while appearing to advocate consumer choice. Such a rationale is difficult to reconcile with empowerment for less able pupils.

Guidelines attempted to compensate for earlier omissions, emphasizing that *all* children were entitled to equal curricular access to the National Curriculum, including children with profound and multiple learning difficulties (PMLD) (NCC, 1989). Ware and Peacey (1993) saw the extension of staff expertise as broadening access, and the provision of science and modern foreign languages was generally welcomed. Perhaps the most dramatic improvement has been in that most fundamental area: the teaching of reading. Robinson and Robinson (1976 : 374) believed that children with SLD needed only a social sight vocabulary 'since traditional academic skills are unlikely to be functionally useful to them', a perception which persisted, and was reflected in the low priority reading was afforded during the 1970s and 1980s (Leeming *et al.*, 1979; Harris, 1987). Conversely, reading was always seen as fundamental for children with moderate learning difficulties (Brennan, 1979). This is a clear example of an arbitrary classificatory system denying access to disabled people, for it is now known that many people with learning difficulties can learn to read (Bird and Buckley, 1994) – a right codified in law by the

ERA and given expression in the National Literacy Strategy in 1998. However, despite a reduction in National Curriculum content resulting from the Dearing Report (SCAA, 1994), its subject-based format is significantly at odds with the process model of curriculum accepted as fundamental by many (Halpin and Lewis, 1996).

The pragmatics of entitlement

For entitlement to be effective, delivery must be appropriate for each child. Jordan and Powell (1992) contend that far from enhancing participation in the education system, the National Curriculum may have resulted in significant disadvantage for *some* children. They examined the experiences of Calvin, a child with PMLD, who was integrated into an age-appropriate mainstream leaver's class and attended subject-based lessons. They wrote:

> These opportunities meant that Calvin moved from (his) familiar environment, . . . the pace of the curriculum meant that there was little time [for new staff] to learn about his needs. . . . He attended cooking lessons where he could not even taste the food let alone assist in its preparation. The rich and full curriculum meant that there was insufficient time to give him the physiotherapy he needed to keep his joints flexible. He frequently returned home fitting profusely, his chest rattling and his joints rigid. (1992 : 29)

Jordan and Powell asserted that concepts of education must differ because the needs of individuals vary. If empowerment for pupils with PMLD should include opportunities to experience autonomy and self-esteem, along with gratifying and pleasurable experiences (Wilkinson, 1994), then clearly Calvin's access to the National Curriculum has been extremely disempowering.

Stainback and Stainback highlighted an example of 'good practice' in full inclusion:

> During a map reading activity, one student may be called upon to discuss the economic system of a country, . . . while another student *may simply be requested to grasp and hold a corner of a map* (1990 : 11, our emphasis)

This falls into the category of what PMLD children can do, rather than what they need to do. It is not an example of 'meaningful' learning as the authors claim but a shallow trick which demeans both the child and the concept of inclusion. Other similar examples can be subsumed under the convenient umbrella of experiential learning, as in: 'John will experience: an experiment to demonstrate Boyle's Law', etc.

More positive alternatives will be considered under 'The inclusive school' below. Further independent case studies are needed to assess the impact of the National Curriculum on exceptional children.

Kelly (1990) stressed that modifying National Curriculum guidelines to allow for the slower rate of progress of pupils with learning difficulties is to misunderstand the nature of their fundamental needs. He argued that they may require a different curriculum, not merely the same curriculum at a different pace.

The whole curriculum: a panacea?

The notion of a 'Whole Curriculum' (NCC, 1990) was intended to address the concerns of many educationalists who believed that essential areas of learning for SLD pupils were underrepresented in the National Curriculum. The NCC later accepted that some pupils need access to developmental work such as fundamental social, communication and physical skills, and specialist therapy (NCC, 1993). While considering such elements 'essential' (p.3) to the education of some pupils, the NCC nevertheless conceived of them as *additional to* the National Curriculum. Given that the teaching of the National Curriculum has to take up 80 per cent of schools' timetable, these 'essential' elements must apparently be taught during the remaining 20 per cent of time, which will be clearly insufficient for many young, or less able, pupils.

Fletcher and Gordon (1994) suggested that Personal and Social Education (PSE) can be taught within the National Curriculum; indeed, Sebba *et al.* (1993) stressed that cross-curricular skills (NCC, 1990) could be viewed as a core curriculum for pupils with learning difficulties. Within the current inspection framework, however, schools do not appear to be at liberty to do this, and some have encountered an unfavorable OFSTED response to curricula which do not correspond with statutory orders. One school, catering primarily for children with PMLD, was criticized for failing to build the sequencing of beads into the early stages of an algebra programme. To suggest these children are working towards an understanding of algebra is to devalue their developmental status and needs. Although the purpose of publishing OFSTED reports is to compare individual schools, it also serves to highlight inconsistencies among OFSTED teams. Reports reveal a worrying variability of interpretation of regulations, something which the new independent OFSTED Adjudicator might well address. Kelly (1994) argued that PSE should assume a higher priority. In Scotland, it has. Guidelines state:

> PSE is a fundamental aspect of the education of the whole child . . . [and] will be a core area of the curriculum for those pupils who need to acquire the skills essential for taking care of basic social needs. (Scottish Office Education Department, 1996 : 1)

However, in England and Wales OFSTED reports on PSE are currently limited to generalities about the social atmosphere and staff/pupil relationships.

The government has indicated that preparation for adult life and relationships will be an important element in the revised National Curriculum due to be implemented in September 2000. In our view PSE should contribute to a *compulsory core area* in an Inclusive National Curriculum.

Improved standards for pupils with learning disabilities

Ostensibly the *raison d'être* for the National Curriculum was to raise standards, but there is a distinct lack of evidence in relation to SLD students (Lewis, 1995; Halpin and Lewis, 1996). Indeed, 'standards' are not clearly defined, so any objective assessment of them is problematic

(Kelly, 1990). Ware (1994) emphasized the difficulty of assessing against attainment targets pupils who may be working within Level One for long periods during their schooling, without ever reaching those targets – a fundamentally disempowering situation.

Porter and colleagues have provided important new data on the impact of the National Curriculum on deaf-blind children. Significantly the 57 teachers involved found it necessary to supplement the National Curriculum with *eleven* curricular areas to meet the pupils' needs. They concluded:

> There was little consensus between (teachers), with a variety of additional curriculum areas provided and much cross curriculum delivery. In consequence the curriculum appears fragmented with little way of ensuring continuity and progression. (1997 : 75)

It seems unlikely that the educational standards for the pupils would be raised in those circumstances. The curricular 'fragmentation' reported appears to be a direct result of the inability of the existing National Curriculum to meet the pupils' needs.

Fundamental doubts have not diminished. Carpenter and Ashdown (1996) reported that many teachers continued to believe that the National Curriculum focused on average children in mainstream schools and was not inclusive. Similarly, Lloyd found that many teachers perceived it as 'narrowly prescriptive, relevant for only a minority of children' (1997 : 175) and, of 1434 primary teachers surveyed, 80 per cent saw the National Curriculum as 'unmanageable', leaving the whole curriculum 'ineffective' and 'overcrowded' (Times Educational Supplement, 1997).

Significantly, the Labour Government appears to accept that the National Curriculum may not be the most appropriate vehicle for the raising of standards in at least some situations. 'Education Action Zones' (DfEE, 1998) have been introduced in designated areas to raise standards. A key feature is to allow for the suspension of components of the National Curriculum to focus on its core areas, but schools outside the zones will continue to be constrained, a situation which is logically and ethically indefensible. (For further information on empowerment the reader is referred to Chapter 21A–C.)

The National Curriculum: a gateway to inclusion?

What of the impact of the National Curriculum on mainstream inclusion for SLD pupils? The NCC (1989) promised a common structure to enhance curricular compatibility and facilitate integration, but the amount of differentiation needed in a mainstream classroom for some pupils could highlight differences. Kelly (1994) reported that exclusions have actually increased since the introduction of the National Curriculum, while Lloyd (1994) observed that some mainstream teachers were less willing to integrate pupils because of the focus on standard assessment of reading, writing and numeracy. Clearly, further objective evidence is needed regarding the impact of the ERA on inclusion. A start has been made by the government promising to stop exclusions being used to boost school performance table scores.

Towards an inclusive national curriculum

One implication which could be drawn from this review is that some children with complex learning difficulties should have a separate, parallel, curriculum outside the National Curriculum. We reject this as dangerous negativism, which could easily lead to the exclusion of these children from the educational system, as has happened in some European countries. What is needed is a more radical and creative solution which can meet the needs of *all* children in the new millennium.

First, the balance of time devoted to the elements of the curriculum should be relevant to the assessed needs of the individual child, rather than dictated by crude statutory percentages. The curriculum should fit the child, not vice versa (Whittaker, 1990); this is an issue being addressed at last by the development of access statements (DfEE, 1998b). The child's individualized curriculum would be regularly reviewed and open to scrutiny.

Secondly, an additional core area should be included for *all* children to form an Inclusive National Curriculum. This would secure the curricular centrality of Personal Autonomy and Self-determination as an educational goal. It could contain elements currently subsumed under the PSE banner, although it would have little in common with the old idea of self-help skills (Gunzburg, 1968), and it would go much further than PSE as currently envisaged.

The principles of self-determination (Wehmeyer, 1997) would have an important place. The components are:

- autonomous functioning
- self-regulation
- psychological empowerment
- self-realization.

Having outlined some principles which would underlie an Inclusive National Curriculum, we will now examine where it would take place.

What is inclusive education?

Lusthaus and Forest (1989) defined inclusive education as every student being educated within a mainstream class in their local mainstream school. This conceptualization of inclusive education is related to, but different from, integration/mainstreaming where the focus is on the assimilation of excluded outsiders, often through the largesse of the powerful. Inclusion can be seen as an advanced formulation of the argument as it does not start from a basis of difference but from one of equality. Both Ramasut (1989) and Barnes (1991) stressed that education for all in a mainstream environment is a human rights issue, for there is clear evidence that segregated education results in unequal status and opportunities for disabled people.

The evidence on inclusive education

For those, such as Barnes (1991), who believe that it is the inalienable right of all children to be educated in inclusive settings, the question of the advantages and disadvantages of inclusion is a spurious one. But the issue of who benefits, and how, pervades the literature, and needs to be evaluated in arguing for fundamental changes to the educational system.

A commonly perceived benefit for disabled children is the proximity of typical role models and enhanced opportunities for interaction (Lewis, 1995). Other advantages include: integration into the local community (Wade and Moore, 1992); reduced stigmatization (McHale and Simeonssen, 1980); better prospects in adulthood (Stainback and Stainback, 1990); and evidence that the social behaviour of mainstream pupils matures in inclusive settings (Whitaker, 1994).

Attitudes to inclusive education

The success of any innovation is dependent upon the attitudes of those most closely associated with its implementation. Often these reflect, rather than lead, attitudes within society. Although there has been some improvement in societal attitudes towards people with learning difficulties, there is still widespread ignorance and irrational fear. Less extreme, but still worrying, levels of prejudice are apparent among those who would implement inclusive education.

Evidence indicates that the more removed professionals are from having to implement inclusive education the stronger they advocate it, with classroom practitioners being less enthusiastic than headteachers or academics (Houck and Rogers, 1994). Balanced against this is the finding that the more experience teachers have of inclusion the more positive they are about it (Scruggs and Mastropieri, 1996).

We will briefly examine evidence on the attitudes of some of those closely affected by inclusion: teachers, parents and the students themselves. Scruggs and Mastropieri (1996) reviewed studies on the attitudes of mainstream teachers towards inclusion. Overall, 60 per cent of the teachers were supportive of the general concept of inclusion, but these figures dropped dramatically in relation to pupils with learning difficulties (Diebold and VonEschenbach, 1991). Willingness to participate in inclusion did not vary between primary and secondary teachers but was low if it would lead to additional responsibilities (Houck and Rogers, 1994).

The perceived benefits varied according to the degree of inclusion. Overall, 15 per cent of general, and 66 per cent of special, educators believed that some degree of integration could lead to some benefits, but:

> ... only a minority of teachers agreed that the general classroom was the best environment for students with special needs, or that full-time inclusion would (lead to) social or academic benefits. (Scruggs and Mastropieri, 1996 : 65)

Most studies referred specifically to students with a mild disability – depressing findings for those who advocate full inclusion for all. Seventy per cent of mainstream teachers surveyed believed that they had insufficient expertise to cope with inclusion. Even with the possibility of further training, 83 per cent of the teachers in one study (Coates, 1989) felt that they would not be able to meet the educational needs of all disabled children.

Attitudes of student teachers showed a similar negative pattern. Wishart and Manning (1996) surveyed 231 teacher trainees about inclusive education for pupils with Down's syndrome. The concept of inclusion was widely accepted, but again there was little support for it to be implemented. A significant majority (87 per cent) of the trainees did not want to teach in an inclusive setting, and 96 per cent believed that they had not been prepared by their training. This is not perhaps surprising. Statutory guidelines for the training of teachers in England and Wales focus increasingly on the core areas of the National Curriculum. Special Educational Needs, and Child Development, are often expressed as cross-curricula issues, or given tokenistic slots in an overcrowded programme, while Disability Studies is only rarely offered.

Parental attitudes towards inclusion are fundamentally important. McDonnell (1987) found that parents of children in special schools predicted that mainstream placement would be a negative experience for their children, while parents of integrated disabled children were extremely positive. McDonnell concluded that parental fears may be an influential factor in the continued support for segregated education.

Whitaker (1994) examined college students' attitudes to the inclusion of learning disabled people. Seventy per cent had very positive attitudes, with those who had actually shared classrooms being most positive. This is a recurring theme: shared experiences leads to more open, less stereotyped attitudes.

Both the Children Act 1989, and the Code of Practice (DfEE, 1994), set out the rights of disabled children to be involved in decisions concerning their educational placement, but Hegarty (1993) found that their voices were heard rarely in research. In a single-school case study, Swain (1993) pointed out the 'central paradox' of able-bodied professionals deciding if students should participate in educational decision-making processes. Recently, attempts have been made to rectify this exclusion.

Beveridge (1996) sought the views of teenagers with learning difficulties who attended their local comprehensive on a link scheme. Care was taken to get to know the pupils well before interviewing them, and non-verbal cueing supplemented the questions. Pupils were significantly more positive about the social opportunities for making friends and interacting with peers at the comprehensive compared with their special school. Wade and Moore (1994) explored the perception of 160 children with learning and related difficulties, reporting their need for work matched to their capabilities, greater freedom of curricular choice, and a desire for more responsibility to enhance their self-perception.

Some people with learning difficulties have been given the opportunity to record their own perceptions. Robert said:

> I remember being very upset because I found arithmetic difficult and I couldn't cope with it. . . . I was angry because nobody let me do anything that I wanted to do. I used to run away from the hospital, most of the time during the night. (Atkinson and Williams, 1990 : 213).

Researching the views of young people with learning difficulties needs to develop rapidly to provide an important perspective on inclusion.

Attitudes to inclusive education: a summary

Professionals and trainees, like the general population, expressed more negative attitudes towards people with learning difficulties when they have had little contact with them. Teachers who have worked in inclusive settings tended to be enthusiastic about the benefits. Parents who had experience of inclusion were far less anxious than those who had not. Most encouragingly, students with experience of inclusion were the most positive. We should not minimize the long-term prospect that growing up together in inclusive schools will lead to a more harmonious view than that shown by current generations.

There is an obvious need for sensitive, ongoing consultation with all of those affected by inclusion, along with carefully targeted training. We believe, however, that there is a need to go further – to reconceptualize the nature of schools.

The inclusive school

True inclusion requires the reorganization of the system, with the closure of existing special *and* mainstream provision and the creation of new schools with a fresh ethos. Arbitrary and derogatory labels such as severe and moderate learning difficulties which limit expectations and fail to recognize the social construction of disability would be removed. Teaching approaches which recognized the sociocultural context of development and the transactional nature of learning (Mallory and New, 1994) would define the professional environment. A continuum of need would be matched by a continuum of provision within school, with flexible learning environments replacing the concept of the traditional classroom.

Inclusive schools would be based on the principle that every child has the right to be educated in a neighbourhood school alongside their peers, with individualized access to an Inclusive National Curriculum designed to meet the needs of every child. Although a range of provision would be offered within the school to meet these needs, all decisions would be based on the principle of *maximum access to full inclusion for all children*, with any variation on this having to be carefully justified, regularly reviewed and open to external scrutiny.

Inclusive schooling would retain the educational advantages of social integration, while providing the impetus for appropriate academic inclusion. For example, children with PMLD can benefit a great deal from learning alongside mainstream peers in an inclusive school: one where their curriculum objective *match* rather than *mimic* each other. We have observed situations where typically developing children, as part of their PSE syllabus plan, then take part in supervised interactive play sessions with their PMLD peers, and reflect on the experience afterwards. The PMLD children benefited from appropriate one-to-one work with a wider range of people. Inclusive schools would promote a natural environment for this joint learning. A key element in realizing inclusive schools is the phasing out of most segregated provision.

Ending segregation

We can see few valid arguments for the continued existence of the majority of segregated education. The moral and ethical case against segregation, already outlined, is overwhelming. From an economic perspective it has been claimed that special schools can provide dedicated resources not available in mainstream. With devolved budgets to schools, however, it is easier to see the true costs of maintaining segregated provision, while economies of scale in inclusive schools could make the purchase and wider use of many material resources more cost effective.

The specialist design of segregated schools is no longer a tenable argument for their retention, now that legislation requires public buildings to have access for all. Government funds have been allocated for improving disabled access to existing mainstream schools from 1998/99. It is equally important to consider the full market value of unwanted school sites when budgeting for change. The real economic problem is to ensure that capital released flows back into the education system, and that per capita spending is not reduced in inclusive settings. Too often the language of integration has been usurped by officials interested only in financial rationalization to cut expenditure.

It has been suggested (Dessent, 1987) that special schools staff have expertise that would be lost in inclusive settings, but since the closure of full-time specialist courses in the mid-1980s the numbers of trained staff have reached worryingly low levels. There is a clear need for extensive in-service training and the development of innovative new courses to prepare high-quality teachers who have the skills and credibility to teach, and support others, in fully inclusive schools. It will be necessary to safeguard against the replacement of teachers by auxiliaries or some new para-educational grade – an attractive option for administrators cutting costs. We would otherwise face the invidious situation of children with SLD having achieved inclusion, being denied full access to suitably qualified teachers.

The new Education Action Zones could be ideal for the piloting of inclusive schools, but, as we have learnt from the USA, only legislation will ensure widespread adoption of the principle.

Therapists and inclusive schools

Therapy has traditionally played a pivotal role in an interdisciplinary service for many children in special schools. But one of the most radical thinkers in the Disabled People's Movement has questioned the ideological basis of this work. Oliver is scathing about attempts by professionals to exhort physically disabled people:

> ... to approximate to the walkie-talkie model of living, where physical and social environments remain unchanged and unchanging. (1989:189)

The Disabled People's Movement has challenged professionals to consider their role in creating disabling barriers and perpetuating power elites (Abberley, 1987; Swain et al., 1993) and therapists need to closely examine how received beliefs and accepted practice contribute to this. But we believe that it is possible to differentiate therapy designed to maintain and extend the mobility of joints, improve posture, and give access to communication and educational activity, from an approach which devalues wheelchair use by promoting walking as a goal to be pursued to the detriment of educational opportunity. Postural drainage is necessary to maintain life for some children, while the prevention, or limitation, of contractures is a basic right. Developmental delay can lead to the late onset of walking in children capable of doing so for the rest of their lives; therapeutic help, here, is crucial. For these reasons we would see therapy as an integral part of the educational curriculum for children with PMLD. Rather belatedly this is now the DfEE's acknowledged position (NCC, 1993). The SCAA has stated that therapists should be involved in

> ... defining the curriculum for a pupil with PMLD. Therapists and sensory support services will have a role in specialized assessment leading to the identification of specific needs. (1996 : 10)

However, they then assume that therapeutic intervention can be integrated within the present National Curriculum and delivered in the mainstream classroom:

> Priority skills such as physiotherapy can be addressed continuously across the curriculum and through all key stages. (1996 : 13)

But can they? McWilliam and Bailey (1994) found that physiotherapists were least likely to favour integrated services in mainstream classrooms compared to other therapists. This may be because others tend to employ less obtrusive table-top activities, while the physiotherapy programme can encompass floor-work and exercise routines. It is difficult to argue that the intimate physical contact, and relaxed atmosphere, which is at the heart of the professional relationship between child and therapist, should be set in the public arena of the mainstream classroom. Discreet help with positioning might be carried out there, but intensive work would require a more private setting – which would have to be accurately budgeted into inclusion plans.

Whether therapy is seen as an integral element within the curriculum or a separate service, therapists have a vital role, ranging from awareness raising of the implications of minor motor problems, to specific therapeutic intervention and support. Therapists may also contribute to the recognition of neurological difficulties in mainstream children which might otherwise have been misunderstood (Whittaker, 1997). A new multi-agency pilot programme has been announced (DfEE, 1998a), to support early assessment and intervention for disabled children, which should further enhance the therapist's role.

Resourcing therapy

Experience in the USA has indicated that inclusion requires more resources for therapy than segregated provision. Gregory *et al.* (1992) found the same for physically disabled children in inclusive settings in Dundee – occupational therapy needs in particular were underestimated. If all children with learning difficulties were taught in inclusive schools, then further resources for travelling time between schools would be needed. Accommodation and some equipment would have to be duplicated for each setting. Vigilance would be required to ensure that adequate resourcing was built into proposals for inclusive schools.

Conclusion

We have reviewed a daunting range of potential impediments to the inclusion of pupils with learning difficulties in their own neighbourhood schools. But we have also highlighted the successes and the positive effects these can have in changing attitudes and dissipating prejudice. A challenging agenda has been proposed: to reconceptualize the core National Curriculum giving weight to self-determination and individual needs; this will help to expedite a move to inclusive schools based on the principle of maximum access to full inclusion for all children.

Therapists need to examine their own belief systems and how these impinge on their practice; and to enter into constructive dialogue concerning their important role in supporting young people with learning difficulties in their right to inclusive schooling.

References

Abberley, P. (1987) The concept of oppression and the development of a social theory of disability. *Disability Handicap and Society*, **2**(1), 5–19

Atkinson, D. and Williams, F. (1990) *Know Me As I Am: An Anthology of Prose, Poetry and Art by People with Learning Difficulties*, Hodder and Stoughton, London (in association with the Open University Press)

Barnes, C. (1991) *Disabled People in Britain and Discrimination: A Case for Anti-Discrimination Legislation*, Hurst, London.

Beveridge, S. (1996) Experiences of an integration link scheme: the perspectives of pupils with severe learning difficulties and their mainstream peers. *British Journal of Learning Disabilities*, **24**, 9–19

Bird, G. and Buckley, S. (1994) *Meeting the Educational Needs of Children with Down's Syndrome: A Handbook for Teachers*, University of Portsmouth

Brennan, K. (1979) *Curricular Needs of Slow Learners*, Methuen, London

Brown, F. and Cohen S. (1996) Self determination and young children. *Journal of the Association for Persons with Severe Handicaps*, **21**(1), 22–30

Carpenter, B. and Ashdown, R. (1996) Enabling access. In Carpenter, B. *et al.* (eds), *Enabling Access: Effective Teaching and Learning for Pupils with Learning Disabilities*, David Fulton, London

Coates, R.D. (1989) The regular education initiative and opinions of regular classroom teachers. *Journal of Learning Disabilities*, **22**, 532–536

Coupe O'Cane, J. and Smith, B. (eds) (1994) *Taking Control: Enabling People with Learning Disabilities*, David Fulton, London

Cunningham, C. and Sloper, P. (1978) *Helping Your Handicapped Baby*, Souveinir Press, London

Dessent, T. (1987) *Making the Ordinary School Special*, The Falmer Press, London

DfEE (1994) *Code of Practice on the Identification and Assessment of Special Educational Needs*, HMSO, London

DfEE (1998a) *Education Action Zones*, HMSO, London

DfEE (1998b) *Policies for Excellence*, HMSO, London

Diebold, M.H. and VonEschenbach, J.F. (1991) Teacher educator predictions of regular class teacher perceptions of mainstreaming. *Teacher Education and Special Education*, **25**, 221–227

Fletcher, W. and Gordon, J. (1994) Personal and social education in a school for pupils with severe learning difficulties. In Rose, R. *et al.* (eds), *Implementing the Whole Curriculum for Pupils with Learning Difficulties*, David Fulton, London

Gardner, J., Murphy, J. and Crawford, N. (1983) *The Skills Analysis Model*, BILD Publications, Kidderminster

Gregory, J.W., Fairgrieve, E.M., Anderson, D.M. and Hammond, H.F. (1992) Therapy needs of children in mainstream education. *British Journal of Occupational Therapy*, **55**(7), 271–272

Gunzberg, H.C. (1968) *Social Competence and Mental Handicap*, Cassell, London

Halpin, D. and Lewis, A. (1996) The impact of the national curriculum on twelve special schools. *European Journal of Special Needs Education*, **11**(1), 95–105

Harris, J. (1987) *Language Learning in Schools for Children with Severe Learning Disabilities*, Croom Helm, London

Hegarty, S. (1993) Reviewing the literature on integration. *European Journal of Special Needs Education*, **8**(3), 194–200

Hogg, J. (1975) Normative development and educational programme planning for severely educationally subnormal children. In Kiernan, C.C. and Woodford, F.P. (eds), *Behaviour Modification with the Severely Retarded*, Elsevier, Amsterdam

Hogg, J. (1987) Early development and Piagetian tests. In Hogg, J. and Raynes, N.V. (eds), *Assessment in Mental Handicap. A Guide to Assessment Practices, Tests and Checklists*, Croom Helm, London

Houck, C.K. and Rogers, C.J. (1994) The special/general education integration initiative for students with specific learning disabilities: a 'snapshot' of program change. *Journal of Learning Disabilities*, **27**, 435–453

Jordan, R. and Powell, S. (1992) Stop the reforms, Calvin wants to get off. *Disability, Handicap and Society*, **7**(1), 85–88

Kelly, A.V. (1990) *The National Curriculum: A Critical Review*, Paul Chapman, London

Kelly, A.V. (1994) Beyond the rhetoric and the discourse. In Blenkin, G. and Kelly, A.V. (eds), *The National Curriculum and Early Learning*, Paul Chapman, London

Kiernan, C., Jordan, R. and Saunders, C. (1978) *Starting Off*, Human Horizon Series, Souvenir Press, London

Leeming, K., Swann W., Coupe, J. and Mittler P. (1979) *Teaching Language and Communication to the Mentally Handicapped*, Schools Council Curriculum Bulletin, Methuen Educational, London

Lewis, A. (1995) The code of practice, the national curriculum and children with special educational needs. *Education*, **23**(1), 3–13.

Lloyd, C. (1994) Special educational needs and the early years. In Blenkin, G.M. and Kelly, A.V. (eds), *The National Curriculum and Early Learning: An Evaluation*, Paul Chapman, London

Lloyd, C. (1997) Inclusive education for children with special educational needs. In Wolfendale, S. (ed.), *Meeting Special Needs in the Early Years: Directions in Policy and Practice*, David Fulton, London

Lloyd-Smith, M. (1992) The education reform act and special needs education: conflicting ideologies. In Jones, N. and Docking, J. (eds), *Special Educational Needs and the Education Reform Act*, Trentham Books, Stoke-on-Trent

Lusthaus, E. and Forest, M. (1989) Promoting educational equality for all students. In Stainback, S. *et al.* (eds), *Educating All Students in the Mainstream of Regular Education*, Paul Brookes, Baltimore

Mallory, B. and New, R.S. (1994) Social constructivist theory and principles of inclusion: challenges for early childhood special education. *Journal of Special Education*, **8**(3), 322–337

McConkey, R. (1981) Education without understanding? *Special Education: Forward Trends*, **8**(3), 8–10

McDonnell, J. (1987) The integration of students with severe handicaps: an analysis of parental perspectives. *Education and Training in Mental Retardation*, **22**(2), 98–111

McHale, S.M. and Simeonssen, R.J. (1980) Effects of interaction on non-handicapped children's attitudes towards autistic children. *American Journal of Mental Deficiency*, **85**(1), 18–24

McWilliam, R.A. and Bailey, D.B. (1994) Predictors of service-delivery models in center-based early intervention. *Exceptional Children*, **61**(1), 56–71

NCC (1989) *Curriculum Guidance 2: A Curriculum for All*, National Curriculum Council, York.

NCC (1990) *Curriculum Guidance 3: The Whole Curriculum*, National Curriculum Council, York

NCC (1993) *Special Needs and the National Curriculum: Opportunity and Challenge*, National Curriculum Council, York.

Oliver, M. (1989) Conductive education: if it wasn't so sad it would be funny. *Disability, Handicap and Society*, **4**(2), 197–200

Porter, J., Miller, O. and Pease, L. (1997) *Curriculum Access for Deaf-Blind Children*, HMSO, London

Ramasut, A. (ed.) (1989) *Whole School Approaches to Special Needs*, Falmer Press, Hove

Robinson, N.M. and Robinson, H.B. (1976) *The Mentally Retarded Child. A Psychological Approach*, 2nd edn, McGraw-Hill, Maidenhead

SCAA (1994) *The National Curriculum and its Assessment: Final Report*, School Curriculum and Assessment Authority, London

SCAA (1996) *Planning the Curriculum for Pupils with Profound and Multiple Learning Disabilities*, School Curriculum and Assessment Authority, London

Scottish Office Education Department (1996) *Curriculum and Assessment in Scotland. National Guidelines: Personal and Social Development, 5–14*, HMSO, Edinburgh

Scruggs, T.E. and Mastropieri, M.A. (1996) Teacher perceptions of mainstreaming/inclusion, 1958–1995: a research synthesis. *Exceptional Children*, **63**(1), 59–74

Sebba, J., Byers, R. and Rose, R. (1993) *Redefining the Whole Curriculum for Pupils with Learning Difficulties*, David Fulton, London

Stainback, W. and Stainback, S. (1990) *Support Networks for Inclusive Schooling in Interdependent Integrated Education*, Paul Brookes, Baltimore

Swain, J. (1993) Taught helplessness? Or a say for disabled pupils in schools. In Swain, J. *et al.*, (eds), *Disabling Barriers: Enabling Environments*, Sage, London

Swain, J. Finkelstein, V. French, S. and Oliver, M. (eds) (1993) *Disabling Barriers: Enabling Environments*, Sage, London

Times Educational Supplement (1997) *Curriculum 'Unmanageable'*, 5th December, 6

Wade, B. and Moore, M. (1992) *Patterns of Educational Integration: International Perspectives on Mainstreaming Children with Special Educational Needs*, Triangle, Oxford

Wade, B. and Moore, M. (1994) Feeling different: viewpoint of pupils with special educational needs. *British Journal of Special Education*, **21**(4), 161–165

Ware, J. (1994) Implementing the 1988 act with pupils with PMLDs. In Ware, J. (ed.), *Educating Children with Profound and Multiple Learning Difficulties*, David Fulton, London

Ware, J. and Peacey, N. (1993) We're doing history – what does it mean? *British Journal of Special Education*, **20**(2), 65–69

Wehmeyer, M. (1997) Self-determination as an educational outcome: a definitional framework. *Journal of Developmental and Physical Disabilities*, **9**(3), 175–209

Whitaker, P. (1994) Mainstream students talk about integration. *British Journal of Special Education*, **21**(1), 13–16

Whittaker, C.A. (1985) Enhancing conceptual generalisation in the profoundly retarded: guidance towards solutions or imposition of end states? Paper to the American Academy of Child Psychiatry, San Antonio, USA, October.

Whittaker, C.A. (1990) The Whole Curriculum subsumes the National Curriculum: a case study of a school for children with severe learning difficulties. Paper presented to the International Special Needs Congress 'Special Educational Needs: Created or Met?', Cardiff, July

Whittaker, C.A. (1997) Key issues in the psychological development in the child: implications for physiotherapy practice. In French, S. (ed.), *Physiotherapy: A Psychosocial Approach*, 2nd edn, Butterworth-Heinemann, Oxford

Wilkinson, C. (1994) Teaching pupils with PMLD to exert control. In Coupe O'Cane, J. and Smith, B. (eds), *Taking Control: Enabling People with Learning Difficulties*, David Fulton, London

Wishart, J.G. and Manning G. (1996) Trainee teachers' attitudes to inclusive education for children with Down's syndrome. *Journal of Intellectual Disability Research*, **40**, 56–65

Wood, S. and Shears, B. (1986) *Teaching Children with Severe Learning Difficulties: A Radical Reappraisal*, Croom Helm, London

Zigler, E. (1969) Development versus difference theories of mental retardation and the problem of motivation. *American Journal of Mental Deficiency*, **73**, 536–556

Further education and employment

Jenny Corbett

13

Introduction

In any examination of the opportunities for people with learning difficulties in further education and employment it is necessary to explore the support they might receive at each stage of development and what obstacles they are likely to encounter. The impact of recent legislation needs to be carefully considered, as does the effect of changing attitudes to disability and to youth unemployment.

It is important to consider what exactly constitutes a learning difficulty. The term is generic in covering a wide range of degrees of difficulty, with different requirements for support. There are some learners with profound difficulties who require a sensory curriculum and others who are unable to read or write but who have significant social skills which help them to manage in community activities. There are others who have the label of 'autism' or 'Asperger's syndrome', which might mean they are able to cope with difficult subjects like mathematics but find real problems in social interactions.

While the term 'learning difficulties and disabilities (LDD)' has become commonly used in the further education sector, it is not a term favoured by national organizations like Mencap and the British Institute of Learning Disabilities (BILD). The political campaigning groups within the Disabled People's Movement argue that those who used to be called someone with a learning difficulty should be called a learning disabled person because it is not they who have a difficulty but society which creates difficulties for them, and the term 'disability' aligns them more powerfully to the Disabled People's Movement, of which they are a part. In this chapter, the term 'learning difficulty' will be used to maintain continuity in the overall text, although its use reflects an educational convention rather than a political stance.

For some years there have been various attempts to define transition from childhood to adulthood. The 1986 Organisation for Economic Cooperation and Development (OECD) version was that it combined the following goals:

- employment, useful work and valued activity;
- personal autonomy;
- independent living and adult status;

- social interaction, community participation, leisure and recreation;
- adult roles within the family including marriage.

In their evaluation of the transition process, McGinty and Fish asked, 'What are the performance criteria by which young people will be assessed for training and employment programmes? How is individual progress through a transition programme evaluated?' (1992:16). These questions also require contextualization into the economic climate of unequal opportunities, professional prejudices and limited social horizons (Corbett and Barton, 1992).

The impact of recent legislation on practice and provision

The major report on practice and provision in further education for students with learning difficulties and/or disabilities is *Inclusive Learning* (FEFC, 1996) which presents the findings of the Tomlinson Committee. The emphasis upon inclusion is powerful and pervasive:

> Central to all our thinking and recommendations is the approach towards learning, which we term 'Inclusive learning', and which we want to see adopted everywhere. Put simply, we want to avoid a viewpoint which locates the difficulty or deficit with the student and focus instead on the capacity of the educational institution to understand and respond to the individual learner's requirement. This means we must move away from labelling the student and towards creating an appropriate educational environment; concentrate on understanding better how people learn so that they can better be helped to learn; and see people with disabilities and/or learning difficulties first and foremost as learners. (FEFC, 1996: 4)

This is a most positive and progressive response, yet it is extremely challenging without being prescriptive or presenting immediate access to additional resources. Like much recent government rhetoric, the Tomlinson Report may be seen as being full of inclusive ideologies but short of practical hints.

There have been various responses to *Inclusive Learning* and it is interesting to compare a response from a college principal with one from a college lecturer. Ruth Silver, the Principal of Lewisham College, sets out a management agenda based on this report, which asks other principals to

> ... get this work to your governors and staff, establish your policy of inclusiveness with all students and staff, read and disseminate this report with other professional colleagues; discuss the report and plan, both inside and outside the organization; see how close you are and how far away from inclusiveness; 'hoover' the curriculum for barriers. (1997: 33).

This concept of 'hoovering' the curriculum for barriers is novel but pertinent. It implies that sorting out barriers to inclusive practices and provision is a relatively easy process, much like cleaning the house. However, as Hatton's (1997) reflections testify, it is actually more like demolishing the house and rebuilding it to new specifications – altogether a very different and much more challenging task!

The barriers to participation within transition to further education

Most students with learning difficulties which could be termed 'severe' are placed on segregated course provision in further education colleges, having generally come from the special school sector. This is still the case in most colleges in Britain and the Tomlinson Report is now challenging segregated practices and calling for more inclusion on mainstream courses.

In her account of the implications for staff and students at Solihull College of dismantling the discrete (segregated) two-year full-time programme for school leavers from the schools for pupils with moderate and severe learning difficulties, Sue Hatton (1997) found that there were mixed feelings at the prospect of change:

> I feel petrified, I know we can make it work because we will put the effort in, but what if there is not enough, support?
> *Member of support staff*

> I will manage. I do one day a week now with the Health and Social Care lot, but I will need Pat to keep helping me. I will need Pat every day or I won't be able to keep up and my folder will get in a mess and I will get it all wrong. [Pat is a member of staff already supporting on an infill basis].
> *Student currently on discrete programme*

> I don't want to do that, thank you. I want to do Social Mobility with Kay and my Core Skills with you and Cookery with Macrina.
> *Student currently on discrete programme*

> I think it is a great idea but I am not very sure about having teaching staff across college who will cope. I do have one or two in the area I manage who will be OK, but generally speaking I think you will face some major problems.
> *Curriculum manager*

> If we do this, what about my teaching? There will only be so much you need me to do in terms of support for students. What about my actual teaching hours? Will I really be needed any more?
> *Member of teaching staff within supported learning.*

(Quoted from Hatton, 1997: 23)

These various responses to the plans to dismantle existing segregated systems are interesting in that they reflect the outstanding tensions within the integration/inclusion debate. There is a fear of change and anxiety about the loss of former roles and specialist status. Some students want to be protected and given additional support, while others are so used to being in segregated provision that the thought of being in mainstream classes becomes awesome.

It is most important to recognize attitudinal barriers to change and to the inclusion of students with learning difficulties. Unless these barriers are addressed, support will tend to remain the responsibility of the learning support staff rather than being considered an issue of shared ownership taken on by all staff and, most significantly, by fellow students.

Available support for college participation and progression

The terminology of further education is not that of 'special educational needs', still commonly used in schools, but that of 'learning support'. Dumbleton describes the role of learning support staff as being a combination of:

Core Roles
(a) Offering support to students who are experiencing learning difficulties that cannot be resolved by the class teacher. This support may be offered in a number of ways: indirectly by consultation with the teacher concerned; by cooperative working with the teacher concerned in the classroom; and directly by working with the student.
(b) Offering support to staff who are concerned with preventing or overcoming learning difficulties in their students. This support may be offered in a number of ways: by consultation; through formal staff development sessions; and by joint curriculum planning activities, and

Wider roles
(c) Cooperating with admissions staff to ensure that students are not enrolled on inappropriate courses. Cooperating with admissions staff to ensure that equal opportunities policies are implemented . . .,
(d) Cooperating with other guidance support staff to ensure that, for example, students with physical or sensory impairment receive adequate support. (Dumbleton, 1993: 112)

Thus, learning support provided for students with learning difficulties in further education can be seen to offer a comprehensive approach to broad learning, social and institutional goals. The occupational therapist could be called upon to advise on appropriate classroom aids and to help develop suitable strategies to cope with the physical demands of getting around on a large college campus and enhancing the daily quality of life in a challenging setting.

Peer integration: the inclusion of students with learning difficulties

I am going to describe the work on peer integration at Richmond Tertiary College undertaken by Helen Hayhoe (1998). This is an excellent model for the kind of support which really can create an inclusive institutional culture within the current context of restricted funding, for the following reasons: it is student-centred; it used available human resources; it changes attitudes by the *process of* inclusive practice, rather than by policy alone; it enables students with learning difficulties to participate at a level which offers them increased opportunities and new challenges. I regard this as an example which exemplifies the ways in which *inclusion* differs markedly from *integration*. In my own doctoral case study of integration in a college of further education, the emphasis was upon the students with learning difficulties having to adapt to the existing courses or to remain within discrete provision, as there was no peer support available to them and they had to rely upon goodwill and generosity which was always an unpredictable variable (Corbett, 1987). I find it interesting to reflect that in the 10 years since my research and that of Hayhoe, there has been a major ideological shift from integration to inclusion in all sectors of education.

Integration, as I observed it in the mid-1980s, was a piecemeal, unsatisfactory arrangement in which students with learning difficulties had to cope with tremendous obstacles which often led to a high risk of failure. The failure tended to be seen as their problem, not the result of institutional inertia or ineptitude. Hayhoe's research shows that actual, directed and monitored peer support can and does make a huge difference to all concerned. Inclusion is proactive and about changing the institutional culture; integration tended to be individual-focused and about learning to fit in to the status quo. The late 1990s offers a very different scenario to students with learning difficulties.

The initiative at Richmond Tertiary College is particularly valuable as a model of good practice in the wake of the Tomlinson Report, when other colleges are looking for examples of how they might make steps towards full inclusion for their students. I use the term 'make steps' with care, as it seems important that we recognize that inclusion as an ideology has to be translated into actuality in easy stages if it is to be seen as viable.

At Richmond College, mainstream student volunteers are selected either to work alongside students with learning difficulties in class or to join in recreational activities or lunchtime socializing with students from the discrete courses. The scheme is committed to the

> ... contact hypothesis: that structured opportunities for contact between students will result in positive attitudinal changes among mainstream students which will benefit the students who have learning difficulties. Specifically, the opportunity to get to know people who have learning difficulties should allow mainstream students to see them as individuals and the experience of engaging with the practical details of facilitating integration should give mainstream students a realistic grounding which will make them more welcoming of integration in the future. (Hayhoe, 1998: 44)

Such an approach has to be recognized as a valuable step towards a more inclusive institutional and societal culture.

Transition to employment

There has developed an established impetus to prepare young people with learning disabilities for employment or for satisfying alternatives in various ways. One example is that of the Team Enterprise Programme which operates in a structured framework to help students with learning disabilities to set up, run and eventually wind down their own company over two academic years, supported by college staff and local business advisers (Hewitson, 1996). Not all people with learning disabilities are either seeking conventional employment opportunities or are likely to find them, but this does not mean that there is no valued social role for them. The advocacy movement has meant that more professionals now value the contribution that adults with learning difficulties can make to the learning experiences of those who are training to work in this field.

Kirkpatrick and Earwaker (1997), for example, as tutors at King Alfred's College in Winchester, offer a three-year degree course in social and professional studies in learning difficulties in which they involve people with learning difficulties at all stages of the process: in designing the format of the course; in delivery and contribution to some lectures; as course representatives; on interview panels. Members of the Eastleigh Advocacy Project, a local self-advocacy group for people with learning difficulties, felt that their involvement included these benefits: 'the opportunity for real, paid and diverse work; a perceived rise in status as lecturers, interviewers, advisors and committee members; the perception of equal status' (Kirkpatrick and Earwaker 1997: 20), all of which can be seen as empowering and appropriately adult in scope and challenge.

In a recent analysis of employment opportunities for people with various disabilities, Thornton and Lunt said of the process of transition from sheltered employment to the open employment sector that

> ... mechanisms for encouraging transition range from withdrawal of state funding [in Australia] to financial compensations to sheltered employers. Some countries are beginning to facilitate support services to help effect such a move. The action plan in Spain sees a new role for sheltered employment in training and in promoting transition ... (1997: 311)

thus illustrating that there are still stages required in this transition into potential employment.

Steele (1996a, 1996b) has made extensive studies of supported employment and has concluded that there are certain barriers which arise. One is the dilemma of the benefit system. She quotes the words of a manager of a successful recruiting agency in the North West who says:

> Our agency is high profile, serving learning disabled people with high support needs. They are referred to us by social services. Many do get part-time jobs and do very well. The feedback from employers is almost always positive. Our staff are highly skilled, hard working and fully committed to the inclusion of these people who are, quite frankly, very difficult to serve. I should be able to say we are doing fine but we can only be as successful as the system allows us to be. All of the people we have found jobs for are working part-time in the 'therapeutic earnings' category because they live in residential group homes. They are not free to work because if they earn over £15 a week they lose the funding for their accommodation. Some of the obstacles that appear to be so overpowering are problems we created ourselves. I don't know how we are going to undo the damage but we cannot continue to pretend that these are real jobs. We've got to tell the truth about the situation we find ourselves in or somebody will tell it for us. If that happens, supported employment will be finished and all the good work wasted. (Quoted in Steele, 1996b: 16–18)

Steele sets this dilemma into the current context of the contract culture, in which she says that for people who are able to fast-track through the service, getting out to work with the minimum of support, there are many sources available to assist their passage. However, for those with high support needs, the assistance is fragmented and opportunities limited. She reflects that it takes creativity, skill and resilience on the part of staff and, in the worst scenario, the jobs are not real and the staff burn out quicker.

If we are to consider young people in their transition to adulthood as truly empowered, we need to listen to their views on supported employment. Recent research has indicated that people with learning difficulties like to work in integrated community settings where they can meet new people and keep active (Di-Terlizzi, 1997). Yet, cuts in funding are preventing the continuation of vital support structures like the Pathway service, which supports people with learning difficulties into work. North East Lincolnshire Social Services, for example, have cut the £30 000 funding for the Mencap service in the area. This meant the loss of a Pathway Officer to support the 35 people with learning difficulties in jobs and the 33 clients preparing for work.

Some of the difficulties in making the move into employment are illustrated in the example of Emma McAuley, a young woman with Down's syndrome. Getting her working meant:

> . . . abolish the 'Sixteen Hours Rule' which prevents people getting Incapacity Benefit from working for more than 16 hours; allow someone to try working without jeopardizing their benefits, e.g. allow someone to pick up their claim if work does not suit; restore the original value of the Income Support Disregard which has been frozen at £15 for several years; ease local authority treatment of earnings in assessing liability to pay for support, more employment advisers such as Pathway officers so that employers and workers get the support they need. (*Viewpoint*, 1997: 9)

This comes at a time when the potential of people with learning difficulties like Down's syndrome is just being fully understood and when the individuals themselves are speaking up for their civil rights.

Life skills and quality of life

Anya Souza, a young woman with Down's syndrome, reflected upon her transition phases in a most powerful way. After much struggle to move into further education from school, she says:

> I was accepted onto a course training me up in office work. I was interviewed for the course and got in on my abilities. They looked upon me as a person and saw my value and potential, just like the eleven others who were taken on. Their confidence in me was not misplaced because I passed the course and became proficient in typing, duplicating, filing, phone skills and so forth. (1997: 9)

This indicates that people with learning difficulties like Down's syndrome vary considerably in their capabilities and it is important to take each person as a unique individual and to assess them without prejudice or stereotyping.

Anya went on to take a City and Guilds course in the Catering and Food Industry at a well-known college in London and enjoyed all aspects of it but, after the two years of the course, she was disappointed in the response of the careers adviser when she visited the group. It was to rebuff her enthusiasm for seeking a job in France. Anya reflects that '. . . her immediate response was: "No, there isn't a chance of that", made in a very rude manner followed by her walking away from me', and she goes on to reflect: 'This careers officer seemed to react to me on the basis of her prejudice. She did not see the qualified cook, like the other students, but a person with Down's Syndrome'. (1997: 10). Anya's testimony offers a challenge to professionals who so easily fall into the pattern of observing the category before we get to know the personality and the potential.

Sometimes it is most helpful for us, as health and education professionals who support people with learning difficulties in community living, to look and to learn from other countries. In Sweden, for example, the culture of normalization has firmly established an ethos in which people with learning difficulties are seen to have a community role. Gustavsonn (1998) refers to 'the integration generation' in Sweden as those adults with learning difficulties who have grown up to expect they have a *right to services* and not just to have *a need for services*. This includes support into employment and help in keeping the job. In Gustavsonn's research, he found that one of the men with learning difficulties, when told by his employer that he was cleaning the tables in the cafe too slowly, said to him that he had to expect this as he had learning difficulties. The notion of a 'right to services' includes the assumption that employers will make allowances and recognize differences without negative stereotyping. In this scenario, the health and education professionals offer practical support to ensure that the required skills are developed, while acknowledging that pace and accuracy will reflect levels of capability and concentration. If there is an attitude of 'rights' rather than 'needs', the difficulties experienced by individuals can be honestly addressed without diminishing their status as valued citizens. For therapists who work with young adults with learning difficulties in the community, a focus on their 'can do' skills is essential.

In his recent report on qualifications for 16 to 19 year olds, Dearing (1996) suggested that appropriate training for young people with learning difficulties was related to home management, learning to use recreational facilities and to budget carefully. It is interesting to speculate as to whether this helps them to fit into the role of active citizenship or to manage their time effectively without paid employment. Where there is no longer stigma attached to young people in general being unemployed, it is a fair assumption that this can include young people with learning difficulties. I would suggest that if they are alone in addressing daily living tasks as their main training goal, this seems to be oppressive to them as citizens with choices (Corbett, 1998). There is a real role for the therapist in supporting their choices of daily occupation, however unorthodox these may appear to be.

Conclusion

In this chapter I have examined the phases of transition from school to college and from college to supported employment and employment opportunities. Inevitably, this includes addressing the barriers at every stage of progression. It is easy to become pessimistic at a time of funding cuts in further education and cut-backs in supported employment. However, it seems important to me that we acknowledge the remarkable progress we have made in recognizing the potential in people with learning difficulties and in encouraging their active social participation through further education and employment.

For therapists, there is a role to support empowerment by recognizing individual choices and devising practical strategies for progression. The balance is between setting high expectations and in aiming for realistic stages of attainment.

References

Corbett, J. (1987) Integration in further education. *PhD thesis*, Open University, Milton Keynes

Corbett, J. (1998) *Special Educational Needs in the Twentieth Century: A Cultural Analysis*, Cassell, London

Corbett, J. and Barton, L. (1992) *A Struggle for Choice: Students with Special Needs in Transition to Adulthood*, Routledge, London

Di-Terlizzi, M. (1997) Talking about work: I used to talk about nothing else, I was excited and it got a bit too much for my parents. *Disability and Society*, **12**(4), 501–511

Dumbleton, P. (1993) Learning support in further education: putting policy into practice. In Lloyd, G. and Watson, J. (eds), *Meeting Special Educational Needs: A Scottish Perspective*, Moray House Publications, Edinburgh

FEFC (1996) *Inclusive Learning*, Further Education Funding Council, Coventry

Gustavsonn, A. (1998) The politics of defining difference: Swedish experiences. Paper presented at '*Policy, Failure and Difference*' Seminar, University of Sheffield, 13th–15th February

Hayhoe, H. (1998) Peer integration in a Further Education College: evaluating the outcomes for mainstream students and their peers with severe learning difficulties. *PhD thesis*, Institute of Education, University of London

Hatton, S. (1997) Responding to Tomlinson: the realisation of a vision. *Skill Journal*, **58**, 22–23

Hewitson, C. (1996) Team talk: creating curriculum materials on tape for students with learning difficulties. *Skill Journal*, **54**, 22–24

Kirkpatrick, K. and Earwaker, S. (1997) Advocacy, empowerment and participation: turning words into actions. *Community Living*, **10**(4), 20–21

McGinty, J. and Fish, J. (1992) *Learning Support for Young People in Transition*, Open University Press, Buckingham

National Committee of Inquiry into Higher Education (NCIHE) (1997) *Higher Education in the Learning Society*, The Dearing Report, HMSO, London

Silver, R. (1997) Inclusive learning: the college principal's perspective. *Skill Journal*, **57**, 32–34

Souza, A. (1997) Everything you ever wanted to know about Down's syndrome but never bothered to ask. In Ramcharan, P. *et al.* (eds), *Empowerment in Everyday Life: Learning Disabilities*, Jessica Kingsley, London

Steele, D. (1996a) Supported employment: we have all the ingredients . . . so let's bake the cake! *Community Living*, **9**(3), 26–27

Steele, D. (1996b) Supported employment: is the honeymoon over? *Community Living*, **10**(2), 16–18

Thornton, P. and Lunt, N. (1997) *Employment Policies for Disabled People in 18 Countries: A Review*, Social Policy Research Unit, University of York

Viewpoint (1997) Editorial. July, 2–3, Mencap, London

14 Community and people with learning difficulties

Jan Walmsley

Introduction

The word 'community' has been and remains of considerable significance for people with learning difficulties. It carries with it symbolic statements about inclusion or exclusion. Indeed, one political theorist has defined citizenship as 'membership of the community' (Norman, 1992: 35). If we accept this definition, then when people with learning difficulties are included in 'the community', they can be regarded as citizens. If excluded, as they so often have been, then they are equally excluded from citizenship. Viewed in this light, debates about including people with learning difficulties in the community through policies such as community care acquire an importance beyond practical measures and resource constraints.

This chapter explores the significance of the idea of community for people with learning difficulties from two perspectives, one historical, the other practical:

- how the history of people with learning difficulties can be read in terms of exclusion from community;
- how health care and other professionals can contribute to making community inclusion a reality for people with learning difficulties.

The significance of the idea of community for people with learning difficulties

Community has been a significant concept in policy and practice relating to people with learning difficulties, because the history of this group can be seen in terms of their exclusion from the sorts of community taken for granted by most people. For this reason, an exploration of the significance of community can provide a fruitful perspective.

The most obvious connection between people with learning difficulties and community can be seen in ideas about community care. Bayley (1973) saw community care as having two main strands: care by the community – meaning family and family networks – and care in the community – meaning state and/or voluntary sector provision. On the one hand, 'community care' can be seen as a shorthand description for care by the community or care in families; on the other hand, community care is a policy associated with de-institutionalization, a policy concerned with relocation in spatial terms from one type of residential care to another. The philosophy of the White Paper Caring for People, precursor to the NHS and Community Care Act 1990, developed the meaning of community care as

> ... providing the right level of intervention to enable people to achieve the maximum control and independence over their own lives so that they are able to live as independently as possible in their own homes or in 'homely' settings in the community. (Department of Health, 1989:2)

Whatever the reality on the ground, it is important to recognize that this conception of community care is a firm statement that it is more than family care or state-provided care. It represents an aspiration that people who are not able to function without support from others should still be individuals in their own right. This, as I demonstrate below, is a significant development of the concept of community care.

Community care, as a modern policy phenomenon, emerged for people with learning difficulties as a reaction to institutional care, the dominant policy of the early and mid twentieth century. But it is helpful, when considering the role 'community' has played, to delve a little further back into the past to discover what the reality was prior to the era of institutionalization.

The continuing role of the family

One of the most enduring characteristics of policy relating to people with learning difficulties is the continuing role of the family. It is easy to see the history of people with learning difficulties as the history of those obvious monuments, the hospitals and hostels, built to house large numbers economically and, at least in theory, safely. Yet this is only the visible tip of the iceberg. Deep down, under the surface, is the other meaning of 'community', care by the community, or, as Finch and Groves (1983) persuasively argue, care by the family.

Little is known of life for people with learning difficulties before the twentieth century. Recent scholarship points to a significant degree of continuity in the apparent ups and downs of policy changes – the actual or residual expectation that ultimately it is the responsibility of the family to supply care. Peter Rushton (1996), who studied provision for people with learning difficulties in the eighteenth century in England, coined the memorable phrase 'buried in the family' to describe the situation. When emergencies arose, and families looked outside for help, there was, according to Jonathan Andrews, a fairly sophisticated set of responses open to the authorities, including, in Scotland at least, 'boarding out' in households. But parish assistance was strictly time limited, for example 'often comprising arrangements to see mentally disabled children through infancy' (1996: 67). Andrews observes: 'In the majority of cases, and in a notably larger proportion than others identified as "lunatic", the family was relied upon to provide.' (1996: 74). He illustrates his argument with examples: 'Commonly, parochial aid was sought and granted following the death or illness of a family member. Parochial provision for Harry Southern, the "fool" of Coleman Street, for instance, commenced only after the death of his elderly father.' (1996: 79).

These extracts from Andrews's work have been included here because they indicate the remarkable continuity in basic assumptions about families carrying the ultimate responsibility of care for people with learning difficulties, a tradition discernible as threaded through the history of provision. For example, until the NHS took over the management of mental deficiency hospitals in 1948, families were means tested for their ability to contribute to the costs of keeping their relatives with learning difficulties in an institution, and much energy was expended in chasing up arrears (Walmsley, 1995).

In terms of community membership, then, people with learning difficulties were seen, if considered at all, as adjuncts to their families, not as individuals in their own right.

The emergence of institutional care

The big push for institutional care for people with learning difficulties came at the beginning of the twentieth century. This is not to say that people with learning difficulties had not been put into institutions prior to this, but the early twentieth century campaigns were characterized by two main arguments: first, that all people with learning difficulties would benefit from institutional care; and second, that they should be put into specialist facilities. People with learning difficulties, it was argued by those campaigning for a change in legislation, needed to be protected for their own good, from exploitation, neglect and abuse by the community. But, at the same time, the community was also believed to need protection from them. The two impulses, care and control, are neatly summed up in this scenario, painted by proponents of the Mental Deficiency Act, 1913, legislation which set up mental handicap colonies as the 'solution' to the contemporary problems of mental deficiency:

> HR, a little feeble minded girl. Turned into the streets by her father. Found by the School Attendance Officer and placed in safe keeping. Was actually starving and filthy – verminous. Horribly disfigured by burns. Her feeble minded brother, an adult, had put her on the fire and kept her there. (Quoted in Jones, 1972: 196–197)

In the quotation, the girl (portrayed as an innocent) has been neglected by her father, who turned her onto the streets to starve, and victimized by her 'feeble minded brother' who put her on the fire. The messages are that she needs protection by the authorities, but that the brother, also 'feeble-minded', may also need control because he has violent tendencies. Whichever way you look at it, the message is that the community is not the place for either victim, or victimizer.

The history of learning disability in the twentieth century has been dominated by the institutions set up under the Mental Deficiency Act 1913, which was enacted subsequent to the campaign of which the above quotation was a part. The solution to the perceived problem of mental deficiency was segregation from the community. Local Authorities were put in charge of seeking out, certifying and providing for 'mental defectives', preferably in institutions, subsequently termed 'colonies'. The regimes in such places are now well documented in publications such as Ryan and Thomas's *Politics of Mental Handicap* (1990), Potts and Fido's *A Fit Person to be Removed* (1991) and Atkinson's *Past Times* (1993). The emphasis was on containment, punishment, and 'care' of the most basic nature. Mixing of the sexes was forbidden, visitors were strictly controlled and visiting times limited to once a month, time on leave with families was granted not as a right but as a privilege, and leaving was at the discretion of the authorities. It is this history of segregation which makes the idea of community membership such a powerful one, as a contrast to the punitive, soulless and often abusive care characteristic of institutions.

The development of community provision

The institution casts a huge shadow over the history of the lives of people with learning difficulties in the twentieth century. However, it is probable that the majority did not live in institutional care, or spent only part of their lives in public care facilities. They remained, like their eighteenth century predecessors whose lives were researched by Jonathan Andrews, cited above, buried in the family, considered by those who researched their situation as 'burdens' (Voysey, 1975). The emergence of 'care in the community' can be seen in part as a move to relieve that burden.

Initially, however, the growth of community facilities was prompted principally by a realization that the colony solution to mental deficiency was ultimately too expensive. As early as the 1920s local authorities were being urged to set up arrangements for people with learning difficulties to be supervised in their own homes, to appoint Mental Deficiency Officers to oversee such arrangements, to open Occupation Centres, to build hostels. Although few Local Authorities showed much energy in complying with these exhortations before World War II (Jones, 1972), the attraction of doing so was soon proved. Cecil French, writing about Bedfordshire, described how those families whose children were admitted to the county's first Occupation Centre, set up in a converted egg-packing factory for 16 children in 1946, rapidly removed their children's names from the waiting list for hospital care (French, 1971).

As hospital places were at a premium, such investments in community services which enabled families to care for longer were very attractive and cost effective. The growth of the parents' movement through the spread of branches of the National Association for the Parents of Backward Children (later to become Mencap) in the decade 1945–55 was an additional spur to the type of services known as community care, and 'the family' came to be seen as the ideal environment for the person with learning difficulties. As a fairly recent text had it: The most positive environment for mentally handicapped people is to live in their parental home' (Hattersley *et al.*, 1987:99).

Thus, in the second half of the twentieth century, provision for people with learning difficulties outside of hospitals began to develop throughout the UK, motivated by the sheer impossibility of financing enough institutional places, and accompanied by an ideology which asserted that family care was best, and family care should be supported.

Human rights

However, there were impulses other than adminstrative convenience behind moves to community care. Human rights ideas began to permeate the debates on people with learning difficulties and community. It is a matter of shame that the colony solution to the 'problem' of intellectual impairment drew no discernible criticism on principle from its official inception in Britain in 1913 to the 1950s, a period of almost 40 years. The first major challenge was launched by the National Council for Civil Liberties (NCCL) in 1951. In a pamphlet entitled *50,000 Outside the Law*, the NCCL argued that segregation of people with mental handicaps constituted fundamental breaches of human rights:

> Not only is the mental defective under orders deprived of his liberty and of the opportunity of obtaining an education . . . but the standards of care, protection and health facilities often leave much to be desired. (Quoted in Stainton, 1994: 132)

Their final paragraph sums up their principles:

> The idiot, the imbecile, and feeble minded are an integral part of the human race; their existence constitutes an important demand on us. The extent to which we guard their right to the fullest and most useful life, the extent to which we guarantee to them the maximum freedom which they can enjoy and the extent to which we help their families to give them the love they need is a measure of the extent to which we ourselves are civilised. (NCCL, 1954, quoted in Stainton, 1994: 132)

The campaign by the NCCL demonstrates the implicit equation which has been fundamental to the meaning of community for people with learning difficulties – membership of the community is a prerequisite for the rights of people with learning difficulties to be regarded as fully human: exclusion is a denial of basic human rights.

It could be said that the NCCL's campaign set in train the current philosophy of community care. It was a precursor to the 1954 Royal Commission which investigated provision for people 'who are, or are alleged to be, suffering from mental illness or defect' (quoted in Jones, 1972: 304), which resulted in the Mental Health Act 1959 which sought 'the re-orientation of the mental health services away from institutional care towards care in the community' (Jones, 1972: 307). The impetus for de-institutionalization was maintained by the publication of research studies revealing the limitations of institutional care (Goffman, 1961; Morris, 1969; Oswin, 1971) and subsequent well-publicized hospital scandals (Donges, 1982) which were precursors to the 1971 White Paper *Better Services for the Mentally Handicapped*, another legislative landmark in the slow progress towards reversing the institutional imperative. The modern shift towards community care was officially born, though its progress has been extraordinarily slow and patchy. The 1959 Act and the 1971 White Paper may have instituted the modern rhetoric of community, but it is now over a quarter of a century since the publication of the latter, and approximately 15 000 people still live in mental handicap hospitals (Ward, 1995: 4). Old practices live on well into the 1990s. In 1992 I met 'Bert' who had been put into a mental handicap hospital in the 1960s, following a minor criminal offence; 30 years later he was still there, shut away, and with no definite prospect of release. 'Mike' had been admitted six months earlier, following a violent outburst in his hostel after hearing of the death of his father. He, too, had no idea of how long he was to stay.

However, for the majority of people with learning difficulties things have changed. Government decisions to close the large institutions was only a first step. There followed a period where community care meant relocation of residential provision, the building of hostels often on the outskirts of towns, or in new housing estates. Once it was accepted, however reluctantly in some quarters, that the long-stay hospitals had had their day, the practical consequences of providing for people living in hostels or group homes fed the growth of other specialist services – adult training or social education centres, sheltered workshops, special schools – which, if they did nothing else, made people with learning difficulties slightly more visible in their communities, no longer totally buried either in the family or in institutions.

So, historically speaking, community has been seen for people with learning difficulties as: a place of danger, from which they need protection; somewhere, or some people who need protection from them; or it has been somewhere to be 'buried in the family'. As far as is known, however, the idea of people with learning difficulties finding a place of their own in communities is of relatively recent origin. For further information on historical aspects of learning difficulties the reader is referred to Chapters 2 and 3.

Normalization and *An Ordinary Life*

Accompanying the policy changes which favour community care over institutional provision have come visions of what life in the community might look like. 'Normalization' is the name given to a philosophy which has been deeply influential. Briefly summarized, it is seen as 'utilization of means which are as culturally normative as possible in order to establish and/or maintain personal behaviours which are as culturally normative as possible' (Wolfensberger, 1972: 28). Obviously, 'culturally normative' means and behaviours are highly unlikely to be found in specialized large-scale institutions where people with learning difficulties are housed *en masse*. Normalization requires that people are included in mainstream community life.

The ideas of normalization have been translated into a checklist – the Five Accomplishments (O'Brien and Lyle, 1987) which can be used as a yardstick to judge how far services enable people with learning difficulties to belong in communities. These are:

- physical presence
- choice
- contribution to the lives of others
- dignity
- relationship

Only the first of these is concerned with *where* people actually live. The other four are more to do with the quality of their lives.

Perhaps the most influential of the visions inspired by normalization principles in the UK is *An Ordinary Life* (King's Fund, 1980). This envisages

> . . . the opportunity to live in a small home, ideally with a companion or companions of one's choice, in an acceptable neighbourhood, with the support that is needed to lead an ordinary domestic life and make use of the facilities available nearby. (Ward, 1995: 5)

It is, indeed, a modest ambition, an image of the sort of cosy community life portrayed in idealistic studies of working class community life, such as Young and Willmott's Bethnal Green (1957), recreated in the late twentieth century in TV soap operas like 'East Enders'. Modest it may be, but it is an alternative conceptualization of the idea of community for people with learning difficulties to those which have prevailed through-out the twentieth century – segregation from the community, or membership through belonging to the family of origin. The commitment in the NHS and Community Care Act 1990 that services should enable people to live as independently as possible, is in line with the vision of *An Ordinary Life*. In principle, the building blocks are in place.

The first part of this chapter has explored the historical significance of the idea of community in considering the lives of people with learning difficulties. In it, I have suggested that belonging to an ordinary community has come to be seen as synonymous with full human status. Conversely, forcibly excluding people from their communities constitutes a denial of basic rights. That is not to say that choosing in a fully informed way not to belong to the mainstream community is reprehensible. For some people with learning difficulties it is a positive choice to remain in a hostel rather than move to more 'ordinary' living in a one-person flat, or to attend an adult training centre in preference to low-paid work or community leisure pursuits. Choice is, however, the key issue here. (For further information on normalization the reader is referred to Chapters 6, 8 and 10.)

Choice and Community Living

Choice is quite an abstract concept. What does it actually mean on a day-to-day level, and why is 'choice' associated with community living? To answer this question it is useful to examine what people with learning difficulties say about their lives. I have selected accounts by two people who have moved to become full community members: one, Jackie, from hospital and the other, Doretta, from her family home.

Jackie Heyworth recorded her thoughts on the contrasts between her life in her own flat with her husband, Billy, and her previous life in Prudhoe Hospital, Northumberland for *Know Me As I Am* (Atkinson and Williams, 1990), an edited anthology of contributions by people with learning difficulties. Here is how she described her present life in her own flat:

> I like to do my own housework. Sometimes Billy helps. I cook in my own slow cooker. I got it as a wedding present from staff at the hospital. . . . Cook mince and chicken. Do shopping on Thursday mornings. . . . I go in the car. Brenda takes us. She's a care worker. . . . I pay all my stamps: my light stamps, my gas stamps, my rent and my TV stamps, telephone stamps. (1990:108)

In another extract she recalls the past:

> The hospital was dreadful. My mam's got me in there. First I was in Ryton Hospital near Prudhoe. That's for the handicapped. I was nervous when I first been.
>
> Billy was on E villa and I was on B villa. . . . I didn't like it. There was fighting everywhere, them patients. They'd be doing arguing. A person would tell them off. I used to have to go outside until I calmed. I'd be sent outside. I'd have to calm myself. I got told off. (1990: 108)

Jackie's contrasting accounts highlight the differences between her life in the community and the institution she had left. Now she is married; then she and Billy lived on separate villas. Now she controls many aspects of her life; then she had no privacy and no autonomy. Now she is calm; then she was nervous. Her life in her own flat incorporates all the Five Accomplishments (O'Brien and Lyle, 1987).

Doretta Adolphine, contributing to the same anthology, describes her own move from her family home to her own home. Doretta uses a wheelchair and 'speaks' by means of a small word processor on its arm:

> My name is Doretta and I am 25 years old. Last year I decided that I wanted a home of my own so that I could have more freedom. My mother was quite ill when I made my decision so we could not really discuss what I wanted to do. Even now, I am not sure how she feels about it.
>
> I now do all my own shopping. . . . I can also go out if I want to, we have a nice pub nearby where I can take friends for a meal and a drink. . .
>
> I am very glad I decided to get my own flat. I control my own life and no one makes decisions for me. I am much happier now in my own home. (1990: 94)

Like Jackie, Doretta emphasizes control, autonomy, making her own choices about small and large aspects of life. Such testimonies give meaning to the ideological and theoretical battles that have been fought over the idea of community membership for people with learning difficulties.

For Jackie and Doretta, community living is more than merely moving house, from hospital or family home. It is about making choices, and having control over day-to-day activities. Not everyone has been so fortunate. In many cases, while the setting changed, the practices were all too familiar. The institution lives on in the community, dispersed, not dismantled (Collins, 1993). Sinson (1993) coined the term 'micro-institutionalization' to describe the transfer of institutional practices to homes in the 'community'. She draws attention to the impact of contracted services – catering, cleaning, laundry and the like – on the 'ordinary life' of group home residents. Health and Safety Regulations are cited as a reason to forbid the use of kitchen facilities by some group home residents. Private use of a telephone is unheard of, single bedrooms a privilege, not routine, and doors without locks are common. All too rarely in such establishments are residents enabled to take part in the life of the neighbourhood in anything but the most superficial way. People like Jackie and Doretta show that more is possible, even for people with relatively severe impairments.

Ordinary life: extraordinary needs

As more people with learning difficulties become members of ordinary communities as citizens or householders in their own right, questions arise as to how best to provide for them. The normalization and ordinary life principles discussed above strongly imply that people with learning difficulties should use the services that are used by 'ordinary' people. However, to lead an 'ordinary life' many people with learning difficulties require more than ordinary support. This applies to schooling, jobs, leisure pursuits, relationships, transport, budgeting, health care and frequently, basic domestic tasks such as cooking, cleaning and hygiene.

If we take health care as an example, the ideal is for everyone to use local primary health care facilities. There are, however, some alarming statistics emerging on the poor standards of care that people with learning difficulties receive in primary health care contexts. Christine Nightingale investigated cervical screening for women with learning difficulties in Norfolk in the early 1990s (Nightingale, 1997). Although the Health of the Nation targets explicitly apply to people with learning difficulties (Department of Health, 1995), she found that none of the 78 practices consulted had any strategy to make cervical screening available to women with learning difficulties specifically: almost all relied on letters to call people for screening, and appeared not to have considered the needs of non-readers; and very few had any systematic knowledge of women with learning disabilities on the practice lists. In addition, some health care practitioners expressed doubt about the usefulness of cervical screening for women with learning difficulties. One practice manager said: 'These people should be removed from our targets' (1997: 156), and several GPs seemed to believe that women with learning difficulties were not sexually active ('like nuns') and therefore were not susceptible to cervical cancer. The only professionals who emerged in this study as having any understanding of the circumstances of women with learning difficulties were learning disability nurses, suggesting that there is a continuing role for special expertise to build a bridge between generic services and people with learning difficulties.

In another research study, Lois Greenhalgh (1994) investigated health information for people with learning difficulties living independently in the community. She found that the women she interviewed had very poor levels of health information, and that 'traditional' modes of providing health information were inadequate to remedy this lack. The limitations of leaflets for people whose literacy skills are poor was a fairly obvious finding, but others were more surprising. For example, the use of video to provide health information seemed superficially attractive, but few of the group had ready access to individualized use of a video recorder. Videos were invariably in shared lounges; some women did not know how to work the controls, a problem exacerbated by poor sight; and there was no local facility for loan of suitable videotapes. Greenhalgh also found that verbal information from health professionals was risky. 'Shakira' had been told to avoid spicy foods. However, she did not know what this meant, and named chilli con carne as her favourite dish.

Relocation either from the family home or from large-scale institutions to homes in the community means that in theory people with learning difficulties should enjoy equal access to primary and secondary health care, and health information, but much of the research to date reveals huge gaps between theory and practice. To a certain extent, ideas about normalization can be blamed for this. There has been a tendency to interpret 'normalization' as *carte blanche* for doing little (Brown and Walmsley, 1997). A crude equation drawn to say 'we treat them as we would anyone else' is discernible in the responses, particularly of untrained care workers who are often the main day-to-day contact in community care services. Greenhalgh observed of the staff involved in the lives of the women she worked with:

> . . . it emerged that they were working to a model of normalization which prohibited them from taking any sort of pro-active role with clients. The philosophy was 'They are independent adults now. We can't interfere with what they do'. In other words, they admitted that if a client had a very obvious problem they might suggest a doctor's appointment, to which they would accompany the client if asked, but beyond that they did not feel they could go. This seemed to the researcher a very narrow interpretation of normalization, but one which was implicitly if not overtly, promoted by higher management. (1994: 77)

To some extent one can see that such a minimalist approach is a response to circumstances. Most of the women involved had only a couple of hours a week scheduled with the 'rehabs' as they were known. If any crisis arose, time had to be borrowed from other clients' timetables (1994: 76). For higher management the crude misinterpretation of normalization exhibited here is convenient in resource terms. It is also comprehensible in terms of a teamwork approach. The untrained 'rehabs' believed that the Community Learning Disability Teams were responsible for health, though members of the local CLDT saw their role as confined to quite specific interventions – behaviour modification programmes and the like. However one explains the absence of health monitoring from the working agendas of untrained staff, it is clear that unless staff who work on a day-to-day basis with people with learning difficulties see their role as monitoring basic health needs, large numbers of minor and not so minor ailments will go untreated.

Home at last

A detailed example shows that even for people with quite complex health and care needs, community living can be successful, but that the input of specialists is a necessary part of the service provision. Victoria Willson has tuberous sclerosis. Her medical condition is described thus:

> This has affected the development of her brain, so she has severe learning and physical disabilities, and her skin [is covered] with white skin patches on her trunk, arms and legs. From the age of 6 weeks she has had convulsions ranging from slight tremors to salaam seizures to total clonic fits. . . . At age eight she developed scoliosis of the spine and has had to wear a body brace for 23 hours. (Fitton *et al.*, 1995: 135)

Her story is told in a book entitled *Home at Last* co-written by her mother, Jean (Fitton *et al.*, 1995). Victoria was born in 1970. The first 21 years of her life were spent either at home, with her parents struggling to manage her condition, or in residential care, far away from her home in Islington. In residential care, Victoria's special needs were managed through what Jean calls 'over reliance on drugs' and she spent her days in front of a TV with 30 other residents (1995: 9). Her family fought for provision in her own home, near to them in Islington. The National Health Service and Community Care Act 1990 set up the legislative framework for a care package to be put together to enable Victoria to have her own home. In 1991, Victoria moved into her own place, with rotas of staff to support her and another woman, also with considerable support needs.

One area that has received a lot of attention is Victoria's health. The staff working in Victoria's home are not trained in health care, but her condition gives rise to many special considerations. As staff change frequently, Victoria's parents have worked with health professionals to put together a 'Care Book' covering different aspects of her care needs – unusual behaviour, toileting, use of a brace, wheelchair, splints and boots, exercise programmes devised in conjunction with chartered physio-therapists, skin care, management of fits, drugs and how to administer them, along with names and telephone numbers for key specialist personnel to consult as necessary. (The description of her medical condition above is extracted from the Care Book.) In this way, Victoria has been enabled to live in the community with a considerable degree of success, and without undue risk to herself. Jean Willson is adamant, though, that access to the whole range of paramedical support, including occupational therapists, physiotherapists, community nurses, continence service, dentistry and chiropody are vital to the success of this pioneering example of community living – not to mention a sympathetic GP who knows Victoria personally.

It has not been all plain sailing. High staff turnover and lack of attention to induction procedures have meant that at times staff are not told of the existence of the Care Book. The local council has been slow to respond to minor repairs until they become major problems. Nevertheless, the authors argue that the costs of this home are lower, and the quality of life immeasurably better than comparable institutional care:

> There can be no doubt that the quality of life for the women who have been involved in the project has improved overall. They have been treated more as individuals and given a higher status than they ever had in the various institutions in which they previously lived. . . . The fact that they are living in their own home and not a 'home' is of great importance. (1995: 77)

Victoria's situation shows that arguments over generic versus specialist services are to some extent misplaced. Victoria does use generic services, but those services have had to take on board her unique needs, and have had to be supplemented by specialist professional expertise. (For further information on the health care needs of people with learning difficulties the reader is referred to Chapters 7 and 21.)

Conclusion

This chapter has examined the concept of community in relation to people with learning difficulties. In it I have suggested that community is a key idea, associated with human rights for people with learning difficulties. Affording people with learning difficulties the opportunity of being members of the community in their own right, rather than being confined to their family of origin or an institution, is a development of very recent times. Facilitating full participation in community life, beyond mere physical location, is a challenge to all concerned, and it is easy to be overwhelmed by the difficulties. However, it is important to remember the fundamental importance of persevering against the odds, and keeping in mind what can be achieved. It is easy to equate 'community care' with resource shortages and systems constraints, but the ideas behind it are worth holding on to. The last word goes to Jenny Trim of Highbridge, Somerset, who reflects on life since she and her friend Margaret moved out of a hostel into their own flat:

> We feel proud of what we have achieved. That we could actually move out of a hostel and live in a flat by ourselves. We have been here for more than ten years now. We like being independent. We have our ups and downs but we manage all right. We would not wish to live anywhere else. (Atkinson and Williams, 1990: 181)

References

Andrews, J. (1996) identifying and providing for the mentally disabled in early modern London. In Wright, D. and Digby, A. (eds), *From Idiocy to Mental Deficiency: Historical Perspectives on People with Learning Disabilities*, Routledge, London

Atkinson, D. (1993) *Past times*, private publication, Open University, Milton Keynes

Atkinson, D. and Williams, F. (eds) (1990) *Know Me As I Am: An Anthology of Prose, Poetry and Art by People with Learning Difficulties*, Hodder and Stoughton, London

Bayley, M. (1973) *Mental Handicap and Community Care*, Routledge, London

Brown, H. and Walmsley, J. (1997) When 'ordinary' isn't enough: a review of the concept of normalisation. In Bornat, J. *et al.* (eds), *Community Care: A Reader*, 2nd edn, Macmillan, London

Collins, J. (1993) *The Resettlement Game*, Values Into Action, London

Department of Health (1989) *Caring for People*, HMSO, London

Department of Health (1995) *The Health of the Nation: A Strategy for People with Learning Disabilities*, HMSO, London

Donges, G. (1982) *Policy Making for the Mentally Handicapped*, Gower, Aldershot

Finch, M. and Groves, D. (1983) *A Labour of Love: Women, Work and Caring*, Routledge and Kegan Paul, London

Fitton, P., O'Brien, C. and Willson, J. (1995) *Home at Last*, Jessica Kingsley, London

French, C. (1971) *A History of the Development of the Mental Health Services in Bedfordshire*, Bedfordshire County Council Health Committee, Bedford

Goffman, I. (1961) *Asylums*, Penguin, Harmondsworth

Greenhalgh, L. (1994) *Well Aware: Improving Access to Health Information for People with Learning Difficulties*, Anglia and Oxford RHA

Hattersley, J., Hasking, G.P., Morron, D. and Myers, M. (1987) *People with Mental Handicaps: Perspectives on Intellectual Disability*, Faber and Faber, London

Jones, K. (1972) *A History of the Mental Health Services*, Routledge and Kegan Paul, London

King's Fund (1980) *An Ordinary Life*, King's Fund, London

Morris, P. (1969) *Put Away*, Routledge, London

Nightingale, C. (1997) Issues of access to health services for people with learning disabilities: a case study of cervical screening. *PhD thesis*, Anglia Polytechnic University

Norman, R. (1992) Citizenship, politics and autonomy. In Milligan, D. and Miller, W.W. (eds), *Liberalism, Citizenship and Autonomy*, Avebury, Aldershot

O'Brien, J. and Lyle, C. (1987) *Framework for Accomplishments: GA Workshop for People Developing Better Services*, Responsive Systems Associates, Decatur, Ga

Oswin, M. (1971) *The Empty Hours*, Penguin, Harmondsworth

Potts, M. and Fido, R. (1991) *A Fit Person to be Removed: Personal Accounts of Life in a Mental Deficiency Institution*, Northcote House, Plymouth

Rushton, P. (1996) idiocy, the family and the community in early modern north east England. In Wright, D. and Digby, A. (eds), *From Idiocy to Mental Deficiency: Historical Perspectives on People with Learning Disabilities*, Routledge, London

Ryan, J. and Thomas, F. (1990) *The Politics of Mental Handicap*, Free Association Books, London

Sinson, J. (1993) *Group Homes and Integration of Developmentally Disabled People*, Jessica Kingsley, London

Stainton, T. (1994) *Autonomy and Social Policy: Rights, Mental Handicap and Community Care*, Avebury, Aldershot

Voysey, M. (1975) *A Constant Burden*, Routledge and Kegan Paul, London

Walmsley, J. (1995) Gender, caring and learning disability. *PhD thesis*, Open University, Milton Keynes

Ward, L. (1995) equal citizens: current issues for people with learning difficulties and their allies. In Philpot, T. and Ward, L. (eds), *Values and Visions: Changing Ideas in Services for People with Learning Difficulties*, Butterworth-Heinemann, London

Wolfensberger, W. (1972) *The Principle of Normalisation in Human Services*, National Institute on Mental Retardation, Toronto

Young, M. and Willmott, P. (1957) *Family and Kinship in East London*, Penguin, Harmondsworth

15 Families: participation advocacy and partnership

John Swain and Carole Thirlaway

Introduction

Most people with learning difficulties live with their families and even for those who do not, members of their families can play an active role in their lives. Professional intervention in general, and therapy in particular, impacts on the individual as a member of a family and on other family members who care for and about, and are cared for by, people with learning difficulties. Furthermore, the impact of therapy can be mediated through the family as a whole. Thus the family context is an important starting point for therapists working with people with learning difficulties.

Statements about families, however, belie a much more complex and diverse picture, in so far as they have connotations of a person with learning difficulties living with two biological parents. Some variations from the stereotype of the nuclear family are commonly recognized, such as single biological parents living with their children, though it is perhaps less well known that only approximately one-third of such families involve unmarried mothers. Other variations include foster and adoptive families, and family units with partners of the same gender. The picture becomes even more complicated by the notion of extended families, including grandparents, aunts and uncles, and for many people with learning difficulties the notion of family includes people with whom they have no familial relationship, such as people living in a group home.

In more recent years, some presumptions about families with members with learning difficulties have been increasingly challenged. First and foremost is the denigrating and pathologizing of the parents of children with learning difficulties as 'unrealistic', 'guilt-ridden', 'denying', 'depressed', 'overprotective' and/or 'rejecting' (Dale, 1996). As Thomson states: 'There is now increasing emphasis on *coping processes and positive adaptation* rather than a continued search for signs of dysfunction' (1997: 22). Furthermore, the presumption that people with learning difficulties are solely the 'cared-for' by and within families of origin has been increasingly countered. People with learning difficulties can be in reciprocal caring relationships (Walmsley, 1993), and can and do form new families in which they are partners and parents (Booth and Booth, 1994).

In this chapter we hope to contribute to this challenging of presumptions by focusing our discussion on what Walmsley (1993), referring to relationships within families, calls interdependencies. We look first at the broader context, that is, the participation of families in society, particularly the barriers to participation. This provides a basis for our discussion of interdependencies, particularly in understanding potential for conflict and disequilibrium in families. Finally we turn to another form of interdependency, that is, between families and professionals, again exploring potential differences in views and priorities, and also the potential for partnership.

To help us we conducted a small-scale study involving interviews with seven parents of children who have both learning difficulties and physical impairments. The interviews were conducted by Carole Thirlaway, who is a deputy headteacher, and took the form of open-ended discussions around: the barriers/difficulties faced by people with learning difficulties, and their families, in accessing and fully participating in every aspect of daily life within our society; and the support provided within and for families in overcoming or coping with these barriers to access. This research built on our previous published studies, which we shall also draw on in this chapter. These studies involved interviews with parents, young people themselves and therapists, covering issues relating to family transitions and sexual identity and development (Swain and Thirlaway, 1994, 1996). We shall use quotations from the interviews to illustrate and illuminate our discussions.

Families participating in society

Traditional approaches to understanding the functioning (or more likely, perceived dysfunctioning) of families with members with learning difficulties is as a direct and inevitable consequence of learning difficulties, such as increased social isolation, perceived lower social acceptance of family, parents and siblings, and perceived lower life satisfaction (Barr, 1996). An alternative basis for understanding takes account of the 'whole family' within the wider social context. This is perhaps clearest in the substantial additional expenditure (clothes, travel, etc.) and reduced options for gaining income in employment (through mothers working, overtime, etc.) (Baldwin and Carlisle, 1994). Single parents and families from Black and ethnic minority communities can be particularly disadvantaged (Baxter *et al.*, 1990).

Barriers to participation has been a major theme in the research that we have undertaken. In the following four extracts, parents talk about access to leisure facilities, communication, travel and shops:

Would you believe Pleasure Beach at Blackpool? We went there, he wasn't allowed to go on anything. We found the Astral Ride, and a very nice lady, 'Yes of course he can go on, you can't'. Well how's he going to get up the stairs in a wheelchair? 'Oh if he can't go up he can't go on.' So we went right round Blackpool Pleasure Beach and he couldn't go on a single thing. They wouldn't even let me take him on the dodgems.

Well we talked about this in some depth and we both agree that we could fill a book on the barriers alone, but we consider the main barrier the barrier of communication. It often becomes a unique pattern of communication between the carer and those in daily contact with the person with learning difficulties. There is a pattern of communication, but sadly this pattern of communication is useless in society, in a lot of cases it doesn't extend further, so the contact with society for those with learning difficulties is very much restricted to those in regular contact.

Even the easy access busses, she's had an accident on them. She was thrown from one side to the other and she was in the wheelchair place. She was secure, it's just that he wouldn't stop his bus. She fell forward right on to the other side, on top of this old lady, and the old lady hurt her leg, and he still wouldn't stop his bus. So even though you have got a decent access bus, which are brilliant, there's still not care there. Know what I mean, and they are supposed to take extra care if they've got wheelchairs on. He just went flying round the corner that fast she went on to the other side of the bus. Her brakes was on and everything. She hurt her head. I had to get her to hospital and had her hip x-rayed.

Then I've got to find shops you can actually go into and within the W area I know of only two shops I can take the buggy in. The Hypermarket, the Co-op, is the only one I can do, but then the difficulty is the aisles. They put the displays in the middle of the aisles. I have to keep stopping and shifting the displays, then putting them back.

Another set of frequently mentioned barriers were social attitudes, as illustrated in different ways in the following three quotations, the first being from an interview with a group of parents:

We all have friends outside this group but you can't talk to any of them about your particular child's problem. I've lived in the village I live in for two years and there is very few people in the village even know I have a daughter, you know, because she is never out in the village life or whatever.

That what's wrong with society as a whole: they don't see the person.

And you do get verbal abuse, which is rather shocking. A lot of people have very very little contact with people with physical or learning difficulties. I think that is wrong. I think the normal curriculum should involve some integration with children with learning and physical difficulties, so that children in mainstream school grow up and they learn that these people are there and that they can be respected members of our society, with rights, and its going to have to start in mainstream school and there is a lot of work to do.

The wider social environment is no more evident than in the period and processes of transition to adulthood. Transition represents the interplay between, on the one hand, political social and economic change, and on the other hand, change for the individual. It is a process which is experienced differently depending on such factors as race, class and disability. Certainly, people with learning difficulties experience consider-able restrictions and barriers which limit and dis-able transition to adulthood (Riddell, 1998). The significance this has in families was summarized by a parent as follows:

> I think those things, the transitions, were mind-boggling . . . unlike my other daughter and other people's sons and daughters, you are full of hope and expectation, because usually they are going to fly the nest. They are going to go on to university, or they are going to get a job. They're going to leave home, and you've done a good job. Right. Your role is being affirmed for you. There they are. They are going, and I'm pleased to let them go. . . . We know there isn't going to be anything when she leaves school. There's nothing. There's a huge empty void, and that's terrifying. And living with that fear for a long time, a lot of parents, it traumatizes you. (Swain and Thirlaway, 1994: 162)

Advocating in families

We focus next on interdependence in relationships within the family, concentrating particularly on the potential for conflict and disequilibrium. However, as we have already begun to argue, the problems and stresses within families with members with learning difficulties need to be understood within a wider social context, as indeed do experiences of families generally. As Brotherson *et al.* (1988) point out, for instance, the transition into adulthood can be one of the most stressful life-cycle transitions for any family. It can be argued that families in which there is a member with learning difficulties struggle with the same issues as other families (Thomson, 1997), but have added stresses, particularly in the face of the barriers to participation and the inadequacies of support for families.

Furthermore, our research suggested that the relationships within families of people with learning difficulties should not be characterized as inherently stressful and problematic. One father, for instance, stressed that, '. . . we are essentially a happy family. . . .' A similar picture emerged in the Bristol Advocacy Project (Simons, 1992). Most of the people with learning difficulties interviewed had something positive to say about their family lives, for instance emphasizing contributions to the household: 'I help Mum. . . . I make coffee, and the beds, a bit of drying-up and washing up.'

We also found similar sources of possible tensions as in the Bristol Advocacy Project, that is, disagreements over options open to the person with learning difficulties, particularly in terms of personal relationships. As illustrated in the following quotations from interviews with three adolescents with learning difficulties, points of transitions are again significant.

> *Int.*   . . . so you'd like to get married . . .
> *Ann*   Yeh, but my mum wouldn't let me. . . . I told my mum I want to get married and she said I don't think so . . . .
> *Int.*   Would they let you have a flat of your own when you get older . . . .
> *Ann*   No, they don't want me to leave home at all. My dad goes away and that and my mum gets lonely, so I can never leave home.

Ben   It should go very well, I've got the feeling. . . . By 21 I might be moving out . . . independent living by myself . . . that's why I have to learn to budget my money, because if you don't budget your money you can't do it. . . . I got loads of friends that I go out nightclubbing with and that . . . I can't go out as much as I want.

Int.   In the future what type of things do you worry about, about becoming an adult?

Bill   Don't know, like . . . you don't get holidays do you . . .?

Int.   And what are you looking forward to?

Bill   Getting money.

Int.   Where might you be living?

Bill   In a flat, near my home, not far from my mum and dad.

Int.   What will mum and dad feel?

Bill   Glad . . . as soon as I get a girl and money.

In interviews about their feelings regarding their son or daughter developing, parents talked about possible conflicts from their viewpoint. These quotations also illustrate something of the diversity of parents views:

I suppose I'd have to meet that one if it came, but I can't really see that it would be appropriate or possible because of his profound handicap really. I don't . . . even as an advocate I don't think you could really advocate that it would be a) appropriate and b) possible because you'd be involving somebody else as well. I think in terms of his need for comfort, and cuddling and physical contact, I think that's very important, and I would always want it to be the case that he had that and had it appropriately I suppose.

I suppose really the idea of giving young people more choices in their lives, despite their handicap, is opening a can of worms really in terms of sexuality because I don't know how you act as an advocate for that. I don't know how, just how far you'd be able to go morally . . . .

My attitude is, if in the future Cath is aware of man-woman relationships and she is able to understand about sex as part of relationships then I would have no qualms about it at all. Obviously there would be a very high risk, I wouldn't want a pregnancy because Cath no matter how far she develops is never going to be capable of looking after a child on her own. And I don't think it is fair to let these young people go through a pregnancy and then withdraw that child.

It's a difficult question. I personally don't have problems with Susan having a sexual relationship. But if that's going to happen then we as parents have to make sure . . . and the only way you can do it, to be absolutely certain, is sterilization.

And actually recognizing her as a woman, and she has a woman's needs not a child's needs. And actually letting go. When she was 18 we said we're going to let go and we had a plan. But it's one thing to do it and another thing to cope with the feelings.

We have concentrated in our discussions so far on relationships between people with learning difficulties and their parents. Clearly relations between other members of the family are important, though once again these are best understood in the wider social context. For example, the mother (of two disabled children) who talked above of the problems of access in shops, went on to explain why she turned to her father for support:

> I mean just to get about it is actually easier to get them looked after. I mean I drive down and get granddad, it takes five minutes, bring him back, go do the shopping and then take him back. If I'm shopping with both children there it takes me four hours – a nightmare.

Few of the parents we have talked to, however, could rely on support from the extended family. The myth that Black and ethnic minority families can and wish to rely on extended families is used as a rationale for the lack of use of services by such families. The following extract from our research illustrates some of the diversity within extended families:

> There isn't the support from Paul's [her husband's] family at the moment. There's a complete breakdown of communications, mainly because of a lack of understanding and a lack of wanting to know. We got no support there, and when it was there it was more hindrance than anything else. They've never ever had him for an hour. So it is quite heavy on me and quite heavy on my mum and dad as well, because my mum works. They do the best they can. They come over in the morning. My dad's not getting any younger, and he's in ill health. He's a help, but you can't be very far away.

Families in partnership

In a written statement about his work with families, a physiotherapist told us:

> It should be that the relationship is a partnership in providing the wherewithal to overcome barriers. This means a long-term relationship needs to be developed and be adaptable to the changing needs of the client. A coordinated approach by all involved helps to reduce inconsistencies and engenders trust and understanding. Recognition of the needs of the carers as well as the client should be each professional's aim and a holistic approach to problems fosters trust.

He is expressing a widely-held concern to improve the effectiveness of professionals working together with families, to create a system in which there is openness, effective communication and negotiation about priorities for young people with learning difficulties and their families. However, as Jones points out: 'The rhetoric of parent – professional partnership is often based on shared stereotypes of what families should be like and how they relate to their children' (1998: 50).

Previous research has recognized major differences in the concerns and priorities of parents/carers and professionals (Brown, 1987). Our research suggested that professionals and parents identify different barriers to partnership. First we shall outline some of the concerns of professionals.

Some professionals recognize that services and the work of professionals can deny young people and their parents opportunities and circumstances in which they can have control over their own lives. The system itself creates dependency in that young people and their families are passed from the hands of one professional to another, pressurized by the demands of each professional discipline and have their 'needs' determined by others:

> I think they have very little say from the point of diagnosis to treatment, or anything. They are made very dependent on a variety of specialists for information and advice . . . and in fact so are the parents. They're forced into a position of dependence and, in fact, how do you expect a disabled child to be independent when even their parents aren't?

Such thinking underpins calls for improvements in multi-professional working and communication:

> I think the important thing is that we do establish with the other professionals a real understanding about what we are trying to achieve, an agreement and, as far as possible, a sharing of values between us as to what we are trying to achieve with these youngsters and their families.

From the viewpoint of professionals, it can seem that there are certain ways in which young people can be helped: regimes they should follow; treatments that are essential to their well-being; and risks from which they need to be sheltered. Non-cooperation or non-compliance is a major barrier to partnership:

> The greatest problem that I as a professional face is getting the families to verbalize their problems and a lack of realism about long-term care for their relatives. For example, a mother with a daughter who has severe physical and learning disabilities continually refused moving and handling aids until eventually she began to suffer from stress incontinence and severe back pain. There is still a lack of willingness to talk over long-term future care of her daughter.

> If they followed the regime like some of the other young people, they would be a lot more mobile and more well generally, because the implications of not doing some things affect not only the mobility but the actual kidney function, digestion and other things.

Another related barrier recognized by professionals is that parents do not understand the consequences of non-compliance:

> To say to the family, if you're not going to be able to cooperate with that [i.e. the advice of professionals] or don't feel that that's important, what do you feel is important? . . . Spell out to them the consequences of their choice, but put the decision with them, so there is discussion of what will happen if a particular line is not taken, deterioration of the condition.

It can also seem from the viewpoint of professionals that parents think they know best:

> Relationships between families and professionals in providing support
> for people with learning difficulties are fraught with danger. The families
> by necessity become 'experts' regarding their charges and are some-
> times loath to accept a differing professional viewpoint.

On the other hand, from the point of view of parents, it can seem that it
is the professionals who think they know best:

> But the biggest barrier and difficulty seems to be the fact that the
> therapists say they know best. . . . You take a stop-watch and measure
> the time the speech and physio actually spends with each child each day
> when they're in. That's the biggest barrier, the fact that the therapists
> spend so little time with the kids and they're saying they know them
> better than anybody else. It's ridiculous.

Related to this view is that professionals do not listen to the views of
parents:

> Whenever we meet a new professional we feel that our views is often
> downgraded. We feel as if our social integrity is minimal. We learnt to
> start asking questions and you have got to put across your knowledge
> otherwise you tend to feel as if you are getting wiped aside. In other
> words you have got to accept what information you are being told
> without question. As you grow older with your children that holds some
> sort of a qualification that you should at least be listened to, and quite
> often they don't. Because we don't have letters after our name we get
> ignored.

> When Jan is about 5 or 6 I could well see her with a harness about her
> and I could well see that as a way of getting about. But they won't do it
> for safety reasons. My suggestions aren't taken into consideration at
> all.

The sense of frustration at not being listened to, and having to
repeatedly explain things, was a recurring theme in the interviews:

> I don't want support like that. I just want me and Gwen [her disabled
> daughter] to lead a normal life, not have everybody interfering all the
> time. You get sick. You have to go through everything with everybody.

As Barnes (1997) states, parents make frequent reference to the
significance of the detailed knowledge they have of their sons or
daughters and claim that their detailed knowledge is ignored. This
detailed knowledge, from the viewpoint of parents, provides them with
a better understanding of their child:

> I think parents think of it on a more individual basis and professionals
> tend to think of the subject and people fit into it. I think with individuals,
> with Julie, for example, she is sexually aware in certain areas, the
> problem is she can't express herself, her needs, and we're closer than
> professionals in trying to interpret what she is trying to tell us.

Another major barrier, as far as parents are concerned, is the lack of
services in the first instance, coupled with the need to repeatedly demand
services:

I've seen her once when she first started. That's a few years ago. That's when I mentioned about her brace and it marking her back, and she said she would get things sorted and I sent that many notes in. I thought this was getting dealt with. When you let too many months go by well you get back in touch and you say what's happening to her brace, are you getting something sorted, you know. They just don't get back to you. It's a losing battle. You just don't get any response from any of them, well not from her anyway, the one that started two years ago.

We have the biggest problem, and that is that we worked, I worked and Albert [her husband] worked, and because Albert is on a good wage now we have to go through the grant system to get anything, and we don't qualify for a grant. Because they always take account of your income . . . so it's your fault you know, if you've been a good husband and you've got yourself a better home or a better car, a better life style, and what they take into account is your ability to pay on your own – stair lift, alterations, guard rail and ramp – you have to pay. My children are actually discriminated against because we have worked so hard. We are being discriminated against. What we are having to do at the moment is bid and bid and bid.

Standard argument. . . . And parents are basically made to feel like selfish bastards for trying to get a decent service for their kids.

You see you get that used to it, you just get used to toddling along with what you've got. It doesn't occur to you to think that there's something more you could have, you know. You just cope with what you've got. I mean an electric wheelchair would be nice, but we know a family that's had a lot of bother getting one.

This theme of being listened to as a prerequisite for working in partnership with professionals can also be found in parents' descriptions of effective professionals:

The best support that I have had is Bea, the O.T. She come through for me with everything. Like she got me this house. I'd just come back from holiday when she came to me and said she's got me this bungalow. She's even had a letter typed up and taken to mobility stating about this vehicle and everything. She come through for us. She got that electric hoist. She got the changing bench made to go down on the bath, so I could just slide her (Cath) along. . . . She had a wooden pine bench made as well that sits on top of the bath, where I can just take her up out of the bath and slide her along and dry her in the same place.

But there is some of the professionals that we have, they are more friends than anything else. They are great with the children. We've seen both sides. We've seen professionals that push their point of view and are not prepared to listen to you at all, but we have also got some professionals that are very good.

Finally, the importance of being listened to is also apparent in parents' suggestions for improvements:

I think just somebody to talk to, a counsellor or somebody that's been trained to give you relevant advice for any problems that might crop up with different things – somebody who knows how to help you deal with the situation.

What would be best, is that parents of disabled children are consulted, say somebody whose child is still in nappies but in a wheelchair. They won't come out and consult us because basically what we would need for Simon is way over the top from what they want to provide.

Conclusion

The 'Negotiating Model' of partnership, as proposed by Dale, seems to recognize that dissent may be a major factor in the parent – professional relationship. She describes this model as follows:

... a working relationship where the partners use negotiation and joint decision-making and resolve differences of opinion and disagreement, in order to reach some kind of shared perspective or jointly agreed decision on issues of mutual concern. (1996: 14)

We would argue that partnership will remain at the level of rhetoric if parents are pathologized, no account is given to the wider social context, and parents' views are ignored. Furthermore, there are dangers in this notion of partnership. In their study of parents, Booth and Booth also found that services were, 'failing to involve parents in decisions affecting their lives or to respond to parents' concerns' (1994: 55), though in this study it was the parents who had learning difficulties. The crucial challenge to therapists in working with families of people with learning difficulties is building negotiated partnerships with parents of children with learning difficulties, but also, particularly through the period of transition to adulthood, building negotiated partnership with people with learning difficulties.

References

Baldwin, S. and Carlisle, J. (1994) *Social Support for Disabled Children and their Families: A Review of the Literature*, HMSO, Edinburgh

Barnes, M. (1997) Families and empowerment. In Ramcharan, P. *et al.* (eds), *Empowerment in Everyday Life: Learning Disability*, Jessica Kingsley, London

Barr, O. (1996) Developing services for people with learning difficulties which actively involve family members: a review of recent literature. *Health and Social Care in the Community*, **4**(2), 103–112

Baxter, C. (1995) Confronting colour blindness: developing better services for people with learning difficulties from Black and ethnic minority communities. In Philpot, T. and Ward, L. (eds), *Values and Visions: Changing Ideas in Services for People with Learning Difficulties*, Butterworth-Heinemann, Oxford

Booth, T. and Booth, W. (1994) *Parenting Under Pressure: Mothers and Fathers with Learning Difficulties*, Open University Press, Buckingham

Brotherson, M.J., Turnbull, A.P. and Bronicki, G.J. (1988) Transition into adulthood: parental planning for sons and daughters with disabilities. *Education and Training in Mental Retardation*, **23**(3), 165–174

Brown, H. (1987) Working with parents. In Craft, A. (ed), *Mental Handicap and Sexuality: Issues and Perspectives*, Costello, Tunbridge Wells

Dale, N. (1996) *Working with Families of Children with Special Needs: Partnership and Practice*, Routledge, London

Jones, C. (1998) Early intervention: the eternal triangle? Issues relating to parents, professionals and children. In Robinson, C. and Stalker, K. (eds), *Growing Up with Disability*, Jessica Kingsley, London

Riddell, S. (1998) The dynamic of transition to adulthood. In Robinson, C. and Stalker, K. (eds), *Growing Up with Disability*, Jessica Kingsley, London

Simons, K. (1992) *'Stick Up For Yourself': Self-advocacy and People with Learning Difficulties*, Joseph Rowntree Foundation, York

Swain, J. and Thirlaway, C. (1994) Families in transition. In French, S. (ed.), *On Equal Terms: Working with Disabled People*, Butterworth-Heinemann, Oxford

Swain, J. and Thirlaway, C. (1996) 'Just when we thought we had it sorted': parental views of sexuality and profound and multiple impairment. *British Journal of Learning Disabilities*, **24**(2), 58–64

Thomson, S. (1997) Family aspects. In O'Hara, J. and Sperlinger, A. (eds), *Adults with Learning Difficulties: A Practical Approach for Health Professionals*, John Wiley, Chichester

Walmsley, J. (1993) Contradictions in caring: reciprocity and interdependence. *Disability, Handicap and Society*, **8**(2), 129–141

16

How can therapists help to promote the sexual well-being of adults with learning difficulties? A risk management dilemma

Bob Heyman and Elizabeth C. Handyside

Introduction

Therapists are practical folk. Faced with human or health needs, their inclination and training incline them to seek out interventions which will 'work' with a defined problem. Because sexuality relates to so many other aspects of human life, therapists contemplating their potential sphere of operation in relation to people with learning difficulties are faced with an awesome range of issues, including: sexual behaviour, pleasure and display rules; biological knowledge; communication and interpersonal relationships; self-assertion; prevention of abuse; fertility management; sexual variation and morality; sexual health; marriage, independent living and parenthood.

Therapists may relate to clients in various modes: as facilitators of self-expression, e.g. through interactive drama; as advocates, counsellors or self-help facilitators; as educators or trainers; and as direct providers of support or referral to other zones of the health/voluntary/social services jungle. The 'targets' for all this activity may include people with learning difficulties, a heterogeneous category, family carers and other professionals. Therapists, thus, find themselves facing a three-dimensional typology of needs, modes of operation and target groups.

The present chapter will not seek to survey this huge field, and the reader is referred to the extant literature (Dixon, 1986, 1998; Craft, 1987a, 1987b; Fraser, 1988; Craft, 1994). Instead, it will focus on a sometimes neglected strategic question: namely, what are all these interventions for? This question will be considered in relation to research which has investigated the views of people with learning difficulties, and carers.

We will draw both upon published studies and our own research (Heyman and Huckle, 1995; Heyman *et al.*, 1997; Handyside and Heyman, 1997). These three studies were all based on detailed qualitative interviews with people with learning difficulties and their families and paid carers. The first two studies focused on the perspectives of people with learning difficulties about their own lives, with themes involving sexuality explored as they emerged. The third, hitherto unpublished, study was designed specifically to explore the sexual attitudes, knowledge, behaviour and relationships of 14 people with learning difficulties. In total, 52 case studies have been carried out with adults with learning difficulties, mostly aged 20–40 years. Family carers, parents in all but one case, were interviewed separately wherever possible and appropriate. A focus group was held with four parents at the end of the third study to obtain feedback on the research conclusions. Professional carers providing day services have also been interviewed.

Research into the sexuality of people with learning difficulties requires careful management of a number of difficult ethical issues: obtaining genuinely informed consent; avoiding harm to informants; confidentiality; responding to abuse, if identified; and managing relationships with carers. Space limitations prevent a detailed analysis of these issues, which have been more fully discussed elsewhere (Swain *et al.*, 1998).

A decade ago, Heshusius (1987) criticized the dearth of studies considering sexuality from the perspectives of people with learning difficulties, and offered two explanations for this lacuna. First, stigmatization has generated the implicit assumption that such individuals cannot speak for themselves. Secondly, the prevailing positivist methodology treated research participants as 'subjects' whose behaviour could be measured and manipulated, rather than as informants whose views could be articulated. Although supporting methodological pluralism, we share Heshusius's strong preference for qualitative over quantitative methods in this field, given the difficulty inherent in exploring a taboo topic with individuals who may have communication problems over and above those of other groups.

Since sexuality cannot be defined in a social vacuum, our analysis of the need for interventions in the sexual sphere will be preceded by a brief exploration of the wider cultural context. We will then present a typology which highlights differences in the sexual attitudes of people with learning difficulties, and locates them in their micro-social context. This material provides the groundwork for our central thesis: that differences in attitudes towards the sexuality of people with learning difficulties can best be understood as arising from responses to the risk management dilemma of balancing safety against autonomy.

The cultural context for the sexuality of people with learning difficulties

All cultures attempt to regulate sexuality. In multicultural, rapidly changing, modern societies therapists and other professionals must cope with cultural, subcultural, familial and personal variability. Policies which work against the grain of deeply-held convictions will simply be rejected. In the mainstream, secular culture, a set of sexual beliefs and practices can be identified which is characterized by confusion, contradiction and gaps between expressed attitudes and behaviour with respect to: nudity; commercialized sex; sexual display rules; marriage; fidelity; homosexuality; abortion; and disease prevention.

One reason why some may prefer the term 'learning difficulties' over 'learning disabilities' is the former term's neutrality about the source of problems. A learning difficulty may arise out of various combinations of disability and poor learning opportunities. Cultural uncertainty almost guarantees that slow learners will become muddled, as illustrated in the following quotation:

> Peter grew up with us just wandering around, and he got used to what women look like, and what men look like, not in a furtive way, but in an open way. And we perhaps pay the price now that Peter does not know that you reach an age where discretion. . . . He cannot understand, now, why you say, 'You mustn't, now you are a man you don't walk round naked in front of people'. (Father, parental group discussion)

Americanized, mass media-dominated cultures associate sexuality with physical attractiveness. People with learning difficulties, along with most of the population, don't necessarily display this characteristic, and the association of disability and sexuality arouses additional ambivalence. Adults with learning difficulties may be seen as 'really' children, despite their physical maturity:

> I think they would have the sexual feeling, but, to my mind, they would not have the capability of the love. They could have it physically without any sort of emotion. I think it would be best if they weren't encouraged at all. (Mother, parental group discussion)

The danger of slipping into simplistic and punitive thinking about 'normality' (Chappell, 1992) may be reduced if the sexuality of adults with learning difficulties is considered in terms of citizens' rights rather than normalization. Craft (1987) proposes that adults with learning difficulties have six main rights relevant to their sexual being: to be treated with the respect and dignity accorded to adults; to have access to as much information about sexuality, social behaviour and interpersonal relationships as they can handle; to be sexual, and to make and break relationships; not to be dependent on the sexual attitudes of individual care-givers; not to be sexually abused; and to live in humane and dignified environments.

A commitment to citizens' rights provides an appropriate ethical starting point for professional intervention, but certain caveats must be noted. First, policy statements endorsing human rights should not be confused with their achievement in practice. Secondly, the right of people with learning difficulties to choose *not* to be sexually active must be acknowledged. Thirdly, rights should be considered to provide powerful but not absolute grounds for entitlement, which must be balanced against the welfare and safety of the person and others.

Considerable debate has taken place about managing the competing principles of beneficence and autonomy, and defining the circumstances in which a carer may ethically override the wishes of a dependent person for his or her own good, or to protect the legitimate rights of others (Veatch and Fry, 1987; Beauchamp and Childress, 1994; Cook and Procter, 1998). Many, but not all, parents of an adult with learning difficulties believe that she or he cannot safely exercise sexual rights. Because the social label 'learning difficulties' covers a wide variety of phenomena, judgements can only be made in particular cases. Therapists need to understand the perspectives of both individuals with learning difficulties and their family carers.

A typology of sexual attitude

Sexual attitude encompasses a range of issues, e.g. relationships, behaviour, contraception, health. Individuals can only be located on a single dimension of conservatism/liberalism (Brantlinger, 1983) at the price of considerable simplification. We have found it useful to loosely categorize respondents' attitudes as positive, negative and uncertain, but only as a means of exploring the views of specific persons.

Positive attitudes were mostly expressed by adults in our sample who were involved in a relationship, and were associated with feelings of love:

Interviewer What do you think of when I say the word sex?

Dean Just nice, nice loving feeling, you know, I mean if anybody wants sex, done in a nice way to love people . . ., not just, like, going out and raping.

Such favourable attitudes were often hedged with caveats, for example that sexual intercourse should only take place in marriage, or should be linked to procreation:

Interviewer You were saying that sex is a good thing if you want to have children. Might you have sex for any other reason?

Lynn If you were married you may do, but not if you're not.

However, in the sexual sphere, variability rules. One respondent (Heyman and Huckle, 1995) described having sexual intercourse, without contraception, on the lawn outside his adult training centre, and reported enjoying the experience, which he wanted to repeat.

In contrast, those who expressed negative attitudes globally rejected sex as 'bad', 'rude' or 'dirty':

Interviewer OK, so are there any good things about sex?

Edward I don't think so.

Interviewer What are the bad things about sex?

Edward Well, it's just a very, very bad thing.

About 40 per cent of the 52 adults with learning difficulties whom we interviewed expressed negative attitudes to becoming sexually active, while Heshusius (1987) concluded from an analysis of a number of qualitative American studies that about a third of the sample thought in this way. This evidence suggests that, in the UK and USA at least, a much larger proportion of people with learning difficulties reject sexuality altogether than might be expected in the general population. This rejection can be linked to parental attitudes. In our first study (Heyman and

Huckle, 1995), 16 out of 20 parents indicated that their adult son or daughter was not interested in, or could not handle, sexual relationships.

A typology of sexual attitudes can be elaborated in a way which provides a starting point for appropriate therapy interventions if, in addition, the clients' sexual or potentially sexual relationships and the attitudes of actively caring family members are taken into account, as shown in Table 16.1. This typology reflects our own experience of common patterns in 52 detailed case studies. The important issue of prevention of sexual abuse has been excluded from the table since it is considered in Chapter 22d. The interventions should be considered as services which can be offered, rather than as provision which clients definitely need. Interventions should be carried down the table. For example, sex education will benefit many people in established relationships as well as those seeking to acquire a partner, but might be rejected by a client who views sex as 'dirty'.

The typology is designed to bring out some points about the varying appropriateness of services for clients with differing needs. Firstly, adults who clearly reject sexuality generally do not wish to receive further sex education. There may be some value in offering individuals means for self-exploration, for example through drama groups, but the right not to be sexually active must be respected.

Secondly, as in the rest of the population, some adults with learning difficulties would like to meet, but cannot find, a suitable partner. For them, sex education provides no more than theoretical knowledge, and intervention should, in addition, aim to facilitate relationship formation.

Table 16.1 A typology of client need in the sexual sphere

Ideal type	Possible intervention priorities
Incapable of informed consent	Culturally appropriate (private) masturbation, if desired by client
Rejects sexuality	Consciousness raising with clients and family carers, e.g. drama, parental discussion groups
Seeks relationship	Relationship promotion, e.g. through social events, dating agency. Opportunities for privacy. Communication and relationship skills enhancement. Sex education
Has relationship: Family carer opposition	Counselling. Self-assertion. Family carer discussion groups. Advocacy and self-help groups
Has relationship: Family carer support or independent	Practical interventions, e.g. in relation to contraception, sterilization, marriage, independent living, and parenting

The central life project of one young man whom we interviewed (Heyman *et al.*, 1997) was to acquire a girlfriend. His efforts were continually frustrated by limited communication skills and low self-esteem. Over-worked day centre carers treated his silences as evidence of learning disability rather than distress. A therapist could have helped him greatly to increase his confidence and skills.

Thirdly, clients involved in sexual or potentially sexual relationships often encounter family carer lack of recognition or opposition. An approach to sexual development based on citizens' rights would suggest that adults who are capable of informed consent should make their own decision, and that, therefore, therapists should be prepared to support their clients against family carers. Although this stance should not be ruled out, it will rarely work in practice because clients depend upon family carers who, in general, devote their lives to their relative's welfare. Negotiation provides the main way forward in these circumstances. Therapists need to be able to understand the perspectives of both adults with learning difficulties and their family carers.

Finally, variability in family carer attitudes should be expected. For example, one mother of two sisters with learning difficulties supported their sexual relationships, and enjoyed a friendly, equal relationship with them. The attitudes even of parental 'conservatives' are not necessarily fixed in stone. Many value opportunities to discuss sexual issues (Squire, 1989). Parents involved in our research indicated that they would welcome opportunities to participate in carers' groups.

The risk dilemma

Three explanations for the high prevalence of family carer 'conservatism' concerning the sexuality of people with learning difficulties can be put forward. First, it can be viewed as a symptom of parental reluctance about 'letting go' (Richardson, 1989). Secondly, it can be explained in terms of the history of failure and reduced expectation which family carers will often have experienced (Brown, 1987), as illustrated below:

> He was born, obviously, and then you suddenly realized that he's not meeting his milestones. . . . You go to your GPs, and they put you off, and say there's nothing the matter, you know, until it's all started to show itself really at what, twos and threes. . . . And then, well, obviously, he went to an ESN school. . . . He could have done better, but he didn't. He had an aggravated life. . . . If anything goes wrong, well it's Simon to blame. . . . So that was very difficult. (Simon's mother, individual interview)

Although parents may sometimes have difficulty 'letting go', or become fatalistic, they do not usually explain away their own caution in these ways. The carers whom we have interviewed invariably *regard themselves as therapists* attempting to act in the best interests of their relative. Just as professionals sometimes see themselves as thwarted by the 'attitudes' of family carers, so family carers may believe that their efforts on behalf of their relative are undermined by professionals:

> It [advocacy group] was dealing with citizens' rights and things of that nature, which, in principle, sounds great. But it is raising topics, again, in his mind, that would not have arisen in a natural way. This is something you have to safeguard against the so-called professional people. To some extent they are justifying their own existence, their jobs and such, in raising these matters. But it can create a lot of backlash in the family circle. (Father, parental group discussion)

Explaining away a professional's *or* family carer's attitude towards risk-taking *presupposes* the irrationality of the stance taken. For example, describing parents as 'overprotective' precludes detailed analysis of the risks they fear. Mutual understanding may be enhanced if the possibilities of sexual fulfilment for people with learning difficulties are understood to raise the risk dilemma of autonomy versus safety (Heyman and Huckle, 1993; Thorin *et al.*, 1996; Heyman *et al.*, 1998). In general, policies which enhance the autonomy of vulnerable people increase the probability that they will suffer adverse consequences. Although risk can be reduced, for example through training, monitoring and support, some trade-off between risk and autonomy cannot be avoided. No single correct solution can be found which optimizes both.

Those family carers who do not wish their relative to develop sexually, identify a host of associated dangers, for example that the person might be taken advantage of, or might abuse others; that he or she might be unable to cope with an intimate personal relationship, and might end up emotionally damaged; or that an unplanned child might be produced. Some family carer fears may seem trivial from a health perspective, but their seriousness must be understood in its cultural context:

> He still sometimes embarrasses us by coming out with things in conversation that we would not talk openly about. (Mother, parental group discussion)

These parents felt that they had done their best to teach their child display rules which he could not fully grasp, and that the danger of their son embarrassing others could be minimized if he was not introduced to sexual topics.

The following quotation illustrates parental concern about the longer-term risks associated with the development of sexual relationships:

> He had a heart operation or something, but he's been bad a few times. . . . I like them to be girl and boyfriend, but I wouldn't like it to be any more. . . . I know it might be selfish for me, but if they just stay the way they are for as long as they can, I'd be quite happy. It's too much to ask two people to be together when one's not well and the other would have to have the job of . . . You know, I'm always thinking ahead. . . . How would [daughter] nurse or look after somebody if it had to come to the crunch? (Mother, carer interviews)

This quotation illustrates two important general features of risk reasoning. First, complex human actions generate an indefinite number of potential consequences. The outcome of any risk analysis will depend upon which consequences are selected for consideration (Hansson, 1993) when individuals attempt to manage the future. Secondly, assessment of the direction of identified costs and benefits plays a crucial, but often implicit, role in risk appraisal (Heyman and Henriksen, 1998: 42–43). The above respondent, when she mentions being 'selfish' suggests a fear, commonly voiced by family carers, that they, not the couple or professionals, would be left to deal with any ensuing problems. Therapists may focus on the benefit for clients' life quality of them developing sexually. Family carer caution is often reinforced by doubt, based on experience, about the long-term reliability of service support.

Family carer opposition to the sexual progression of their relative was based on rational risk appraisal. However, this opposition regularly produced unintended consequences which they may not have fully appreciated. First, in order to avoid sexual dangers, some family carers restricted their relative's autonomy in other ways, for example restricting interpersonal privacy:

> *Interviewer* Has Cliff ever visited Veronica's [girlfriend's house]?
> *Cliff's mother* No. I wouldn't let him. I would be worried that something might develop. (Quoted in Heyman *et al.*, 1998: 207)

Some adults with learning difficulties are denied 'freedom of the locality' (Heyman *et al.*, 1998) so that sexual risks may be avoided:

> I am happier if she isn't [out on her own]. It is partly the roads, but it is also, partly, this business of, she would go with anybody, she would speak to anybody. She often speaks to people, and I have not got a clue who they are, but she has met them at some do or another. (Mother, group discussion)

Secondly, some family carers considered their relative to be asexual. Such beliefs may provide an apparent way out of the painful dilemma of autonomy versus safety, but at the potential price of denial of experience and restricted communication. One parent explained away incidents in which he had seen his son masturbate during puberty as 'a patch where he was physically aroused without really being aware'. The perspectives of a family carer and the person with learning difficulties can sometimes be directly contrasted:

> *Interviewer* Do you think he has sexual feelings towards [girlfriend]?
> *Mother* I don't know, because she will sit in one chair and he will sit in another, so it's not like they both sit together. And they go upstairs to listen to the radio, and then they are back down to watch the telly. He does not seem the romantic type. (Dean's mother)
> *Interviewer* So, how do you feel when you are on your own with [girlfriend]?
> *Dean* It's a nice feeling.
> *Interviewer* Can you tell me a bit more about that?
> *Dean* Well, when we're alone, sometimes feel things. I want to have a relationship . . . .
> *Interviewer* Do you mean a sexual relationship?
> *Dean* Yeh.

Family carers sometimes waited for the person with learning difficulties to raise sexual topics, and treated their absence as evidence of disinterest:

> In my experience there has never been a need expressed by Edward to know these things, so why then introduce him to it? (Father, group discussion)

Few children learn about sexuality from their parents, but parents do not usually treat this reticence as evidence of disinterest! Family carers who took this line opposed sex education for their relative on the grounds that it would create sexual need, and open up consequent dangers. Levels of understanding of sexuality among our sample were generally poor, with only five of the 14 adults with learning difficulties in the third study judged reasonably knowledgeable about crucial issues such as fertility and contraception. The following quotation suggests an existential level of ignorance:

> *Simon* It's [male penis] sticking up.
> *Interviewer* Why do you think it's doing that?
> *Simon* Don't know.
> *Interviewer* Does that sometimes happen to you?
> *Simon* Yeh.
> *Interviewer* Do you know why that happens?
> *Simon* No.
> *Interviewer* How does it feel when that happens to you?
> *Simon* Don't know.
> *Interviewer* Do you feel happy, do you feel uncomfortable... ?
> *Simon* Happy.

Discussion

Research into the views of people with learning difficulties and their family carers suggests that attitudes towards the sexuality of the former vary substantially. However, most parents, at least within the generation who currently have adult children, can be characterized as 'conservative'.

Although adults capable of informed consent are entitled to make their own decisions about sexual matters, this right is unlikely to be exercised in practice when their quality of life depends upon the devoted care of relatives who do not wish to encourage their sexual development.

Therapists, faced with this micro-political conundrum, may be tempted to fall back on sex education (Thompson, 1991) which at least provides them with an 'intervention' which they can unilaterally control. But sex education will achieve little unless its recipients want to receive it, and can translate its messages into practice. More useful interventions should begin from the starting point that adults with learning difficulties, their family carers and professionals all have rational, but sometimes distinct, perspectives on difficult issues including sexual needs, risk appraisal and individuals' personal growth potential.

Therapists need to distinguish carefully between advising other people to take risks and accepting personal responsibility for risk taking. The present authors support a 'liberal' position, but neither of us has a child with a learning difficulty, and we cannot know how we would define 'safety' if faced with the risk/autonomy dilemma confronting family carers.

Professionals providing direct care appear to behave restrictively (Johnson and Davies, 1989), and some adults with learning difficulties whom we have interviewed reported that day centre staff treat them like children. Parents themselves detect gaps between professional rhetoric and practice:

> If you treat them as normal, then they should always be treated that way. But I find, sometimes, that Peter comes in from the Base and says things to me, and I feel that, on the one hand, they're saying to him, 'You're the same as us', type of thing. . . . And then, another time, they're treating him as if he isn't on their level. And I think this can be very confusing to the likes of Peter, because they end up . . . not quite sure . . . where they are. (Peter's mother, individual interview)

Squire (1989) found that parents of younger children expressed more positive attitudes towards their sexual development than did parents of older children. Although this finding can be explained in various ways, it does suggest that parental 'conservatism' increases, just like that of professionals, when they have to directly confront sexual issues.

A professional stance which seeks to recognize and share expertise will generate greater client and family carer receptiveness than one which claims a monopoly of expertise:

> Glenda's family doctor once called at our house and asked Glenda's advice on a particular case of his, on the basis that he said, 'I know the technical side of how a Down's syndrome child comes about with the chromosomes etc, but you have actually looked after one and brought one up'. . . . And when you get a professional with that approach, then you will endeavour to cooperate fully, to give what help you can in-between. You, then, I think you can achieve something. There does seem to be a tendency that it is 'them' and 'us' (Father, group discussion)

Conclusion

The sexual development of people with learning difficulties should be approached within a framework of human rights and quality of life. Adult citizens are entitled to seek to engage, or not engage, in sexual activities based on informed consent. Some adults with learning difficulties manage to establish sexual relationships, to marry, to live independently and to rear children. Others do not, for a variety of reasons, including disability, disinclination, absence of sexual opportunities, lack of resources and family opposition.

Therapists have a part to play in promoting the sexual development and health of this client group, and we have discussed the range of services which they might offer. These services need to be matched to the varying needs, capabilities and circumstances of individuals. Above all, therapists need to appreciate both the limitations of the long-term resources that they can offer, and of their own expertise. Family carers will have acquired detailed practical knowledge of their relative's capabilities. Therapists can introduce useful outsider perspectives, particularly about individuals' learning potential, but need to take seriously family carers' concerns about the risks they associate with their relative embarking on sexual journeys.

References

Beauchamp, T.L. and Childress, J. (1994) *Principles of Biomedical Ethics*, 4th edn, Oxford University Press, Oxford

Brantlinger, E. (1983) Measuring variation and change in attitudes of residential staff towards the sexuality of mentally retarded persons. *Mental Retardation*, **21**, 17–22

Brown, H. (1987) Working with parents. In Craft, A. (ed.), *Mental Handicap and Sexuality*, Cotello, Tunbridge Wells

Chappell, A.L. (1992) Towards a sociological critique of the normalisation principle. *Disability, Handicap and Society*, **7**, 35–51

Cook, G. and Procter, S. (1998) Risk: a nursing dilemma. In Heyman, B. (ed.), *Risk, Health and Health Care: A Qualitative Approach*, Edward Arnold, London

Craft, A. (1987a) *Health, Social and Sex Education for Children, Adolescents and Adults with a Mental Handicap: A Review of Audio-Visual Resources*, Health Education Authority, Nottingham

Craft, A. (ed.) (1987b) Mental handicap and sexuality: issues for individuals with a mental handicap, their parents and professionals. In *Mental Handicap and Sexuality*, Cotello, Tunbridge Wells

Craft, A. (ed.) (1994) *Sexuality and Learning Difficulties*, Routledge, London

Dixon, H. (1986) *Options for Change: A Staff Training Handbook on Personal Relationships and Sexuality for People with a Mental Handicap*, BIMH Publications/FPA, London

Dixon, H. (1998) *Chance to Choose: Sexuality and Relationships Education for People with Learning Difficulties* – An Educator's Resource Book, Learning Development Aids, Wisbech, Cambs.

Fraser, J. (1988) *Not a Child Any More*, Brook Advisory Centre, London

Handyside, E.C. and Heyman, B. (1997) *Promoting the Sexual Health of Adults with Learning Difficulties*, unpublished Report, University of Northumbria

Hansson, S.O. (1993) The false promise of risk analysis. *Ratio* (New Series), **6**, 16–26

Heshusius, L. (1987) Research and perceptions of sexuality by persons labelled mentally handicapped. In Craft, A. (ed.), *Mental Handicap and Sexuality*, Cotello, Tunbridge Wells

Heyman, B. and Henriksen, M. (1998) Values and health risks. In Heyman, B. (ed.), *Risk, Health and Health Care: A Qualitative Approach*, Edward Arnold, London

Heyman, B. and Huckle, S. (1993) Not Worth the risk? Attitudes of adults with learning difficulties and their informal and formal carers to the hazards of everyday life. *Social Science and Medicine*, **12**, 1557–1564

Heyman, B. and Huckle, S. (1995) Sexuality as a perceived hazard in the lives of adults with learning difficulties. *Disability and Society*, **10**, 139–155

Heyman, B., Huckle, S. and Handyside, E.C. (1998) Freedom of the locality for people with learning difficulties. In Heyman, B. (ed.), *Risk, Health and Health Care: A Qualitative Approach*, Edward Arnold, London

Heyman, B. Swain, J., Gillman, M., Handyside, E.C. and Newman W. (1997) Alone in the crowd: how adults with learning difficulties cope with social network problems. *Social Science and Medicine*, **44**, 41–53

Johnson, P.R. and Davies, R. (1989) Sexual attitudes of members of staff. *British Journal of Mental Subnormality*, **35**, 17–21

Richardson, S.A. (1989) Letting go: a mother's view. *Disability, Handicap and Society*, **4**, 81–92

Squire, J. (1989) Sex education for pupils with severe learning difficulties: a survey of parent and staff attitudes. *Mental Handicap*, **17**, 66–69

Swain, J., Gillman, M. and Heyman B. (1998) Public research, private concerns: ethical issues in the use of open-ended interviews with people who have learning difficulties. *Disability and Society*, **13**, 21–36

Thompson, S.B.N. (1991) Sexuality training in occupational therapy for people with a learning difficulty. *British Journal of Occupational Therapy*, **54**, 303–304

Thorin, E., Yovanoff, P. and Irvin, L. (1996) Dilemmas faced by families during their young adults' transitions to adulthood: a brief report. *Mental Retardation*, **34**, 117–120

Veatch, R.M. and Fry, S.T. (1987) *Case Studies in Nursing Ethics*, J.B. Lippincott, Philadelphia

17

Bereavement, loss and grief

John Swain and Paul Lawrence

Introduction

This chapter focuses on experiences of bereavement, loss and grief as part of the social world in which we all participate. We shall concentrate on bereavement through the death of a significant person, though much of our discussion will be relevant to loss through broken relationships and separations of different kinds, including those that can be seen as part of the transitions through life-cycles.

Our starting point for this chapter is that death and bereavement raises significant and highly complex issues for therapists working with people with learning difficulties. McAteer suggests that many physiotherapists encounter death in their professional lives on an almost daily basis, and the same could be said about occupational therapists, 'since approximately 70% of all deaths occur in public sector facilities of one sort or another' (1997: 169). In some respects, it seems likely that therapists have increasingly encountered people with learning difficulties who have experienced the loss of someone with whom they have had a close association, including their parents. We shall review some of the available literature related to the bereavement process and consider how this corresponds to what is known of the experiences of people with learning difficulties, and illustrate the discussion with extracts from interviews conducted by Paul Lawrence.

Before looking in more detail at the denial and medicalization of death and grief in the experiences of people with learning difficulties, we shall outline some of the research and ideas concerning commonalities in grieving.

Bereavement models: maps and myths

The application of what Bowlby calls 'separation anxiety' in young children to the experience of bereaved adults has been based on the idea that all significant relationships follow the same pattern. Therefore, according to Bowlby's early work (Bowlby, 1961), the loss of a significant other by death will provoke the same patterns of behaviour. The first phase, in which crying and anger is the signature, is followed by the despair or depression phase, with the realization that the recovery of the lost individual is impossible. The third phase sees a reorganization of behaviour involving adjustment and attachment to new people. As with children, separation anxiety produces searching behaviour, but because the bereaved person knows that recovery is impossible, these behaviours are subconscious and can manifest themselves in the bereaved person reporting that they 'feel the presence' of the dead person, or believing that they have heard them speak, and this can also manifest as restlessness.

Later, Bowlby (1981) recognized that this model left out an important phase, namely an initial shock or numbness. What emerges in this model (and others) is an attempt to present bereavement as a process with definable stages which are experienced over a period of time. This formulaic approach to grieving incorporates the danger of rigidity. Sidell (1992) points out this danger, and states that these phases or stages of grieving can be prescriptive rather than descriptive, and that those undergoing bereavement can feel trapped in a model which suggests what they *should* feel, rather than helping them understand how they *do* feel. There is a sense, too, in which suggestions of timings of each phase can place additional burdens of conformity. This danger is not lost on Bowlby himself, and he states:

> Admittedly these phases are not clear cut, and any one individual may oscillate for a time back and forth between any two of them. (1981:85)

Many writers have suggested factors which may determine responses to bereavement, including the following:

- The nature of the relationship between the bereaved and the deceased is one which a number of researchers have suggested could be a determinant of atypical grief. Worden (1991), for instance, suggests that dependent relationships can be difficult to grieve. Other relationships can lead to difficult and mixed feelings, including guilt and feelings of unfinished business.
- The circumstances surrounding the death is also seen as an important factor. Unanticipated deaths are claimed to be more difficult to cope with than those in which the bereaved have time to prepare themselves for the loss (Horn, 1989). Suicides are particularly difficult for the bereaved. On the other hand, death can be a source of relief if the deceased has been suffering from a protracted illness. In this situation the grieving often starts long before the death. The age of the deceased can also be significant, in that the death of an old person can seem less of a 'tragedy', and the funeral can be an occasion to celebrate the life of the deceased.
- One's personal history is likely to influence the outcome of the grieving process, such as previous experiences of bereavement.
- The personality of the bereaved may also affect the outcome of the experience. Parkes and Weiss (1983), for instance, claimed that people who are generally anxious and insecure are likely to react more intensely to the experiences of bereavement.
- Social factors also influence the development of reactions to bereavement. A key factor here is the support available to the bereaved, and

opportunities to turn to others for support are not always there, as Marshall (1993) points out. Social support is most likely to be received if the relationship was conventional. Less social support is likely with the loss of a gay or lesbian partner, for instance. The death of a friend is taken less seriously, in terms of compassionate leave from work, for example, than the death of a parent. It seems to be the perceived intensity of the attachment that is significant.

As mentioned above, the biopsychosocial models of grief that dominate the literature and research have come under increasing criticism. Basically, the danger of the 'models and maps' we have summarized here is that they become a prescriptive, expected pattern of grieving and deviations from the pattern are not only seem as 'atypical', but are pathologized. Hale states:

> . . . there is an urgent need to *stop modelling* and to *stop tidying up bereavement experiences*. Only then can the acknowledged diversity and richness of such experiences be given full expression, and be addressed as a strength rather than as an 'inconvenience' to be overcome through a never-ending process of research. (1996: 118)

Bereavement and people with learning difficulties

Moving on from a general discussion of bereavement to the experiences of people with learning difficulties, Oswin's (1981) four assumptions or principles make a good starting point:

1 There is no reason to think that people with learning difficulties will not go through stages of mourning as others do.
2 People with learning difficulties have as much right as other people to be given consideration when their relatives and friends die.
3 Each person who has learning difficulty is an individual who will grieve as an individual. There is no reason to expect them to react in some particular way because they have learning difficulties.
4 Some people with learning difficulties, as some people without learning difficulties, may need some specific help when they become bereaved.

Though there has been little research in this area specifically relating to the lives of people with learning difficulties, the available literature generally supports Oswin. The evidence suggests that there is a commonality in the processes of grief. In terms of the models of the processes of grief, the responses of people with learning difficulties are no different. In a study in which 43 adults with learning difficulties were interviewed, Harper and Wadsworth concluded that people with learning difficulties 'display grief responses similar to all adults' (1993: 313).

Reports of more detailed single case studies reflect the same sort of findings. O'Nians (1993) traces the progress of Matthew's grieving, a young man with severe learning difficulties, after the death of his mother, through what O'Nians calls the 'natural' stages of grieving. Evidence about the responses of people with learning difficulties, following the death of a fellow resident, consistently suggests that people living in large-scale institutions for many years, progress through the usual processes and stages of grieving (Thrum, 1989).

Though having learning difficulties does not, in itself, affect the processes and feelings associated with grief, it would seem that people with learning difficulties are at risk in terms of the factors which determine responses to bereavement. People with learning difficulties can be denied the right to participate fully in the grief and mourning process and in all of society's support systems and rituals associated with these losses. In the following extract from a group interview with young people with learning difficulties, John is talking about events after the death of his cousin and Diane about the death of her grandparents. Neither, it seems, was given the choice of attending the funeral, and both were given a rationale for why they should not attend:

> *Paul*   Let's talk about who went to the funeral.
> *John*   My mam was there. My gran and grandad, my aunty Judith was there and my uncle John, my aunty Sandra and my aunty Maureen, all the family.
> *Paul*   The whole family was there.
> *John*   Yeah.
> *Paul*   Did you go to the funeral?
> *John*   No.
> *Paul*   Did you want to go?
> *John*   I was at a different school at that time.
> *Paul*   So you stayed at home while the funeral was on did you?
> *John*   No. I was at a different school. I was at S school. My mam had to bring us home early at about quarter past two.
> *Paul*   After the funeral, or to go to the funeral?
> *John*   After the funeral.
> *Paul*   So you were at school and everyone else went to the funeral, then they came and got you from school.
> *John*   Yes. All they do is put the box in and cover it over.
> *Paul*   What about you Diane? Did you go to the funeral of your gran or grandad?
> *Diane*   No. I didn't want to.
> *Paul*   You didn't want to?
> *John*   I was going to go but I didn't because I was at school.
> *Paul*   You would have gone but you were at school.
> *John*   I would liked to have but I was at school.
> *Diane*   It was too upsetting for us.
> *Paul*   Did you decide that? Did you say that you won't go because it is too upsetting or did someone say that to you?
> *Diane*   Me mam said that it would be a good idea if you didn't go. So they just went.

In the following example, the person with learning difficulties, Luke, did attend the funeral. Luke had been through a particularly traumatic experience. While his father was in hospital with a terminal illness, and Luke was living alone with his mother, she died unexpectedly. He returned home from the day centre to find his mother had died. Not knowing what to do, Luke went to bed, and the situation was not discovered until the next morning when his sister arrived. In the following extract from an interview with Luke's care worker, she talks of Luke's and the family's response:

> *Janet*   There was this laid back sort of . . . 'Oh I've been to my mum's funeral. It was a nice day out. I've had something to eat afterwards. I went to church'. But I think the family reinforced that as well. Very much sort of, 'Luke's been to the funeral, they've all had a good time', as if it was wonderful, which I personally found a very difficult thing to cope with because I felt it was a very unreal situation, a very . . . sort of patronizing way to treat Luke. I think the family felt if they were incredibly cheerful, while Luke was there, they could get to a situation where he didn't have to go through the pain and the grief. They try, I think to put on this sort of happy, cheerful front. 'Let's all have a nice day out and everything will be all right', hoping they could maybe cheat themselves through the sad and the real side of losing your mum, even though they must have been feeling emotional.

Understandable feelings of wishing to 'protect' people with learning difficulties can deny them the very recognition of their feelings and the social support they need, as everyone else, to progress through the process of mourning. Luke's story is particularly poignant as his father died shortly afterwards. What basis did he have to cope with this second loss?

French and Kuczaj state:

> Until fairly recently, It has been an accepted myth that people with learning difficulties are not able to understand, or even feel the same as 'normal' people. They are expected to continue their life and daily activities as though nothing has happened. Any alterations in behaviour following loss are usually attributed to the original diagnosis that the person has already. (1992: 108)

From the research undertaken by Paul Lawrence, there is a different interpretation of this denial of bereavement. Though it may be recognized that people with learning difficulties have 'normal reactions', they are thought to need protection from the pain of grief. However, whatever the explanation, the consequences are the same: the denial of bereavement; the pathologizing of the responses of the person with learning difficulties; and the lack of support through the grieving process.

The situation can be exacerbated through other factors determining responses to bereavement. Bereavement can be more difficult if the person with learning difficulties, like Luke, has difficulties understanding the causes of death, how and why his mother died. Also, the relationship may be one of dependency on caring (either by or for the person with learning difficulties). On the evening of his mother's death, Luke had no tea. For whatever reason, this was a dependent relationship in which Luke lost not only his mother as a person, but also the practical help he required in his daily living. In terms of the broader circumstances surrounding the death of his parents, Luke also lost his home and lifestyle as he had to move into a group home. Before the death of his parents, there had been plans for Luke to move into residential care, but these were only at a rudimentary stage. The death of his parents did not allow for careful preparation, and the loss was not only of his parents, which was difficult enough, but also of his home.

Luke's story illustrates two other significant factors. The first is the effect of previous experiences of bereavement. Though Luke's father had a terminal illness, his death was as 'unexpected' and unprepared for, by Luke, as his mother's. The other factor is communication. Luke's abilities in terms of verbally expressing his feelings of grief were limited and this factor was exacerbated by the loss of two people who were well 'tuned in' to his communication. Again there is a danger of pathologizing the responses of people with learning difficulties whose limited communication allows little or no verbal expression of grief, and whose behaviour might be deemed 'challenging' rather than an understandable expression of grief. (For further information on challenging behaviour the reader is referred to Chapter 18.)

It is important to reiterate that all the above factors can be significant in bereavement and the experience of grief irrespective of whether a person has learning difficulties. When the father of one of the authors of this chapter died, for instance, his mother felt she could not continue to live in the same house and had moved within days. She, too, lost her home as well as the most significant person in her life, though the difference in this case is that she chose to move, whereas some people with learning difficulties do not have a choice. Our argument is not that these factors are peculiar to the experiences of people with learning difficulties, but rather that people with learning difficulties are at greater risk from these factors that can make the process of grieving more difficult.

Bereavement and therapy

There are no set formulas that therapists can turn to in helping people with learning difficulties, or people without learning difficulties, through the process of grieving. There are, however, important implications for therapists in their work with people with learning difficulties. One starting point is the recognition, by therapists, that they have a role to play. It may be solely one of showing awareness, sensitivity and availability. The person with learning difficulties may feel more comfortable talking with someone else, possibly someone who is not a professional or service provider, but the therapist still has an important role.

A second starting point is the recognition that grieving is an individual response, notwithstanding the possible commonalities in stages and processes of grieving. Values, expectations and beliefs can underpin social pressures not only to suppress grief, as discussed above, but also to comply to expected patterns of behaviour and phases of grief. It is the differences that need to be explored and provide the basis for the understanding, help and support that therapists can provide: differences in individual responses and differences in the contexts in which people with learning difficulties have lived their lives.

Strategies for helping people with learning difficulties to progress through grieving seem to fall into four categories. Clearly therapists will need to coordinate their approach with that of other professionals, in partnership with carers, and with paramount importance given to the view of the person with learning difficulties about the support he or she requires. The first category of strategies is in the preparation to cope with loss generally or to cope with the impending death of a significant person through a terminal illness. An interesting approach is described by French, an occupational therapist, and Kuczaj, an art therapist, who have run workshops on the theme of loss and change for people with learning difficulties and their keyworkers/supporters. They write:

> Our intentions for the two-day workshop were therefore to confront some of the myths regarding the emotional responses of people with learning difficulties and to explore feelings which may be encountered following a personal loss, or bereavement. We also hoped to look at ways of gaining and giving support in relation to these feelings. (1992:108)

The second set of strategies involves the preparation of therapists themselves. Supporting someone who is grieving the loss of a significant person in their lives requires the therapist, at least to a certain extent, to feel comfortable themselves about bereavement, loss and grief. Supporting people experiencing grief is something of two-way street. As Kübler-Ross (1969) pointed out 30 years ago, professionals who are willing to respond to needs for support can themselves emerge with fewer anxieties about death in their own lives.

The third set of strategies involve facilitating people with learning difficulties through the actual event and subsequent responses and feelings. McAteer (1997) suggests a number of ways in which therapists can provide practical help in promoting the health of bereaved people. These include attention to sleep patterns and the possible use of relaxation techniques. There can be a role, too, for therapists through the use of counselling skills. Some people with learning difficulties require counselling to facilitate the process of grieving, as do some people without learning difficulties, and therapists can be involved in referral processes to ensure the person receives an appropriate bereavement counselling service. Nevertheless, therapists can themselves facilitate grieving through listening and building an open and trusting relationship:

> For therapists this requires an exploration of the nature of relationships and communication by which they seek to help others to help themselves. (Swain, 1995: 1–2)

Acceptance is a major component in the use of counselling skills. Acceptance by others can facilitate acceptance by the person with learning difficulties of their particular feelings and responses. This applies particularly, perhaps, when the responses and feelings might not be expected. They can be mixed or ambivalent and, depending on the relationship with the deceased, grief can be coloured by anger and sometimes feelings of guilt. Guilt and anger can reflect unfinished business in a relationship in which feelings were not expressed. There can be feelings of relief too, when for instance the deceased had experienced an extended period of illness prior to death. Furthermore, grief reactions can still be strong for many years after the actual bereavement, and can be expressed through what are seen as 'challenging behaviours'.

Acceptance by therapists involves reflecting on their own presumptions about bereavement, loss and grief. Crick states:

> Most important of all in working with the dying and bereaved is a willingness to help them and to spend time listening and talking. It is not necessary to be a skilled counsellor. Even those who have no special training in counselling and bereavement can help to guide their clients to an acceptance of their loss and to a new life. (1988: 63)

The following poem was included in an anthology of prose, poetry and art by people with learning difficulties:

Sad

My aunty is dead and my uncle too
They are buried
A long way away
In Wales.
I'm sad
I miss them
I've never been to the grave
I'd like to go
I would cry
I cry in bed
I miss them.

(by Pearl Chilcott, in Atkinson and Williams, 1990: 98)

As this poem illustrates, it is important to remember that talking is not the only way that people express and work through their grief. Creative activities such as writing poetry, painting, drama and dance can facilitate awareness and expression of emotions and needs. (For further information on creative art activities the reader is referred to Chapter 24.)

The fourth set of strategies are those involved in facilitating the person with learning difficulties through problems and changes arising through loss, such as moving into residential accommodation. Baxter and colleagues suggest that continuity in the bereaved person's life is essential following the death of a parent. They state:

> Established routines, norms and experiences should not suddenly cease. This can only be ensured by obtaining detailed information about the bereaved person's life. Where the person with learning difficulties is from a black or ethnic minority community, difficulties in communication between professionals and relatives could entail that loss of important detail. There is also a risk that professionals will not appreciate the significance of a particular activity or possession in the bereaved person's life. (1990: 166)

Conclusion

As with many topics covered in this book, bereavement, loss and grief is a wide-ranging arena of social life that can only be touched on in a chapter of this length. The complexities and individual nuances speak against easy definitions of 'problems' and 'solutions'. However, bereavement and loss can have a crucial significance for us all in relation to feelings and understandings about ourselves, our relationships, our behaviour and our lives. The dominant response when a person has learning difficulties is the denial of the significance of bereavement and loss. Such denial only serves to distort and exacerbate experiences that are a natural part of social life.

References

Atkinson, D. and Williams, F. (eds) (1990) 'Know Me As I Am': An Anthology of Prose, Poetry and Art by People with Learning Difficulties, Hodder and Stoughton, London (in association with the Open University Press)

Baxter, C., Poonia, K., Ward, L. and Nadirshaw, Z. (1990) Issues and Services for People with Learning Difficulties from Black and Ethnic Minority Communities, King's Fund Centre, London

Bowlby, J. (1961) Processes of mourning. International Journal of Psycho-Analysis, **42**, 317–340.

Bowlby, J. (1981) Attachment and Loss: Loss, Sadness and Depression, Penguin, London

Crick, L. (1988) Facing grief. Nursing Times, **84**(28), 61–63.

French, J. and Kuczaj, E. (1992) working through loss and change with people with learning difficulties. Mental Handicap, **20**, 108–111

Hale, G. (1996) The social construction of grief. In Cooper, C. et al. (eds), Integrating Perspectives on Health, Open University Press, Buckingham

Harper, D.C. and Wadsworth, J.S. (1993) Grief in adults with mental retardation: preliminary findings. Research in Developmental Disabilities, **14**, 313–330

Horn, S. (1989) Coping with Bereavement: Coming to Terms with a Sense of Loss, Thornsons, Northampton

Kubler-Ross, E. (1969) On Death and Dying, Macmillan, New York

Marshall, F. (1993) Losing a Parent, Sheldon Press, London

McAteer, M.F. (1997) Death, dying and bereavement. In French, S. (ed.), Physiotherapy: A Psychosocial Approach, 2nd edn Butterworth-Heinemann, Oxford

O'Nians, R. (1993) Support in grief. Nursing Times, **89**(50), 62–64

Oswin, M. (1981) Bereavement and Mentally Handicapped People, King's Fund, London

Parkes, C.M. and Weiss, R.S. (1983) Recovery From Bereavement, Basic Books, New York

Sidell, M. (1992) Bereavement: Private Grief and Collective Responsibility, Workbook 5 of 'Death and Dying', Open University Press, Milton Keynes

Swain, J. (1995) The Use of Counselling Skills: A Guide for Therapists, Butterworth-Heinemann, Oxford

Thrum, A. (1989) I've lost a good friend, Nursing Times, **85**(32), 66–68

Worden, J. (1991) Grief Counselling and Grief Therapy, 2nd edn, Routledge, London

18

Challenging questions

John Swain, Maureen Gillman
and Bob Heyman

Is there a problem?

Therapists, like others who work or spend time with people with learning difficulties, may well encounter what has come to be known as 'challenging behaviour'. Certainly the literature would suggest that this is the case. It has been estimated that between 15 and 20 per cent of the people with learning difficulties in contact with services, at any one time, will present significant challenges to those who live and work with them (Keirnan and Qureshi, 1993). Challenging behaviour is the most frequently cited reason for the breakdown of community placements (Emerson *et al.*, 1987), and people with challenging behaviour have been the most difficult to place in de-institutionalization programmes (Department of Health, 1989). Research into the responses of care staff suggests emotional responses such as sadness, anger and high levels of stress (Bromley and Emerson, 1995). Many people who display challenging behaviour have also been diagnosed as having a psychiatric disorder and responsibility for providing a service to such clients is often unclear (Allen *et al.*, 1991). The scale and complexity of the problems has provided justification for the provision of specialist services which have been the subject of quite extensive evaluation programmes. The Special Development Team of the University of Kent, for instance, undertook research to assist local services plan, set up and support 'high quality' services over a five-year period for 38 people with severe learning difficulties and challenging behaviour.

It would seem, then, that there is 'a problem'. However, this whole arena is one of controversy rather than consensus. Even the use of the term 'challenging behaviour' has been the subject of critical debate. Slevin (1995), for example, argues that it is used as a negative label, often for the purposes of the placement of clients. The meaning of the term 'challenging behaviour' is also itself interpreted in different ways. Some definitions are broad in scope and would allow the inclusion of behaviours such as the use of verbal aggression towards carers and to other clients. Others are narrower, specifying danger to self or others. Furthermore, scales for assessing challenging behaviours have also proved to depend on the viewpoint of the assessor and have low inter-rater reliability (Newton and Sturmey, 1991). What is viewed as 'challenging' is relative to who is doing the viewing, the criteria for judgements and the whole context in which judgements are made. This is the starting point for this chapter. It is the 'challenge' of 'challenging behaviours', rather than the behaviours *per se*, to which this chapter is orientated. While there could be said to be a consensus that there is a challenge, the first fundamental challenge is to understanding. It is this that we shall explore and reflect on – and hence the title, 'Challenging questions'.

What is the challenge?

We shall begin our exploration of the nature of the problem by turning to definitions within the literature, and then summarizing some views of people who work with people with learning difficulties. Clements suggests behaviour should be considered to be challenging or problematic, if it:

1 is unacceptable by the social standards relevant to the person's age, class and cultural background;
2 imposes a significant cost on the person him/herself (such as physical damage, social rejection or limiting opportunities);
3 imposes a significant and unreasonable cost on the lives of others (1997:82).

There are two related ways of answering the question 'What is the problem?' The first, as in the first of the above criteria, lies in the behaviour itself. It is the nipping that is the problem, or the shouting, or whatever form of behaviour is deemed unacceptable. The second and third criteria specify the consequences of behaviour. Thus the problem is the danger to the person him/herself or others, whether the danger is physical, psychological or emotional. The danger can be in the limitation of opportunities and social contacts for the person with learning difficulties as a consequence of the reactions of others to his or her behaviour. Defined in this way, then, challenging behaviour is the behaviour of some people with learning difficulties that challenges formal and informal carers and the services provided.

In a research project we conducted at the University of Northumbria (Heyman *et al.*, 1998), care workers were interviewed about their experiences with people with learning difficulties who they thought had challenging behaviour. We found that both the above ways of defining challenging behaviour were reflected in their views, but also that the whole picture of different understandings of challenging behaviour was complex and, in a word, messy.

The most common behaviours thought to be challenging involved some form of violence or aggression towards staff or other service users. However, a wide range of behaviours were deemed to be challenging including, as in the following quote, sexual assault:

> He put his hand upon my breast, and said, 'I'm sick of this place'. I took hold of his hand, removed it and said, 'Leave it', or something like that. And because I had removed his hand, he sort of nipped us quite badly on the arm.

One interesting point about this statement, in the light of the present discussion, is that such sexual abuse is referred to as 'challenging'. If this had been an example of abuse perpetrated by, rather than upon, staff, it would not have been regarded as 'challenging behaviour'. The next example underlines this point. Here expressions of dislike for a day centre is seen as challenging:

> We had experience here of a behaviour which was quite challenging, that the person concerned would come in, she is from a different cultural background, so that had a bearing on it. But she would come in, and would wail and scream, and would be totally inconsolable. ... She wouldn't even attempt to propel her wheelchair, even though, to all attempts and purposes she appeared to be capable of doing so, but would really drown out any attempt that you had to talk to her.

Again, similar defiance by staff would not be deemed 'challenging' as such, however unacceptable it is thought to be. Another question arising from this quote is whether over-compliance would be seen to be as challenging as behaviours that might be said to resist the status quo.

The consequences of behaviour were also referred to in defining what is challenging, particularly dangers to the person him/herself or others:

> I think it is not taken seriously unless there's physical contact, someone actually is violent towards you, or furniture, whatever. The everyday somebody screaming all day, you'd say that is challenging, but it's not taken really seriously unless people are hurt.
>   Something that puts them or others in danger basically seems to be the main criteria.

Perhaps, inevitably, one factor in whether behaviour is seen as challenging or not is whether it is manageable, and this depends on a variety of considerations, including predictability:

> The two people I've got, one of them, there's trigger points, you can actually see the signs of him building up. And you know that there's going to be an outburst, for want of a better expression, you know, well, towards you. The other person shows no signs at all. There's no trigger points, nothing, and she can just become very very violent towards you for no reason at all.

Though the care workers found it easy to identify examples of challenging behaviour and people whose behaviour was seen as challenging, they also talked of the difficulties of defining what is challenging, suggesting, for instance, that such judgements are relative to individual values: 'it depends how people see it. ... What I might see as a challenging behaviour you mightn't.'

We end this brief exploration of what is challenging with an observation. The term 'challenging' has certain connotations when applied to the behaviour of people with learning difficulties, all of which are negative and problem related. This is in stark contrast to the more general uses of the word 'challenging' as exemplified by the definitions offered within the Oxford Dictionary, which include:

> take exception to (evidence, juryman), dispute, deny; claim (attention, admiration, etc.); offer interesting difficulties (*a challenging problem*).

Is the challenge behaviour?

In the next three sections of our exploration of understandings of challenging behaviour, we turn to three particular viewpoints: behavioural; humanistic; and social. They are not the only relevant perspectives we could discuss. Certainly a biological perspective, particularly with the widespread use of drugs such as largactil, has played a major part in the lives of many people with learning difficulties, and another notable perspective is the psychodynamic approach. However, the three perspectives we have selected are more consistent with the aims of the present volume and, we suggest, have more to offer therapists in their work with people with learning difficulties.

Though challenging behaviour can be approached from a range of perspectives, the behavioural approach has been dominant, directly and indirectly orientating the literature and the development of policies and provision. This is apparent within the very term 'challenging behaviour', as compared to, say, 'challenging communication' or 'challenging relationships'. In one recent text the basics of the perspective are summarized as follows:

> . . . all behaviour is learned in response to the reinforcing properties of the environment; that behaviour must be observable and therefore measurable; that behaviour is the central focus and there is a downplaying concerning feelings and the nature of self. (Gates, 1997: 139)

In terms of service provision, the behavioural perspective puts the emphasis on goal setting, and systematic and consistent procedures for attaining goals, as illustrated by McCool *et al.*:

> Experience to date indicates that if people with severe mental handicaps and challenging behaviours are to be involved in constructive and purposeful activities in all aspects of their daily lives, both within and outside the home, then it will be necessary to: implement and operate effective procedures for planning both service user and staff activity through setting long and medium-term goals and developing the structures and systems to monitor and implement these in the short-term; have consistent and systematic ways of working with service users and agreed strategies for coping with known behaviour problems. (1989: 60)

Remington (1993) argues that there has been what he calls a 'sea-change in emphasis' in behavioural approaches. This newer emphasis on behavioural analysis can be found in two recent practical texts for nurses working with people with learning difficulties, by Birchenall *et al.* (1997) and Gates (1997). Basically this new approach involves keeping detailed **ABC** records of: **A**ntecedents, or the situation and events before an incidence of challenging behaviour; Behaviour, i.e. a detailed description of what the person with learning difficulties does (i.e. the challenging behaviour); and Consequences, or what happens immediately after as a result of the behaviour of the person with learning difficulties. As Remington explains, intervention can then be based on such an analysis:

> If the client's behaviour is escape motivated, the aim must be to reduce the need to escape, and – should that need arise – to provide some other more efficient method of achieving it. Intervention would involve restructuring the task to reduce its aversiveness or, as in many recent studies, teaching a functionally equivalent response to the challenging behaviour.' (1993: 127)

Though it is difficult to characterize 'a behavioural approach', we conclude this brief overview by critically summarizing a number of basic presumptions:

- Challenging behaviour is a social fact, a function of the individual and a problem. As Lovett states: 'The danger of thinking behaviourally about people is that we focus on the behaviour of others and not our own. Even when we ask why a person acts in a certain way we are led to trivial and demeaning reasons – attention and noncompliance, for example' (1996: 222).
- The ultimate goal for change is that the individual will no longer present challenging behaviour, and where this cannot be achieved, the individual will be as normal as possible. A paradigm which justifies, rationalizes and is instrumental in developing strategies of control seems to have had a particular application in an arena which is defined by 'lack of control', whether the lack is sited within the individual or within service provision.
- The processes of change are environmental and, in particular, through the improvement of professional/provider intervention, service organization, policies and delivery. Choice for the person with learning difficulties in this process of change is not fundamental to a behavioural approach.
- A behavioural approach is directed towards professional and provider concerns rather than the material and structural factors which disadvantage people with learning difficulties.

Is the challenge communication and relationships?

Many more recent approaches to understanding and responding to challenging behaviour emanate from, in general terms, a humanistic perspective. This viewpoint, in comparison to behavioural approaches, focuses on: the person as a unique and valued individual, rather than 'the problem'; the meanings of behaviours, rather than the behaviour *per se*; and the qualities of relationships and communication between people, rather than lack of social skills of the person with learning difficulties.

The approach known as Gentle Teaching (McGee *et al.*, 1987) seems to have increased in popularity over recent years with different groups of professionals, including occupational therapists. As the name of this approach implies, it rejects aversive techniques of any kind, and emphasizes 'a humanizing and respectful posture towards people with severe learning difficulties' (Cheseldine, 1991: 101). Specific techniques include ignoring challenging behaviour, redirecting the person with learning difficulties to another activity, and rewarding the person with learning difficulties by simply remaining with, rather than rejecting, her or him.

The divide between humanistic and behavioural approaches is not always clear cut, and Cheseldine (1991) argues that Gentle Teaching can be seen as a more acceptable value-based behavioural approach. There are indeed similarities between the interventions described by Remington above and Gentle Teaching. However, as Cheseldine herself recognizes, there are fundamental differences:

> Teaching the person, rather than changing the behaviour is the focus. Moreover, this teaching is seen to be a process of mutual change, and therefore requires the person who takes on the role of teacher to continually question his or her values (1991: 103)

Another major avenue for critique of the behavioural approach suggests that challenging behaviours serve specific communicative functions from the actor's own perspective. Allen and colleagues advocate a shift towards understanding the messages a person might be communicating about their needs, and they promote approaches incorporating empathizing, enabling and supporting:

> Historically, services have tended to 'control' challenging behaviour, whether by restraint, medication, or psychological methods. However, services based on respect for the individual focuses much more on understanding the person and valuing them while working out what needs they have and how these might be met. This also leads us to question what messages the person might be communicating about their needs through their challenging behaviour. The approach then becomes one of understanding, teaching empathizing, valuing, enabling and supporting rather than controlling, restricting or detaining – a shift which is evident in the services described here (1991: 49).

Challenging behaviour, then, is not considered as behaviour *per se*, but as having meaning or a function for the person with learning difficulties. Myers (1995) identifies the following as some common messages:

- Stimulation ('I'm bored out of my mind, I need something meaningful to do.').
- Escape ('I want to get out of this task/place/noise/company. I want to stop. I don't understand what you want, the anxiety is unbearable.').
- Attention ('I need some undivided attention, some personal interest, someone to belong to. I feel insecure.').
- Tangible ('I'm hungry/thirsty/tired/cold/in pain. I want the music off/TV on. My mother has not come, I'm disappointed and angry.').

As with the behavioural approach, we shall again conclude by critically summarizing the basis of this approach to understanding challenging behaviour

- It focuses on making judgements and interpretations about people, their needs and their behaviour. As Clements points out, this is a social process of construction and there are, what he calls, 'active blocks to understanding', and 'the greater the imbalance (of power) and the less the contact, the greater the likelihood of dehumanization and prejudicial stereotypes' (1997: 84).
- Notwithstanding the practical possibilities of a functional communication orientation, it shares the same analytical poverty as the behavioural paradigm. The analysis of the functioning of communication has nothing to offer in terms of understanding the power relations between providers and users.

Is the challenge social?

The most radical challenges to a behavioural approach have been social perspectives of disability. In relation to the so-called challenging behaviour of people with learning difficulties, social construction explanations reject pathological and individual models. From this viewpoint, challenging behaviour is neither a social fact nor a dysfunction of communication, but is rather socially constructed between providers and users in social relations structured by a society in which people with learning difficulties are marginalized, disempowered and controlled. It has to be said that there have been relatively few attempts to explore the social construction approach specifically in relation to people with learning difficulties. Clegg (1993), however, discusses a shift of focus from individual models to broader social, interactive and multivariant models encompassing multiple perspectives and different levels of understanding and intervention.

Within a social constructionist perspective, challenging behaviour is not a set of events (behaviours and interactions) or objects (people with challenging behaviour), but is 'constructed by the continuing dialectic of interpretation and action' (Pearce, 1989: 32). Categorization and labelling, then, are important considerations from a social constructionist perspective. To paraphrase Gregory (1996), people with challenging behaviour is a social category, which legitimates, or at the very least condones, the disempowerment of people with particular mental attributes exhibiting particular behaviours. Exclusion can be seen as an example of disempowerment, such as enforced 'time out'.

It is important to recognize that there are a number of social perspectives that can be brought to bear in understanding challenging behaviour. A social constructionist perspective has been contrasted with a social creationist (or materialist) approach. Oliver writes:

The essential difference between a social constructionist and a social creationist view of disability centres on where the 'problem' is actually located. Both views have begun to move away from the core ideology of individualism. The social constructionist view sees the problem as being located within the minds of able-bodied people, whether individually (prejudice) or collectively, through the manifestation of hostile social attitudes and the enactment of social policies based upon a tragic view of disability. The social creationist view, however, sees the problem as located within the institutionalized practices of society. (1990: 82–83)

The development of a social creationist perspective of challenging behaviour will need to address inequalities in power relations, institutional discrimination and social disadvantage.

The problematic dimension of relationships involving people with learning difficulties has been discussed, analysed and researched within two extensive but largely separate sets of literature: under the umbrellas of challenging behaviour (i.e. perpetrated by people with learning difficulties) and abuse (i.e. perpetrated against people with learning difficulties). A creationist approach can incorporate challenging behaviour and abuse within the same framework of analysis, particularly when 'abuse' is defined broadly to include different categories of abuse: physical; sexual; psychological; financial or material; and neglect. (For further information on abuse the reader is referred to Chapter 22C.) A combined analysis addresses the possibility of a two-way relationship between the challenging behaviour and abuse in the face of oppression and denial of rights. That is, the responses of people with learning difficulties experiencing abuse can be challenging of others, and the responses of others experiencing challenging behaviour, by people with learning difficulties, can be abusive.

As with the behavioural and humanistic perspectives, we shall conclude this overview by suggesting some limitations of social perspectives:

- One limitation of social perspectives is the lack of theoretical development in terms of understanding the lives of people with learning difficulties, in general (as argued by Chappell, 1998), and people with challenging behaviour.
- It can be argued that the social perspectives are long on theory and short on specific practical implications. Changes in power relations are long term and, it can be argued, beyond the scope of individual therapists.

Reflecting on challenging questions

The most obvious question for therapists working with people with learning difficulties whose behaviour they find threatening is 'What do I do?' or 'How do I solve the problem?', and questions of intervention have received a great deal of attention in research and the literature. Building on the analysis in this chapter, reflecting on challenging questions provides the basis of intervention and change, rather than the comfort of predetermined recipes.

Nevertheless, some challenging behaviours require an immediate response as well as longer term reflection. 'What to do?' is indeed the first question for all involved when there is a serious risk of physical injury for the therapist, person with learning difficulties or others involved. Clements (1997) suggests that, when challenging behaviour is dangerous, 'behaviour management plans' are required for incident management to minimize the risks. Such plans are directed towards coping with the immediate situation, and need to be considered separately from longer term change. They include details of possibilities for preventing the behaviour occurring, such as situations and ways of working to avoid, and the most effective options for responding to incidents. The plans should also include recording procedures, and should be reviewed at regular intervals.

Even within the formulation and implementation of behaviour management plans, however, are embedded longer term questions such as who is involved in the planning. The possible challenging questions for reflection are extensive, and we can only summarize the main issues. Two general questions arise as starting points from the analysis in this chapter:

● What is the challenge? The formulation of solutions depends on the understanding of problems and, indeed, whether the challenge is seen in terms of 'problems' and 'solutions'. Is the challenge the behaviour of the person with learning difficulties, ineffective communication and relationships, or hierarchical power structures and relations? Or is 'challenging behaviour' not one but many things that have to be understood in different ways?
● What needs to change? Within each perspective for understanding challenging behaviour is embedded the aims of intervention. Is it the behaviour of the person with learning difficulties that needs to change, the behaviour or attitudes of therapists, or the social context of therapy?

Each of the perspectives discussed above also raises its own questions. First, from a behavioural perspective the questions would include the following:

● What precisely is the behaviour causing concern, and what are the patterns of situations or events preceding the behaviour (antecedents) and what happens as the immediate result of the behaviour (consequences)?
● What changes can be made in terms of the antecedents and consequences?

A humanistic perspective raises the following questions:

● Does the person with learning difficulties feel valued as a person?
● What are the possible messages being conveyed by the behaviour of the person with learning difficulties?
● How does the therapist feel towards the person with learning difficulties, and what support does the therapist receive in reflecting on his or her feelings?

And finally, a social perspective:

- What autonomy or power does the person with learning difficulties have in the decision making that shapes his or her life?
- What forms of segregation, oppression and abuse has the person with learning difficulties experienced?

Understanding challenging behaviour is the starting point for change, but the term covers many different situations not one problem. Reflecting on challenging questions is a basis for developing understanding, either as an individual therapist, listening to the person with learning difficulties, or within an appropriate multidisciplinary forum.

References

Allen, D., Banks, R. and Staite, S. (1991) *Meeting the Challenge: Some UK Perspectives on Community Services for People with Learning Difficulties and Challenging Behaviour*, King's Fund Centre, London

Birchenall, M., Baldwin, M. and Morris, J. (1997) *Learning Disability and the Social Context of Caring*, Churchill Livingstone, Edinburgh

Bromley, J. and Emerson, E. (1995) Beliefs and emotional reactions of care staff working with people with challenging behaviour. *Journal of Intellectual Disability Research*, **39**(4), 341–352

Chappell, A.L. (1998) Still out in the cold: people with learning difficulties and the social model of disability. In Shakespeare, T. (ed.), *The Disability Reader: Social Science Perspectives*, Cassell, London

Cheseldine, S. (1991) Gentle teaching for challenging behaviour. In Waston, J. (ed.), *Innovatory Practice and Severe Learning Difficulties*, Murray House Publications, Edinburgh

Clegg, M. (1993) Putting people first: a social constructionist approach to learning disability. *British Journal of Clinical Psychology*, **32**, 389–406

Clements, J. (1997) Challenging needs and problematic behaviour. In O'Hara, J. and Sperlinger, A. (eds), *Adults with Learning Disabilities: A Practical Approach for Health Professionals*, Wiley, Chichester

Department of Health (1989) *Needs and Responses: Services for Adults with Mental Handicap Who Are Mentally Ill and Who Have Behavioural Problems or Who Offend*, Department of Health, London

Emerson, E., Toogood, A. and Mansell, J. (1987) Challenging behaviour and community services: 1. Introduction and overview. *Mental Handicap*, **15**, 166–169

Gates, B. (1997) Behavioural difficulties. In Gates, B. (ed) *Learning Disabilities* (3rd edn), Churchill Livingstone, Edinburgh

Gregory, S. (1996) The disabled identity. In Wetherell, M. (ed.), *Identity, Groups and Social Issues*, Sage, London

Heyman, B., Swain, J. and Gillman, M. (1998) A risk management dilemma: how day centre staff understand challenging behaviour. *Disability and Society*, **13**(2), 163–182

Keirnan, C. and Qureshi, H. (1993) Challenging behaviour. In Keirnan, C. (ed.), *Research to Practice? Implications of Research on the Challenging Behaviour of People with Learning Disability*, BILD Publications, Clevedon, Avon

McCool, C., Barrett, S. and Emerson, E. (1989) Challenging behaviour and community services: 5. Structuring staff and client activity. *Mental Handicap*, **17**, 60–64.

McGee, J.J., Menolascino, F.J. and Hobbs, D.C. (1987) *Gentle Teaching: a Nonaversive Approach for Helping Persons with Mental Retardation*, Human Sciences Press, New York

Myers, M. (1995) A challenge to change: better services for people with challenging behaviour. In Philpot, T. and Ward, L. (eds), *Values and Visions: Changing Ideas in Services for People with Learning Difficulties*, Butterworth-Heinemann, Oxford

Newton, J.T. and Sturmey, P. (1991) The motivation assessment scale: inter-rater reliability and internal consistency in a British sample. *Journal of Mental Deficiency Research*, **35**, 472–474

Oliver, M. (1990) *The Politics of Disablement*, Macmillan, Basingstoke

Pearce, W.B. (1989) *Communication and the Human Condition*, Southern Illinois University Press, Carbondale, IL

Remington, B. (1993) Challenging behaviour in people with severe learning disabilities: behaviour modification or behaviour analysis? In Kiernan, C. (ed.), *Research to Practice? Implications of Research on the Challenging Behaviour of People with Learning Disability*, BILD Publications, Clevedon, Avon

Slevin, E. (1995) A concept analysis of, and proposed new term for, challenging behaviour. *Journal of Advanced Nursing*, **21**, 928–934

Changing policies

Richard Servian

Introduction

How do people with learning difficulties and their advocates influence public policies toward their interests? How policies are influenced is a mystery to most people. This is reinforced through a false but widely-held perception that only certain people have a real right to influence policy. Front-line public servants such as therapists and people with learning difficulties are two groups who rarely see themselves as having this right. But even people who are perceived as appropriate to influence policy (like politicians) rarely are perceived as getting it right.

This chapter is presented in three parts. In the first, some important concepts are explored. In the second, some theoretical perspectives on the importance to personal well-being of being involved in policy formation are presented. The final section looks at how people with learning difficulties have changed policies and the possible role of the therapist in helping this process.

Concepts of democracy and policy

A major issue in a society that declares itself to be democratic is whether elected politicians or a policy élite make policy decisions, or whether the notion of living in a democratic society means that we need to recognize that we can influence policy. By democracy I mean a philosophy of inclusion: of adults participating in choosing how we are to be governed, in potentially being elected representatives, having their say or having some form of control over important influences in their lives. Advocacy is part of the tools that help us claim such rights. These are controversial issues. What democracy includes and what rights we have are not universally agreed. I suggest here that community care policies reflect that diffidence. People with learning difficulties who rely on such policies continue to need the advocacy tool.

What do I mean by 'policy'? Policies affecting people with learning difficulties exist in different forms in different places. Government departments of education, health, social security, and arts, all administer funds and activities that have an impact on people with learning difficulties. Influencing policy, at its crudest, is about influencing how government directs such activities. Policy is also about how laws are to be interpreted or the basis to new laws. Policy will also be formed and laws interpreted locally. Local Health Trusts and senior therapists will have their own interpretation of how laws or national government guidance are to be implemented and this is 'local policy'. The attempt here is to ask therapists to question how local and national policies affecting people with learning difficulties have been formed.

Frequently grand plans are presented as the answer to problems in society. Decentralization and the market are two of the current political solutions to a democratic deficit. Both are presented as improving the say that the individual has. In practice, it is frequently hard to see where individuals have a real say in important policy change. Rather, the grand plans attempt to reshape the individual. Railway passengers are now customers, social services clients are now service users, other public service users are now consumers. The public is reinvented according to the current view of policy makers on whether the public are consumers within a marketplace, users of handed-down services or active participants in a democratic society. As advocates we need to challenge the notion that individuals are merely victims or passive beneficiaries of dominant economic and political ideology and consider which ways they can influence policy and practice.

Theoretical perspectives on involvement in changing policies

Why should advocacy address policy?

A definition of advocacy proposed here is 'speaking up to empower'. There is a health warning about the term 'empowerment'. Empowerment has been a watchword of the last decade. It is not clear that this endeavour is always about empowering disabled people rather than a way government and other decision making is presented and legitimized.

Much of the history of the twentieth century has been around different languages of empowerment: from the universal franchise to civil rights legislation, from shopping to the internet, from improving industrial efficiency to rationing state resources, from financial investment to spiritual experience. The term empowerment has been used in all these contexts.

Not all of these can be said to be wholly about improving the lives of individuals, still less for less powerful individuals. Today's moves to decentralization in local government and markets in public services have been legitimized through notions of empowerment. In practice, many of these grand ideas refer to different perceptions of what empowerment is: perceptions that are not directed wholly or mainly toward people with learning difficulties.

It is not clear what is meant by empowerment. Servian (1996) identified 10 different meanings of the term 'empowerment'. He also argued that empowerment was related to an essential need for autonomy and as such was not something only sought by the powerless. If the new political big ideas superficially support notions of empowerment, there remains a need for people with learning difficulties to capture this concept.

Helplessness

The importance through advocacy of taking measures to improve the self-identity of people with learning difficulties may be seen alongside measures that improve their ability to have control over their lives. Neither are wholly political objectives but important issues for personal happiness. Having an impact on policy decisions affecting oneself is important both personally and politically.

Seligman's (1975) theory of learned helplessness is a theory originally around mental illness. Basically it holds that depression can be learned helplessness. Continued experience of not controlling particular events or being unable to control them, in the context of a tendency to blame oneself, itself a consequence of negative experiences, leads to the perception of not being able to control future events, and basically giving up trying to control them. It is suggested here that such a theory is useful in analysing why few individuals feel they are able to affect policy decisions.

Seligman suggested that there are responses that could be made. This included improving professional responses: reducing the likelihood of negative responses by improving positive outcomes to actions of the individual; to make better use of training and community development to change expectations from one of uncontrollability; understanding that the 'system' may be to blame, not you.

Power and advocacy

Power is a contested concept but is an important issue to understand, as many of the theories about power have been based on studies of how the policy process is influenced. Lukes (1974) saw three sets of theory around power. In the first dimension, power was seen as direct and observable and it was obvious who has caused a policy change. In the second, theories such as that of Bachrach and Baratz (1970) saw that there was also indirect power: issues were 'mobilized' off agendas. Those with power set the agendas; those without had difficulty being heard. Lukes himself added a third not directly observable dimension: people forced by ideology or by their inferior position in the workplace or home to act against their objective interests. Foucault's conception of power can be seen as a fourth dimension, as totalizing and forged through history, effectively dictating our thinking and behaviour.

One problem of all four sets of theory about power is the tendency to see individuals as victims without power rather than having power to influence events. Servian's (1996) study of stakeholders in a service for people with learning difficulties suggested that all stakeholders, including people with learning difficulties themselves, had ways of expressing some power. To some this was challenging behaviour. The study suggested that advocacy was seen as a valued way people with learning difficulties could recognize their power, but also that enabling therapists themselves to empower was important.

A study of power should make us aware of: where power lies; what tactics the powerful use to avoid issues of concern to people with learning difficulties; and the historical processes that have led to particular groups and individuals holding power.

The following is an attempt at a checklist for organizations and for advocates in confronting organizations to become user centred:

- For service users to feel they have some control over decisions.
- For there to be encouragement of users to participate in policy making and changing processes.
- For service users, and the social group of which they are part to feel valued as participants, not token members.
- For there to be encouragement to speak out, complain, participate in democratic processes.
- For choice to be real, not restricted by the market or proxies such as care managers according to rationing priorities.
- For meetings to operate on the basis of openness and equality of access both in terms of what the agenda is and the views and actions of the powerful.
- For all decisions to be open to view and challenge.

People with learning difficulties changing policies

The practice of changing policy

There has been a growing number of disabled people involving themselves in organizations of disabled people and attempting to change public policy in their interests. A national movement as described by Campbell and Oliver (1996) has been growing since the 1970s. It is only relatively recently that people with learning difficulties have began to be involved, through People First. Campaigning around the Disability Discrimination Act 1996 and more comprehensive but unsuccessful civil rights Bills has provided a focus for political action.

Identity and power have been key concepts for participants. Through involvement, positive identities for people with learning difficulties form. These replace traditional identities which are seen as negative, built around stigmatizing notions of disabled people as needing care, reliant on medical or social care professionals and incapable of making decisions of their own.

An early political success for People First was a change of the law to allow people with learning difficulties to become charity trustees and to form their own charity. They were also influential in the decision by government to drop the term 'mental handicap'.

For the Disabled People's Movement generally a strong distinction has been drawn between organizations *of* and those *for* disabled people. The latter, often well-known national charities, managed by non-disabled people, are seen as powerful in the lives of, and having gained wealth on the backs of, disabled people. The former are seen as more positive and controlled by disabled people themselves.

Charities and social care and medical professionals are seen as part of a culture which reinforces the medical or dependency model of disability. The development of a positive culture of people with learning difficulties has been tackled in many ways, through the development of drama, comedy and art alongside formal political action.

But for the lobbying and direct action of the Disabled People's Movement, there would be no Disability Discrimination Act (DDA).

Although the Act as it finally appeared was opposed by the movement as weak and without effective enforcement, the practice of successfully getting something on the statute book represents a major step forward from the ghetto of the medical model and the presumption of the need for professional control.

Current debate on the future of the welfare state is essential to the Disabled People's Movement. Traditionally, the state is seen as complicit in the oppression of disabled people. Oliver talks about 'agencies paid to control us and keep us down' (Campbell and Oliver, 1996: 201). At the same time the disability movement is lobbying for government to change its role to one of opposing discrimination through legislation and providing a minimum level of income that enables equality of opportunity.

The debate on the DDA raised a number of issues: is the prime issue for disabled people access to jobs or a wider issue of combating discrimination and changing attitudes? Should anti-discrimination legislation be restricted to what employers can afford or should both government and employers be compensating disabled people for years of discrimination?

A theme of debate in the Disabled People's Movement is 'does government disempower by intervening?' The issue may be not that state intervention is always bad but what form it takes. Changing policy at local level and attempts to tackle professional control over disabled people may be as important as national policy changes, particularly so to the majority of disabled people who are not involved in organizations but rely on local services.

Therapists and local policy

Power is an issue for therapists as it is for disabled people. In certain situations, therapists will be putting themselves in a difficult position by attempting to influence local policies and practices. While the NHS and Community Care Act 1990 was heralded by the Audit Commission (1992) as providing opportunities for empowerment of disabled people, strict contracts on the role of providers in practice may restrict the scope therapists have to be advocatorial. Advocacy may be restricted to choosing wallpaper rather than involvement in challenging local policy.

This should be seen as a reason why therapists should attempt to influence the policy of their organizations rather than a reason why they should do nothing. Some of the systems that have developed through the introduction of market mechanisms into health and social care potentially divorce the therapist's identification of a need for an advocatorial approach from what is allowed by the purchaser–provider divide. There remains a need for therapists to influence such policies.

Therapists being advocatorial is not new. The notion of normalization has been a central position for many therapists. It is also a notion that has been challenged as, for instance, trying to change the identity of people with learning difficulties to a narrow conception of normality. Developments in the concept have instead emphasized the need for people with learning difficulties to be valued. Therapists have played a large part in these policy changes, with the move away from institutions needed for change to be implemented. Dowson (1997) questions the extent to which policies of local health and social services have addressed the challenges to managerial and professional power implicit to modern formulations of normalization. Larger institutions are seen as replaced by smaller units with similar attitudes and power relationships. Residential care has been preferred to tenancies, and inspection systems and health and social care systems dominate the lives of people with learning difficulties in a way apart from notions of 'ordinary life'. The notion of professional power and domination is seen as continuing to reign unchecked.

Conclusion

In this chapter it has been argued that people with learning difficulties can and should be involved in the policy decisions that shape their lives. There is a major role for therapists in facilitating such involvement. There are examples of people with learning difficulties being helped by professionals to propose, for example, their own tenancy agreements (Servian, 1996) and successful self-advocacy through local People First groups (Simons, 1995).

These are constructive but isolated examples of challenges to traditional power relationships. Therapists are working in a context which is not as empowering of people with learning difficulties that the promises of Community Care policy make out.

I conclude by specifying some possible strategies for therapists in facilitating advocacy:

- enabling the self-advocacy of service users in describing and developing their preferred pattern of support;
- promoting organizational structures that do not reinforce existing discrimination;
- challenging traditions of professional power;
- enabling individuals to develop their own positive identities;
- questioning rather than automatically accepting local policies – do they enable power and identity of people with learning difficulties?
- questioning their own practice.

In essence, the role of the therapist goes beyond empowering people with learning difficulties, to the establishment of policies and processes of policy making within which people with learning difficulties are empowered to empower themselves.

References

Audit Commission (1992) *Community Care: Managing the Cascade of Change*, HMSO, London

Bachrach, P. and Baratz, M.S. (1970) *Power and Poverty*, Oxford University Press, Oxford

Campbell, J. and Oliver, M. (1996) *Disability Politics: Understanding our Past, Changing our Future*, Routledge, London

Dowson, S. (1997) Empowerment within services: a comfortable delusion. In Ramcharan, P. *et al.* (eds), *Empowerment in Everyday Life*, Jessica Kingsley, London

Lukes, S. (1974) *Power; A Radical View*, Macmillan, Basingstoke

Seligman, M.E.P. (1975) *Helplessness*, W.H. Freeman, San Francisco

Servian, R. (1996) *Theorising Empowerment: Individual Power and Community Care*, Policy Press, Bristol

Simons, K. (1995) *Standing Up For Yourself*, Joseph Rowntree Trust, York

Changing lives

Margaret Hutchinson

Incorporated throughout this chapter will be a composite case study written in dialogue form, of Jane, a woman with learning difficulties whose life has been affected by changing policies and her interaction with the professionals that enter her life. Jane's story will follow the history of learning difficulties and the continuities and changes will be traced as we move through her life stages.

Jane's story

Jane was born in 1943 during World War II. There was no help available and a difficult birth left Jane with brain damage. Her eyesight was very poor and she did not learn to walk or talk until she was 5 years old. She walked with a wide gait and was very unsteady. Her understanding and language were both limited. Jane's father was killed at the end of the war and her mother had five children before Jane was born. The local doctor thought Jane would receive better care in the large 'mental' hospital which had just become part of the National Health Service (1948):

> *Doctor* Jane will be much better off at Northlands, you know. She will be with people of her own kind. The staff will be specially trained. You can visit her whenever you wish. I really do think you should think about it.
>
> *Mrs Scott* Yes, doctor. I do find it very hard to manage.
>
> *Doctor* I'll arrange it then.

An ambulance duly arrived and Jane was taken to Northlands. Her mother waved her goodbye, and promised to visit her when the special bus ran from the nearby town once a month. Thus, at 5 years old, Jane began her lifelong relationship with professionals.

Ten years later (1958):

> *Sister White* Come on Jane, go down to the hall and see your mum and sister. It's visiting Saturday today. Don't get lost in the grounds on the way back. [Aside to Auxiliary Nurse Brown]: Her mum's not going to like how she looks now all her teeth have been taken out.
>
> *Nurse Brown* Well, we couldn't let her keep biting people – she was turning into a wild animal. She spent most of her time in the punishment

ward, locked up. She'll settle down now. Mary's still a good friend to her. It will be time for her enema when she comes back. So many of them need enemas now, I'm not sure why. At least we didn't need to use them when that last outbreak of dysentery swept through the ward.

Sister White   I think the food has something to do with it. We always have plenty of fruit when we get home but they don't ever have any. The food is so stodgy here.

Ten years later (1968):

Jane   Lots of people are getting out of here. Can I go?

Sister White   No, the 'high grades' are going out first, and those that don't cause any trouble. You will be way down the list. Mary will probably go to a hostel soon.

Ten years later (1978):

Sister White   Jane, it's your review tomorrow. The social worker, Mrs Leigh, will be coming, but as you're just settling into the hospital factory you won't have to come back to the ward for it. You don't want to do you? No, I didn't think so, it will be just the same as last year checking you've had your eyes tested and so on. Malcolm said you were doing quite well putting the cocktail sticks in the tubes at the factory.

Eight years later (1986). As more people with learning difficulties moved out of Northlands it soon became necessary for redeployment of staff to take place. Sister White took early retirement and Nurse Brown had taken an RNMH (Mental Handicap Nursing) course followed by a 'normalization' course and moved to a newly-opened Community Home as an officer-in-charge. The normalization course taught Nurse Brown that 'normalization' was an evolving idea:

> The utilization of means which are as culturally normative as possible in order to establish or support behaviours, appearances and characteristics which are as culturally normative as possible (Wolfensberger, 1972: 42).

Mary had moved to a hostel in 1975 and now joined this Community Home too, but Jane remained in the hospital. This was a dark, unsettled time for Jane as more and more people moved out; the men and women were put together on mixed wards; and later wards closed. She was moved three times to different wards within the hospital as the numbers contracted.

One year later (1987):

A different social worker   I see from your notes, Jane, that you want to move to a house with people you were friendly with some time ago.

Jane   Yes.

Social worker   Well, I am afraid that's not possible as there aren't any vacancies. How do you feel about going to a new place that is opening soon where you will live in a house next to a work placement? It is a new idea and you won't have to travel to your job. There is a vacancy in the green-house work placement. Do you like working with plants?

Jane   I don't know.

Social worker   Well, shall we go and have a look?

One year later (1988):

Yet another social worker [in a hurry]   Well, Jane, at last the day has come. You will be moving to your new home at Carelands. Oh! Did the nurses not tell you – I've come to collect you. Quickly, let's put your things in a bag and we can go in the car now. Oh dear! No bag. I'll go and get a bin liner. Come on, Jane, don't get upset now, there will be lots of nice people there. You went to visit some time ago, didn't you? What did you think of it?

Jane [close to tears]   I didn't like the man who was in the greenhouse

Social worker   He won't be there now – they've had a change since you had a look round. Come on, I'll go and find someone and tell them you are going.

There were many community schemes like Carelands at this time. They were often positioned outside a town, and incorporated a horticultural/craft workshop with adjoining terrace houses (10 or so), each built for four people to share. The home care managers tried to minimize institutionalization by using community-based professionals to be involved with the residents.

Fragmentation of the workforce

In 1987 the government had given the 14 Regional Health Authorities in Britain over £200 million to develop community services to move people with learning difficulties out of long-stay hospitals.

As Jane's story moves towards the 1990s the NHSCC Act also becomes implemented. For the NHS this meant 'opting out' of hospitals from Regional Health Authority management, who, for 40 years, had a watching brief over long-stay and all other hospitals. Individual hospitals or groups of two or three nearby hospitals became self-managing Trusts. It was a method of breaking up the service into more manageable segments. The NHSCC Act 1990 recognized and endorsed the growing awareness that large hospitals were not a suitable home for people with disabilities, and large-scale 'resettlement' ensued with many long-stay hospitals closing down.

Support services were the first to be put to competitive tendering (even before the Act was implemented) and ancillary staff moved away from the NHS. Many private contractors chose not to recognize the existing health unions. In order to win the contracts the costs were drastically cut; wages went down to already low-paid (mostly female) staff and these staff lost their security of tenure (i.e. pension and sickness rights):

The long term effects of this will be a lowering of standards, as at any one time there will be a higher turnover of staff; higher proportion of new/trainee employees and a lowering of workforce morale as there is less loyalty to the job. (Fletcher, 1989: 27)

This contracting out of services also affected Social Services provision, as the NHSCC Act 1990 enforced the purchaser – provider split. This meant that day and residential services were purchased by a care manager. This introduction of markets and quasi-markets into social care indicated a tendency towards cost saving and decentralization which fitted the model of flexible work patterns. Social services departments became 'enablers' rather than providers. They still often remain the 'lead agency', but increasingly in services for people with learning disability NHS nurses are becoming care managers. Thus, the blurring of social work/nursing roles which happened in long-stay hospitals, is happening again in Community Services.

The establishment of internal markets within the public sector is a rejection of the administrative state. Proper procedures count for less than efficiency in outputs and outcomes, and intangible values connected with the public sector receive less attention. The new demands for increased efficiency in the public sector might counterbalance the strides this sector has achieved in equal opportunities and creating effective relationships between policy makers and service users.

Jane's story continued (1989)

She is very depressed in Carelands and her mental health deteriorates rapidly – she talks to herself constantly. She has a four-month return to Northlands' psychiatric ward and while there, Carelands (owned by the NHS) is sold to a private company. The owner is keen to convert the residential houses into craft workshops and move the residents into staffed community houses in the nearby town – so they can travel to work, rather than live on-site. Jane is approached by the new owner's home-care manager, Mr Roy Carter:

Mr. Carter   Jane, I know you didn't live at Carelands very long and you weren't very happy there, but how would you like to live in the town close by with Jim and Dorothy? We have a new girl now called Mary, who used to live at Northlands and she says she wants to live in your house when you come back.

Jane   Yes, I used to know Mary. We were friends for years at the hospital, but she moved out so long ago and I've never seen her since. I've never forgotten her though – I used to ask to move into her house every day, but no one listened to me.

One week later:

Mary: I am so pleased to see you, Jane. I used to ask the staff in the home to let me go back and see you and they wouldn't let me. They said I would get upset going back to that place and wouldn't settle in the new house.

Jane I am so pleased to see you too. I wanted to write to you but the nurses were always so busy to help me send a letter to you. I can't wait to see this house. Have you seen it?

Mary No, not yet, but Mr Carter has brought some curtain material and wallpaper books for us to look at so we can choose our own. We can also go shopping for our bedroom furniture later on. Sister White wouldn't believe it.

Jane's mood began to lift and she enjoyed the preparations for the new move. She was consulted and involved in the arrangements this time and she looked forward to living in this new house, with Mary in the next bedroom. They soon picked up their friendship which had been broken for so many years. The owner and staff at the new privately-run Carelands scheme were very imaginative in their approach to running the scheme. They actively listened to the residents; spent much time with them; and discovered many different day activities for people with learning disabilities to pursue. Self-advocacy groups within the scheme helped Jane to speak up for herself. She felt happy spending so much time with Mary and the two women learnt new independent living skills. The staff were stable because they enjoyed their work and received good job satisfaction supporting a small number of people in their key-worker group. Mr Carter made sure the residents did not have to attend large reviews of the type to which Jane had been subjected when Carelands first opened. He made sure that informal reviews, involving only three or four people who were most important to the person, were held regularly to ensure that the person's needs were being met as fully as possible. Jane enjoyed these meetings with Mr Carter, Joanne, her key-worker, and Lesley, her care manager. They were able to work out many plans together and take as much time as necessary. Mr Carter made sure that the plans were put into action and Jane really trusted his judgement and ability to make things happen for her.

Jane's life – still improved but other problems (1997)

Jane I do wish Roy (Carter) was still here. He is a real miss.

Mary Yes, I don't think he really wanted to move to Manchester. Joanne and Leslie going at the same time was a real blow, too.

Jane None of the new staff seem to know us very well and they never stay five minutes.

Mary Yes, it's a good job we've got each other now, or we would really feel lonely. I cried the other day because I missed Joanne.

If Mr Carter had stayed he may have engaged Citizen Advocates to support Jane and Mary. Citizen Advocacy has developed in parallel to the self-advocacy movement. It aims to promote an independent form of representation for people with learning difficulties through a competent citizen volunteer or employee, who, with the support of an independent citizen advocacy agency, represents as if they were his/her own, the interests of one or two people with learning difficulties. This role may last for life.

Changing work patterns – the influence on teamworking

Since the 1950s, staff working with people with learning difficulties have been employed by a local authority, i.e. Social Services Department or Health Authority. Since the NHSCC Act 1990, the purchaser–provider split has given the purchasers (local authority care managers) the power to purchase care for people with learning difficulties. This can include a package of care that encompasses many resources from a range of providers. These providers can come from the voluntary sector or private companies. Increasingly, staff in provider organizations are working on short fixed-term contracts.

Halting the rising tide of fixed-term contracts and improving the conditions of those already on them are the key targets of major campaigns by unions against 'casualization' of the workforce. The percentage of staff on fixed-term contracts is rising steadily and some local authorities, voluntary organizations and private care companies have stopped issuing any permanent contracts whatsoever.

For people with learning difficulties, Citizen Advocacy may be the way forward and the way to overcome the problems of an unstable workforce caused by this 'flexible' workforce trend.

The purchaser–provider split in Social Services has encouraged the private and voluntary sectors to purchase their provider units. These are either day or residential services and gradually in the 1990s people with learning difficulties and older people have been moved around to fit into these new services. Some Social Services units have closed altogether and others (like Carelands) have been taken over by private or voluntary organizations. The increased use of short-term contracts, sometimes as little as two months' duration, is causing staff to move much more regularly than in previous years. Regular shortages of staff often causes managers to use a 'bank' system whereby staff are brought in for busy hours or days. These staff do not know the people for whom they are caring or with whom they are working, and mistakes and inconsistencies of care prevail. Good teamwork is impossible.

The future and conclusion

For Jane, the future only looks bright if she can establish stability and continuity in the multidisciplinary teams who support her life and has some control over her services.

She does not wish to return to living with large numbers of people in an institution where she had no voice, even though the staff were stable. Neither does she wish to live in a small community house with huge numbers of professionals gathering at an annual review, planning her life on her behalf. Nor does she wish to be supported by a disintegrating team of people who are constantly changing and do not know her individual needs and who are discontented with no living wage or security of tenure.

The alternative future could be to empower Jane, with the help of a few trusted people or a Citizen Advocate, so she controls her own services with an individual budget which will purchase her own individual care.

References

Fletcher, R. (1989) Competitive tendering of NHS ancillary services. In Ormiston, H. and Ross, D.M. (eds), *New Patterns of Work*, St Andrew Press, Edinburgh

Wolfensberger, W. (1972) *The Principle of Normalization in Human Services*, National Institute on Mental Retardation, Toronto

Part III

Towards Partnership: The Practice of Therapy

Reflective practice and practitioner research

Maureen Gillman

Introduction

This chapter discusses the relevance of reflective practice and practitioner research for therapists working with people with learning difficulties. Professional practice in this field necessitates an awareness of the structural inequalities, institutional discrimination, and oppression, experienced by people with learning difficulties and the extent to which this oppression is inextricably woven into professional discourses and their associated practices (Gillman *et al.*, 1997). By virtue of their professional training and societal recognition of their 'expertise', professionals have the power to assess and categorize people with learning difficulties in order to define treatment and prognosis. Many theories and models of practice are based on the individual or medical model of impairment. They are concerned with achieving independence, or overcoming adversity or deviance in order to measure up to societal norms (Gillman, 1996).

Reflective practice can help therapists 'deconstruct' practice at a number of levels. White defines deconstruction as

> ... procedures that subvert taken-for-granted realities and practices; those so called truths that are split off from the conditions and the context of their production; those embodied ways of speaking that hide their biases and prejudices; and those familiar practices of self and relationship that are subjugating of persons' lives. Many of the methods of deconstruction render strange these familiar and every day taken-for-granted realities by objectifying them. (1993: 34)

At the personal level, reflective practice can help therapists examine the beliefs and values they bring to their practice for signs of stereotypical thinking or prejudice. At a professional level, it can provide a framework for evaluating theories and models of practice in terms of their potential to discriminate against, oppress or marginalize people with learning difficulties. It can help practitioners construct models of practice informed by notions of social justice, and based on collaboration and partnership with people with learning difficulties. At an institutional level, reflective practice can help therapists identify aspects of discrimination within their own agencies: for example, the exclusion of people with learning difficulties from some services or 'treatments' and the inaccessibility of written information or instructions.

Reflective practice can lead to the identification of issues which may form the basis of 'practitioner research'. Such issues have the advantage of being grounded in practice and therefore the outcomes of such research may be more meaningful to practitioners and their patients than that which is generated by 'outsider-researchers'. The term 'practitioner research' can refer to a wide range of activities from case studies an narrative approaches to larger scale projects which seek the views of a number of respondents across a variety of settings. Reflective practice is an important component of the research process. Reed and Procter suggest that there are two types of reflexivity in practitioner research: first there are the practitioner's immediate responses to the research setting which are largely a product of practitioner knowledge. The second type of reflexivity involves a contemplative response which promotes an active questioning of the assumptions behind the immediate responses (1995: 47).

Practitioner research is valuable because it generates knowledge that is grounded in practice. It encourages therapists to develop a critical awareness of practice and research and can also give a voice to a marginalized group who are rarely heard in the research arena (Booth and Booth, 1996).

What is reflective practice?

Reflective practice is the capacity of a practitioner to think, talk or write about a piece of practice with the intention to *re*view or *re*search the interaction with clients/patients and other stakeholders for new meanings, 'theories' or perspectives upon the situation. The expectation is that such reflection on practice will develop and enhance practitioner skill and competence and produce 'knowledge' that is grounded in practice. In addition, it will heighten the practitioner's awareness of the potential of some forms of practice to oppress, marginalize or exclude people with learning difficulties.

Reflective practice involves a process of 'reflexivity', which Mead (1982) described as 'A turning back of one's experience upon oneself.' When practice is experienced by the therapist as unsatisfactory, there is a tendency to view the patient as 'difficult' or 'uncooperative'. Reflective practice provides a 'self-referential' framework for examining what part the therapist played in creating or maintaining difficulties and for identifying what they might do differently in future.

Reflective practice can be carried out in a number of ways; one method suggested by Fook (1996) is to 're-search' a piece of interaction, an interview, or an observation by writing a short account of the incident and asking questions such as:

● What major issues emerge from the account?
● How did your interpretations influence the situation?

- How might the situation have been interpreted differently by someone else?
- Whose voices are missing or marginalized in your account?
- Whose interests are best served by the account?
- What questions arise about your practice as a result of this reflection?
- How might your practice now change?

For a more comprehensive list of questions the reader is advised to see Fook (1996).

Reflection can also be conducted in conjunction with colleagues and Fook suggests that 'There is potential for such an approach to be used for self learning, supervision and peer supervision' (1996: 6).

The exercise described above can also be undertaken with colleagues or managers as part of staff development or supervision. Many therapists find it easier to reflect 'in conversation' with others, rather than alone. The process of reflecting is predominantly seen as something that professionals do (either alone or together). However, Andersen (1987, 1990) has developed an approach in which professionals reflect in the presence of those who consult them and then invite patients to reflect upon their reflections. The reflecting team approach requires that therapists work with one or more colleagues. The therapist works directly with the patient, and the colleague(s) observe the practice either in the same room or behind a one-way screen. The reflecting team listens and observes the session with the patient and then the patient is invited to listen to the team (or the co-worker and therapist) as they reflect upon what has been seen or heard. The patient is then invited to share their reflections on the conversation between the professionals. Reflecting team processes encourage the patient to have a voice and perhaps an influence on what is usually regarded as professional territory. It also allows patients to listen to what professionals have to say about them and it can therefore be argued that it is more equitable than the usual supervision process. Finally, it provides an opportunity for the voicing of multiple perspectives on a situation, including the patient's.

One use of reflective practice is to question the assumptions underpinning and shaping practice. De Bono (1979) asserts that perceptions, or what we choose to see, are based on assumptions. They act as boundaries and help us decide what part of a phenomenon to take into account and what to ignore. The assuming process occurs at an unconscious level and, as such, rarely gets challenged. Reflective practice can play a part in making these assumptions conscious.

This may take the form of questioning one's own assumptions about a patient or a situation. For example, reflecting on the ways in which a diagnostic label such as 'cerebral palsy' may have organized one's communication with the patient. That is, the extent to which assumptions about cognitive impairment may have been used as a justification for offering little explanation about treatment, or not recognizing the patient's ability and right to choose. Research has shown that having a stake in the decision-making process about treatment and rehabilitation is associated with its ultimate success. Mattingly found that

> The patients had to see something at stake in therapy. Otherwise why should they bother to try? If the patient did not try, therapy did not work. This was partly because the therapist required the patient to do things in therapy that the patient did not necessarily feel ready to do or believe to be worth the effort. (1991: 1002)

Practitioner assumptions about a patient's inability to understand or communicate may be more influential in preventing proper negotiation over treatment than the actual cognitive impairment!

Reflective practice can also be useful in questioning the value of formal theories of practice in some situations. Schön (1983) argues that technical rationality based on formal theories of practice are insufficient for good professional practice. The complexities of 'real life' situations often do not lend themselves to the application of theoretical frameworks and techniques and practitioners must then rely on practice knowledge and intuition for guidance. For example, Mattingly, discussing the clinical reasoning of occupational therapists, suggests that 'General treatment goals derived from general knowledge of functional deficits and developmental possibilities were insufficient guides to practice' (1991: 1001). She asserts that therapists must understand the patient's experience of disability (and not just the technical details of impairment) in order to achieve therapeutic goals.

Schön (1983) also notes that there is often a discrepancy between the theories that practitioners espouse (theory-in-use) and what they actually do in practice (theory-in-action). Practitioners may feel inadequate if they are not using formal theories or models to organize their practice. Practitioners construct new theories related to unique cases and situations, yet such 'practice knowledge' is often perceived as inferior to formal theory and technical rationality. As a consequence, many formal theories go unchallenged. Professional theories and practices are seldom deconstructed for their devaluing assumptions about people with learning difficulties. For example, Bender (1993) notes that it is almost impossible for people with learning difficulties to access counselling and psychotherapy services based on the assumption that they lack the insight or verbal skills to benefit from 'talking treatments'. Such assumptions have led to the proliferation and dominance of drug treatments and behavioural techniques (Gillman et al., 1997).

Another example is the theory of rehabilitation, which is an influential discourse in the training of physio- and occupational therapists. The theory is underpinned by the view that people want to be independent, self-sufficient and as 'normal' as possible. Health and welfare professionals tend to perceive physical independence as a central aim of the rehabilitation process (French, 1994). Spencer and colleagues note

> It is important to recognize that not all persons practice or value the personal independence we tend to expect of clients in occupational therapy. (1993: 307)

French (1994) argues that independence is not always in the best interest of a disabled person. She cites Corbett (1989) who describes how people with severe learning difficulties can actually regress if independence is forced upon them.

Dickerson and Zimmerman (1995) have designed a reflective exercise to assist practitioners to understand the effects of thinking about problems from a number of different perspectives. Here the exercise has been adapted to help therapists reflect upon how taking certain positions can organize not only therapist's actions, but also those of the patient or other stakeholders.

Consider the following diagnoses:

- challenging behaviour
- cerebral palsy
- severe learning disability

Taking each diagnosis separately, answer the following questions:

1 What effects does the diagnosis have upon the way you think about the person?
2 What effects might this diagnosis have upon the way the person thinks about herself?
3 What effects does this diagnosis have upon the way you feel you have to respond to the patient?

The next step is to reconstruct the diagnosis as a relational pattern. For example, challenging behaviour as a pattern of frustration, aggression, rejection between the patient and the relative/professional, or in severe learning disability as a pattern of low expectations, low achievement. Then answer the following questions:

What effects does thinking about the diagnosis in relational terms have upon:

(a) The way you think about the person?
(b) The way the person thinks about herself?
(c) The way you feel you have to respond to the person?

Next, think about what dominant cultural discourses might be influencing the situation. For example, the notion that people with learning difficulties are perpetual children and are asexual; or that people with severe learning difficulties are unable to make choices for themselves; or that people with learning difficulties should strive to be as 'normal' as possible. Now answer the same questions again.

Dickerson and Zimmerman found that the implications of seeing the problem as a medical diagnosis located the problem within the person and prompted the therapist to view the person as the target for change in terms of strategies such as behaviour management, and control. This had the effect of disempowering the person while placing the power in the hands of the therapist (1995: 39). Foucault (1977) asserted that the professional disciplines characterize, classify and hierarchize individuals and that such 'disciplinary power' manifests itself in the practices of observation, assessment and diagnosis. Through such practices, people with learning difficulties are often problematized and their lives are defined by treatment plans, behavioural programmes and medication (Gillman *et al.*, 1997).

Dickerson and Zimmerman also found that the effect of constructing problems as patterns was to encourage the perception of problems as separate from the patient. It allowed therapists to notice other opportunities and contexts for intervention, such as the relationship between carer and patient, or the influence of the values and beliefs of significant others on maintaining problematic communication. Therapists were also alerted to the part they may have played in the situation.

> Therapists were alerted to ways they might be behaving with their clients that were not dissimilar to the ways other people in the client's world would behave. They [therapists] became less blaming and more interested in whatever context might have created the problem for the system. (1995: 40)

The construction of the problem in terms of cultural discourses helped the therapist to attend to and appreciate the experiences of the patient. It allowed the therapist to see how dominant societal ideas and norms shape identity and justify excluding and marginalizing practices, thus preventing the patient from achieving their desired lifestyle.

The reflective exercise adapted from that which was developed by Dickerson and Zimmerman (1995), and presented in this chapter, demonstrates the power of dominant discourses such as medical diagnosis, cultural norms and professional models of practice, to construe meaning and shape the actions of stakeholders involved in the enterprise of therapy. It shows that therapists can choose to adopt a variety of 'positions' in the therapeutic process: 'We have a need not only to make sense, . . . but to create sense out of situations' (Mattingly, 1994: 812). Some of these positions are more empowering and collaborative than others. White suggests that

> Therapists can contribute to the deconstruction of expert knowledge by considering themselves to be co-authors of alternative and preferred knowledges and practices, and through a concerted effort to establish a context in which the persons who seek therapy are privileged as the primary authors of those knowledges and practices. (1993: 56–57)

What is practitioner research?

Practitioner research is concerned with issues and problems that arise in practice and that are identified by practitioners themselves. It aims to bring about change, or influence policy in the practice arena. Some common concerns investigated by the researcher/practitioner include: deficiencies in services or resources; conflict between professional values and agency requirements; the impact of innovation or change; the improvement of practice; and the development of practice knowledge.

Reed and Proctor argue that practitioners cannot develop knowledge by simply being in practice for a long time. They suggest that

> Attentive practice . . . is more than simply paying attention to puzzling, unexpected or striking events but involves further contemplation and exploration. (1995: 52)

Practitioner research provides a framework for formulating practice knowledge and allows such knowledge to be disseminated to colleagues, agencies and other professionals. Formalizing practitioner knowledge through research enhances professional credibility and strengthens the influence of practice knowledge in the policy-making arena. Fuller and Petch argue that research can also enhance professional development

> . . . the practitioner, who has acquired research skills and the critical antennae which develop alongside them, will be a more complete professional, better able to challenge organizational or political constraints. . . . (1995: 7)

Many of the skills and competencies associated with practice are transferable to the conduct of research. Practitioners are trained to engage with people in a respectful and meaningful way and to enable patients to communicate their needs and wants. Reed and Proctor (1995) assert that 'Every day, practitioners collect information, develop understanding and create theories which are directed to their practice and are derived from it' (1995: 55).

Such activities are also central to the conduct of research. In addition, practitioners bring professional ethics and values to the research act which can help guard against the exploitation of research participants and ensure that the voices of the researched are represented.

Reflexivity and practitioner research

Hasselkus asserts that

> Each of us as a researcher is 'positioned' in relation to that which we are researching. This positioning is the lens through which every researcher sees his or her research. (1997: 81)

While practitioner knowledge is regarded as an asset in the conduct of practitioner research, it can also be seen as a source of bias that could invalidate it. The researcher practitioner role is potentially confusing for all those involved in the process. For example, the subjects of the research may find it difficult to distinguish between the therapist-as-researcher and the therapist-as-practitioner and may feel puzzled by a therapist's unwillingness to take up a therapeutic concern during a research interview. Similarly, a researcher may find it very difficult to distinguish between the questions that are meant to be about 'collecting data' and those which are aimed at promoting change. Practitioner researchers sometimes feel uneasy about using practice knowledge and insight in their analysis of data, while respondents may well divulge information to a practitioner researcher, on the basis of a close, therapeutic relationship, that they may not have given to a 'researcher'. Swain and colleagues argue that ethical dilemmas in research cannot be dealt with solely by 'ethical codes or even predetermined good practice' (1998: 21). They conclude that

> ... ethical dilemmas and decision making pervade the whole research process ... the lived experiences of participants cannot be divorced from the responsibilities of researchers or from researcher/interviewee relationships. (1998: 34)

Research has the potential to exploit vulnerable groups in society and this can occur under the cloak of the rhetoric of empowerment. Practitioner researchers need to examine their research practice in order to identify whose interests and concerns are being served. Reed and Proctor argue that:

> Practitioner researchers must make explicit their position and the attendant concerns, interests and views that they have so that they can be debated not only by research participants and readers but also by themselves. (1995: 54)

The dilemmas discussed above are exacerbated by the dominant view that researchers should adopt a position of neutrality and objectivity. Post-modernist challenges to positivist ways of researching suggest that it is neither possible nor desirable to do objective, value-free research (Lather, 1991). Social constructionist researchers argue that the findings of research say as much about the researchers as they do about the researched (Atkinson and Heath, 1991). The researcher's biases are inextricably woven into the conduct and findings of research. Such biases are shaped by dominant professional and cultural knowledges or discourses (Burr, 1995), and language practices such as the norms and rules of thinking and writing (Lather, 1991).

Vernon emphasizes the importance of adopting a reflexive stance in disability research:

> Reflexivity, the examination of the ways in which the researcher's own social identity and values affect the data gathered and the picture of the social world produced, is a critical exercise for those researching the experience of oppression. (1997: 159)

More attention needs to be paid to the interpretation of meaning in research; the process of research then becomes a legitimate focus of inquiry in its own right. A reflexive stance needs to be adopted throughout the research process so that researchers can challenge the taken-for-granted assumptions embedded in its production. Rather than 'controlling' for bias, Hasselkus (1997) argues that valuing bias is the only way to make sense of the world.

Research methodology and method

In the last decade, the Disability Movement has argued that disabled people who are the 'subjects' of research are rarely consulted about the topics or issues to be researched, or involved in any meaningful way in the conduct of research and the subsequent knowledge production

(French, 1994; Oliver, 1992). The exclusion of disabled people from research has led to the production of distorted and oppressive findings and the development of inappropriate services. In addition, it has maintained the perception of disability as an individual's 'problem' (French, 1994; Oliver, 1996). Research is usually carried out by the powerful on the powerless and can be a source of maintaining or exacerbating marginalization and oppression (Oliver, 1994). Booth and Booth (1996) argues that people with learning difficulties are frequently the 'subject' of research, but rarely the informants. One reason is that they are not seen as good sources of quotable data because of prejudicial assumptions that people with learning difficulties are poor communicators. Research methods, such as interviewing, privilege the articulate and professionals and carers are often asked to speak for people with learning difficulties. Booth and Booth (1996) challenges this view and suggests that researchers need to adapt their methods so that the voices of people with learning difficulties can be heard in the research arena. Atkinson puts forward the view that

> There is a growing interest in and literature about qualitative research with people with learning difficulties. . . . The conscious move away from hierarchical research relationships and the involvement of participants in studies of their lives have opened up opportunities for people to talk about themselves in an atmosphere that is both constructive and enabling. (1993: 60).

Practitioner reflexivity is just as central to the process and conduct of research with people with learning difficulties as it is to practice within this field. Indeed, Schön suggests that practice and research are inextricably linked through the process of reflection: 'When someone reflects-in-action, he becomes a researcher in the practice context' (1993: 20). Adopting a reflective approach to research allows the practitioner to question the power relations of the process, and influences the choice of research method:

> A reflective approach affirms the importance of experiential and interconnected ways of knowing the world, and favours more emancipatory and participatory research practices. (Fook, 1996: 5).

Disabled people's organizations have proposed an emancipatory and participatory paradigm for disability research (Zarb, 1992). Briefly, participatory research requires that researchers work in partnership with disabled people at every stage of the research process. Disabled people would therefore be involved in generating the topic or issue to be researched; they would have a say in who should be researched, and what methods should be used; they would be involved in the process of analysing the data and the dissemination of 'results'. Zarb (1992) suggests that participatory research is a prerequisite for emancipatory research which must be empowering for disabled people and must address disabled peoples' struggle to overcome oppression. The emancipatory paradigm requires researchers to adopt a non-hierarchical approach to research by, for example, being prepared to share as much information about themselves as they require from the researched. The emancipatory paradigm requires researchers to seek opportunities for self-reflection and mutual understanding between the researcher and disabled people.

The emancipatory and participatory paradigm has challenged traditional ways of conducting research. Writers in the field of disability research recognize the constraints on researchers, such as the interests and priorities of those who are funding research, and the dominant discourses of objectivity and value-free research in academia and the world of work (Oliver and Barnes, 1997). However, French points out that 'practitioners are in a unique position to involve disabled people in research which affects their lives' (1994: 144). Therapists who undertake practitioner research can measure the extent that their research with people with learning difficulties is empowering to participants by answering the following questions taken from French:

1 Who controls what the research is about and how it is done?
2 How far are disabled people involved in the research process?
3 Can disabled people influence future directions?
4 Are there pathways by which disabled people can be critical of the research?
5 Does the research have the potential to empower disabled people? (1994: 144–145).

The emancipatory and participatory paradigms are an overarching framework which can be used to inform research practice and evaluate the process at each stage for signs of oppression and discrimination. A common assumption is that positivist methods have more potential to oppress than interpretivist or qualitative approaches. However, Oliver (1992) argues that qualitative research can be just as alienating as a positivist approach if it is carried out by a group of powerful 'experts' on powerless subjects.

One method of research which is particularly relevant to people with learning difficulties and accessible to practitioner/researchers is narrative and life story approaches. Widdershoven (1993) suggests that life is a story put into practice and that in order to make sense of life, individuals need to have access to the 'stock of stories' that constitute a life. Individuals tell stories about their lives in order to make sense of their lives, and lack or loss of this 'stock of stories' is particularly prevalent for people with learning difficulties who have lost touch with relatives and community (Gillman *et al.*, 1997). There is a growing interest in the use of narrative research across a range of disciplines (Wilkins, 1993; Booth and Booth, 1996; Clark *et al.*, 1997). Narrative research aims to give voice to the silenced or subjugated stories of marginalized groups in society and includes methods such as life history (Rosenthal, 1993; Di Terlizzi, 1994), oral history (Atkinson, 1993) and autobiography (Gergen and Gergen, 1993).

Researchers (and practitioners) are storytellers but, from a social constructionist position, stories are not 'discovered' but constructed (White, 1993, Mattingly, 1991)

Research findings about people with learning difficulties tend to be problem-saturated stories which do not reflect or celebrate the achievements of the research subjects. Narrative research can reverse this process by allowing people with learning difficulties to 're-author' their life stories (White, 1993) and to bring forth the silenced 'counter-plots' of their lives (Gillman *et al.*, 1997). For example, Atkinson describes an oral history project in which she worked collaboratively with a group of people with learning difficulties to record their lived experience. Discussing the rewards and benefits of the venture she states:

> Being an oral historian and contributing to a written history have brought other, less tangible, rewards to the people concerned. Their new roles have increased self confidence and an enhanced sense of self. It is, of course, important to reclaim one's past and have that acknowledged, but to have that past put into a written format which can be shown and shared, is to gain full recognition as a person who matters (1993: v)

Another example of a piece of narrative research is a study that was carried out by a practitioner who was undertaking a Master's degree (Bird, 1997). She conducted a piece of practitioner research with an adolescent boy who has learning difficulties. During her therapeutic practice with Bill (fictitious name), she noticed that he enjoyed telling stories about himself and his family and friends and also invited her to tell him stories about himself and those who worked with him in the therapeutic context. The researcher and Bill decided to record some of these stories in a 'life story book' that would be owned by Bill. He would also have control over who had access to his story. The 'professional' story (case history) was problem saturated in that it spoke of his deficiencies and his 'challenging behaviour'. Some parts of this problem-saturated story had also been adopted by his family, but they also had another story which was constructed on Bill's ability to realize his potential and his desired lifestyle. This story shaped the family's behaviour and their passion to help Bill achieve in a host of different ways.

The construction of the life story book involved Bill and the researcher in visiting places that had emotional significance for Bill. Other stories spoke of achievement and success in ventures that were important to Bill. Eventually, Bill and the researcher decided the book was complete and Bill shared the book with family members. The researcher observed in her thesis that the research had contributed to the family's and the professionals' understanding of Bill's behaviour and gave him a voice to influence the direction of his life.

Such approaches fall within the parameters of the emancipatory paradigm, as they are empowering to those involved and reflect the lived experience of the respondents. Shakespeare *et al.* (1993) observe that

> Recounting is necessarily a self-reflective process and may lead to important changes. People, through reflection, may develop insight and awareness, an enhanced sense of self and, perhaps, some useful self-advocacy skills. (1993: 6)

In keeping with the sentiments of this chapter, the voices of people with learning difficulties themselves will have the last word. The following is taken from a report of a collaborative research project between an able-bodied researcher and people with learning difficulties at the University of Northumbria at Newcastle (UNN). The participatory project emerged from another piece of research that was looking at the autonomy of young adults with learning difficulties (Newman, 1995). A research committee was set up comprising an able-bodied researcher and four people with learning difficulties who had participated in the original research project. The committee participants were involved in interviewing, analysis of data and the production of a written report. One of the participants comments:

> We all wanted different things from the research when we started. We all wanted to try and make people's lives a bit better. Some of us wanted to do this by looking at care plans and others felt the interviews might help. We also wanted to gain independence for ourselves and be respected as people with learning difficulties doing their own research. (Fothergill *et al.*, 1996: 4)

The following comments from the participants about their experience of doing research are taken from the report:

> I interviewed people and helped them think about care plans. I enjoyed doing the interviews best. I felt good helping others and proud that I could do it. (1996: 3)
>   When we first started on our interviews we found it quite difficult for the interviewees to answer the questions they were being asked. So we came up with the idea of using photographs for them to answer questions to. When the interviewees were shown these photographs and were asked questions about them they gave us a much more clear and understanding answer to them. It did take me some time to get these photographs taken but I enjoyed it. ... I went on to take photographs when I started my job. (1996: 18)

And finally:

> I would like to say how important I felt being part of a research project at a university. People didn't think I could do it and I proved them wrong. (1996: 37)

Conclusion

This chapter has attempted to make connections between practice and research by arguing that reflexivity is central to both activities. Research and practice inform each other and share many common features and goals. Practitioner research is important because it is grounded in the everyday world of practice and can reflect the voices of stakeholders in that context. Furthermore, therapists tend to work in isolation and sharing examples of good practice in such circumstances is difficult. Practitioner research offers a framework for disseminating practitioner knowledge across a range of contexts and professional groups. The chapter has also attempted to demystify research by challenging the notion of objective, value-free research. Reed and Procter observe

> Perhaps practitioner knowledge is knowledge which, because it has not been derived through research, is not seen as making an acceptable contribution to research. This undervaluing of practitioner knowledge is more a reflection of practitioners' ideas of research itself. (1995: 59)

To be of value, research does not have to be large scale or 'scientific'. Methods such as case study and narrative approaches are familiar territory for practitioners and are more emancipatory than those methods which do not give patients a voice. In addition, the products of this kind of research are more accessible to practitioners because they are written by and for practitioners.

All research has potential to oppress and exploit respondents if attention is not paid to the imbalances of power between researchers and researched, and the vested interests of those undertaking research. The emancipatory and participatory paradigms represent an overarching framework for informing the conduct, and evaluating the products of practitioner research with people who have learning difficulties.

References

Andersen, T. (1987) The reflecting team: dialogue and meta-dialogue in clinical work. *Family Process*, **26**, 415–428

Andersen, T. (1990) *The Reflecting Team: Dialogues and Dialogues about Dialogues*, Borgmann, Broadstairs

Atkinson, B. and Heath, A. (1991) Qualitative research and the legitimisation of knowledge. *Journal of Marital and Family Therapy*, **24**, 161–166

Atkinson, D. (ed.) (1993) *Past Times. People with Learning Difficulties Look Back on their Lives*, Open University Press, London

Bender, M.P. (1993) The unoffered chair. *Clinical Psychology Forum*, **34**, 7–12

Bird, E. (1997) Unpublished Master's dissertation. University of Northumbria at Newcastle

Booth T. and Booth, W. (1996) Sounds of silence: narrative research with inarticulate subjects. *Disability and Society*, **11**, 55–69

Burr, V. (1995) *An Introduction to Social Constructionism*, Routledge, London

Clark, F., Carlson, M. and Polkinghorn, D. (1997) The legitimacy of life history and narrative approaches in the study of occupation. *American Journal of Occupational Therapy*, **51**, 313–317

Corbett, J. (1989) Cited in French, S. (1994) *On Equal Terms: Working with Disabled People*, Butterworth-Heinemann, Oxford

De Bono, E. (1979) *Future Positive*, Penguin, London

Di Terlizzi, M. (1994) Life history: the impact of a changing service provision on an individual with learning disabilities. *Disability and Society*, **9**, 501–517

Dickerson, V.C. and Zimmerman, J.L. (1995) A constructionist exercise in anti-pathologising. *Journal of Systemic Therapies*, **14**, 33–44

Fook, J. (ed.) (1996) *The Reflective Researcher*, Allen and Unwin, London

Fothergill, S., Hardy, M., Lowther, J., McLean, W. and Miller, P. (eds) (1996) *The Participant: A Collection of Personal Accounts from a Participatory Research Committee*, University of Northumbria at Newcastle.

Foucault, M. (1977) *Discipline and Punish*, Penguin, Harmondsworth

Frank, I. (1995) Is there life after categories? Reflexivity in qualitative research. *Occupational Therapy Journal of Research*, **17**, 84–98

French, S. (ed.) (1994) *On Equal Terms: Working with Disabled People*, Butterworth-Heinemann, Oxford

Fuller, R. and Petch, A. (1995) *Practitioner Research: The Reflexive Social Worker*, OU Press, London

Gergen, M.M. and Gergen, K.J. (1993) Narratives of the gendered body in popular and autobiography. In Jasselson, R. and Lieblich, A. (eds), *The Narrative Study of Lives*, Sage, Newbury Park, California

Gillman, M.A. (1996) Empowering professionals in higher education? In Humphries, B. (ed.), *Critical Perspectives on Empowerment*, Venture Press, Birmingham

Gillman, M., Swain, J. and Heyman, B. (1997) Life history or 'case' history: the objectification of people with learning difficulties through the tyranny of professional discourses. *Disability and Society*, **12**, 675–693

Hasselkus, B.R. (1997) In the eye of the beholder: The researcher in qualitative research. *Occupational Therapy Journal of Research*, **17**, 81–84

Lather, P. (1991) Deconstructing/deconstructive inquiry: the politics of knowing and being known. *Educational Theory*, **41**, 153–173

Mattingly, C. (1991) The narrative nature of clinical reasoning. *American Journal of Occupational Therapy*, **45**, 998–1005

Mattingly, C. (1994) The concept of therapeutic employment. *Social Science Medicine*, **38**, 811–822

Mead, G.H. (1982) *Mind, Self and Society*, University of Chicago Press, Chicago

Newman, W. (1995) Unpublished research report. University of Northumbria at Newcastle

Oliver, M. (1992) Changing the social relations of research production. *Disability, Handicap and Society*, **7**, 101–114

Oliver, M. (1994) Re-defining disability: a challenge to research. In Swain, J. *et al.* (eds), *Disabling Barriers, Enabling Environments*, Sage, London

Oliver, M. (1996) *Understanding Disability: from theory to practice*, Macmillan, London

Oliver, M. and Barnes, C. (1997) All we are saying is give disabled researchers a chance. *Disability and Society*, **12**, 811–813

Reed, J. and Procter, S. (eds) (1995) *Practitioner Research in Health Care: The Inside Story*, Chapman and Hall, London

Rosenthal, G. (1993) Reconstruction of life stories: principles of selection in generating stories for narrative biographical interviews. In Josselson, R. and Lieblich, A. (eds), *The Narrative Study of Lives*, Sage, Newbury Park, California

Schön, D. (1983) *The Reflective Practitioner*, Basic Books, London

Schön, D. (1993) Reflection-in-action. In Walmsley, J. *et al.* (eds) *Health and Welfare Practice: Reflection on Roles and Relationships*, OU/Sage, London

Shakespeare, P., Atkinson, D. and French, S. (eds) (1993) *Reflecting on Research Practice: Issues in health and Social Welfare*, OU Press, London

Spencer, J., Krefting, L. and Mattingly, C. (1993) Incorporation of ethnographic methods in occupational therapy assessment. *American Journal of Occupational Therapy*, **47**, 303–309

Swain, J., Heyman, B. and Gillman, M. (1998) Public research, private concerns: ethical issues in the use of open-ended interviews with people who have learning difficulties. *Disability and Society*, **13**, 21–36

Vernon, A. (1997) Reflexivity: The dilemmas of researching from the inside. In Barnes, C. and Mercer, G. (eds), *Doing Disability Research*. The Disability Press, London

White, M. (1993) Deconstruction and therapy. In Gilligan, S. and Price, R. (eds), *Therapeutic Conversations*, Norton, New York

Widdershoven, G.A.M. (1993) The story of life: hermeneutic perspectives on the relationship between narrative and life history. In Josselson, R. and Lieblich, A. *The Narrative Study of Lives*, Sage, Newbury, Park, California

Wilkins, R. (1993) Taking it personally: a note on emotion and autobiography. *Sociology*, **27**, 93–100

Zarb., G. (1992) On the road to Damascus: first steps towards changing the relations of disability research production. *Disability, Handicap and Society*, **7**, 125–138

Contexts for working in partnership

Sally Donati and Clare Ward

Introduction

This chapter begins by describing the changing attitudes and values of society and how these have affected service delivery, the relationship between practitioners and people with learning disabilities and their carers. These changes have in turn influenced the structures and types of partnership that exist within and between the health and social care professions. It then describes current practice and how this attempts to overcome some of the negative experiences that clients and carers have had as a result of traditional approaches. We have only been able to give general guidance on this and have focused on the principle of the practitioner taking an enabling role. The literature referred to gives more detail for those who would like to explore methods and techniques in more depth. We use the term 'learning disabilities', as in our view this reflects the extent of the barriers experienced by people who come into contact with specialist health care services.

Changing values and models of care

Recent decades have seen a significant shift in society's values and attitudes towards adults with learning disabilities. The traditional approach has been to segregate people with learning disabilities by placing them in institutions to protect both them and society (Hughson and Brown, 1992). These institutions replaced the function of the family, as people with learning disabilities were often seen as a product of family dysfunction (Manthorpe, 1995).

Until now, models of care have been based on educational and medical models. The medical model locates the problem in the individual and has led to a view of this group of people as dependent and incurable (Brechin and Swain, 1989). The educational approach, while recognizing the potential for people with learning disabilities to acquire new skills, has often resulted in a group of people being in the position of lifelong learners, never quite able to achieve sufficient skills to be considered ready to lead ordinary lives (Jones, 1995). These two care models results in the professional being in a position of holding power and knowledge and the person with learning disabilities in a passive and dependent role

(Brandon, 1991). Expectations and goals are thus strongly influenced by professionals, leaving little opportunity for the person with learning disabilities to identify and express his or her own wishes and aspirations, which results in barriers to understanding between professionals and clients.

This imbalance is increasingly being recognized by clinicians. Crepeau (1991) describes the ideal communication process between client and clinician as being an open interchange in which the clinician gains understanding of all relevant factors in a client's life before making plans for intervention. She goes on to describe barriers to understanding and the lost opportunity for mutual learning that occurs when a power imbalance exists, and Peloquin (1993) describes the ways in which some clinicians misuse their power and establish a distance that diminishes and degrades their clients. As a result, when clients do not follow advice because they have been merely passive recipients, they may be labelled non-compliant (Jerosch-Herold, 1996) or have their values and perspectives ignored (Hasselkuss, 1989).

A number of developments in social policy have occurred in response to changes in the value systems of society and as a result of individual rights movements. The concept of normalization (Wolfensberger, 1972), which developed in the late 1960s and early 1970s has been adopted as the underpinning philosophy of learning disability services. This concept recognizes that neither living in an institution as a patient nor being a lifelong student reflects an ordinary life consisting of a range of opportunities and experiences. As a result of disability rights and independent living movements, the traditional view of disability has been redefined as one that locates the barriers within the social and built environment rather than within the individual (Swain *et al.*, 1993).

The impact of legislation and organizational structures on partnership

Significant changes and restructuring have taken place in the National Health Service since its inception. The powerful position held by professional groups and the perceived lack of responsiveness of these groups to changing social attitudes have triggered reform (Holliday, 1995). The introduction of general management in the 1980s took place in order to develop strategic direction and planning in the NHS and to create a service more responsive to social policy. However, it was not until the 1990s that more wide-ranging reform was introduced in the form of the NHS and Community Care Act, the Mental Health (Patients in the Community) Act, Carers (Services and Recognition) Act and, more recently, the NHS White Paper (The New NHS). Greater collaboration has been a constant theme throughout; statutory agencies are encouraged to form partnerships with service users, their carers and the voluntary and independent sectors to provide choice in service provision. Hattersley (1995) describes the benefits of working in this way, but also points out some of the inhibiting factors. Different organizations are driven by different imperatives, both political and organizational. These diverse cultures can impede collaboration.

At the heart of recent legislation is the concept of care management and assessment. The care manager is essentially a purchaser who, together with service users and their carers, assesses need and creates a care package. Apart from aiming to identify care packages that are responsive to individual need, Nocon (1994) describes the fundamental principles of care management as promotion of close inter-agency working and provision of seamless services. The assessment process is aimed at facilitating users and carers to define their own needs. However, as Nocon (1994) points out, a considerable amount of skill is needed not only to engage users and carers in the process in a way that enables them to identify their needs but also to be able to obtain, coordinate and evaluate multi-agency service provision. When effective, however, the process of negotiating contracts clarifies the nature of the service to be provided and also serves additional functions. The process of negotiating individual contracts can lead to changes in patterns of health service delivery. For example, a physiotherapist being located within a GP surgery or a care manager being co-located with a multidisciplinary health care team may lead to a more accessible and coordinated service for the users. Equally, where no service exists to meet an identified need, practitioners may adopt the role of advocate for service users by highlighting gaps in service provision at planning meetings or attempting to address the deficits through service development initiatives.

Another example of legislation that promotes collaboration between services is the Care Programme Approach. Introduced as part of the community care arrangements, it aims systematically to assess risks together with health and social needs, and to provide and coordinate the care received by people with additional mental health problems. In some areas, learning disability services have developed joint commissioning in order to promote closer working relationships between local and health authorities. Without structural incentives such as these from purchasers, providers are more likely to compete than collaborate with each other (Churchill, 1992; Sines, 1992).

Partnership with clients

There are a number of ways in which clinicians can enter into partnership with their clients. The therapist must, for each referral, determine who else will be working with the client and how best to work with the other people involved. Glendinning (1986) lists 19 groups of people that may become involved with an individual with learning disabilities and their family. These groups may include social workers/care managers, day and residential careworkers, teachers, interpreters, advocates, specialist clinicians, volunteers, generic health professionals, other families, service planners or commissioners.

Most clinicians working with people with learning disabilities are employed by local or health authorities. They respond to a range of health and social needs and work directly with the individual or with carers and others who provide a service to the client group. Taking into account changes in social values and policies, it has been necessary to re-examine the methods of work used by the practising clinician. As disabled people have increasingly expressed their needs and wish for greater involvement in planning and provision of services, clinicians have adapted their ways of working. Practice has evolved from one of prescription of treatment to one that facilitates change, encouraging independent use of the therapist as a resource (Nocon and Pleace, 1997; RCSLT, 1996). In order to achieve a satisfactory outcome for the client it is necessary to combine the experience of the client with the skill and knowledge of the therapist, thereby working collaboratively to identify disabling barriers and explore options for solutions together.

Although the traditional view maintains that the disability is located in the individual, with the consequent expectation that the person has to change, develop or adapt (e.g. Young, 1979; Bush *et al.*, 1980; Cumming, 1992), the social disability construct described by Finkelstein and French (1993) locates the barriers in the environment. Baumgart *et al.* (1982) and, more recently, Jones (1995) describe the need for educators and therapists to replace the traditional approaches based on medical and developmental models. They propose a set of principles of partial participation which, when put into practice, enable people with learning disabilities to participate, to varying degrees, in the same activities as the rest of the population. As assessment process identifies the skills needed to participate in the identified activity, the skills and deficits of the individual and his or her potential to develop skills. Options for a range of individualized adaptations are then developed to compensate for skill deficits and/or facilitate further skill development. The principles espoused by Baumgart *et al.* (1982) are based on their experience that adults, particularly those with severe learning disabilities, have limited ability to adapt to their environment. Therefore, the environment needs to be adapted to them.

It now seems widely accepted that the most effective way in which to maximize an individual's functional skills is to identify disabling barriers and find ways of reducing them. This approach is particularly important for adults with learning disabilities, since there is an increased chance that their negative past experiences of participation in daily life will have resulted in under-utilization of skills, lowered expectations by those around them, and a subsequent reduction in opportunities (Money, 1997). Thus the focus shifts from skills training with the individual to adaptation of the environment. This involves working in partnership with a range of people in order to establish how much of the chosen activity the person can do and what other supports or adaptations are required in order for the person to engage successfully in the activity. Individualized adaptations may include adaptations to buildings and activities, specialized equipment and extra personal support. This may lead to a consultative way of working as described by Kemmis and Dunn (1996), which involves people with diverse expertise, perspectives, and experiences working together as equal partners to design a combined approach to intervention.

One way in which the clinician can facilitate the client – whether that is the person with learning disabilities, a paid or unpaid carer, a professional or organization – to clarify the issues and consider options for solutions is through reflective practice. In this way, a combination of the objectivity and skills of the clinician, together with the client's own knowledge and first-hand experience, leads to a partnership that values both parties' contributions and shares responsibility for the outcome. This type of partnership has features of the reflective contract described by Schon (1991). He states that where the client and professional join together to develop a greater understanding of a situation, there is increased involvement and action. Again this contrasts with the traditional approach where the responsibility for finding solutions is placed in the hands of the 'expert', while the client is relatively unengaged in the process and consequently less inclined to feel ownership of the resulting solutions. For the reflective practitioner the client is the expert, as he or she has the knowledge about the issues of concern. Jointly, clients and therapists can identify the focus of enquiry, frame the problem and formulate a range of hypotheses and potential solutions.

Therapists working with adults with learning disabilities may also find themselves involved with any number of other people, as they seek to understand the environment of the individual concerned. Since informal carers provide the majority of community care (Smith, et al., 1996), they can be considered one of the major influences on an individual's environment and may take on a number of different roles, including that of information provider, coordinator and implementor of programmes. It may be helpful to consider a carer as a lay practitioner (Hasselkus, 1989; Gitlin et al., 1995) who receives support and reassurance from the therapist, exchanging knowledge and day-to-day experience for clinical skills. Barnes (1997) suggests that client, carer and clinician enter into a three-way partnership, especially where there is likely to be a considerable amount of involvement on the part of the clinician.

Whatever the structure of the partnership, in order to understand fully an individual's environment it is important that barriers to communication are recognized and explored. There are a number of reasons why these barriers exist. Carers, particularly from within the family, have long reported a lack of understanding on the part of professionals (Fairbrother, 1983; Hasselkus, 1989; Larson, 1996; Maggs and Laugharne, 1996) and often feel that their perspective is undervalued or even ignored. Informal carers appear to feel that it is impossible for professionals to appreciate the pattern and meaning of their day-to-day lives without the personal experience of having a family member with learning disabilities (Barnes, 1997).

Robinson (1993) describes the importance many families place on living a 'normal life', as opposed to one which emphasizes difficulties and problems. In order to develop good working relationships with carers, intervening therapists must first identify the essential components of normal life for each family. If they do not do this, they risk disrupting the family environment with their necessary focus on areas of difficulty and family members may view health care providers' efforts as lack of cooperation or interest. In any case, the goals and priorities of practitioners and carers are often strikingly different (Pool, 1993). The therapist works towards increased opportunities, adaptation and independence which carers may perceive as highlighting an individual's deficits and involving interventions which are risky, dangerous, disruptive to normal routines and unrealistic.

It has been reported that carers prioritize security and safety for their vulnerable son or daughter, getting everyday things done and being a parent (rather than a teacher), and have a tendency to under- or over-emphasize their son's or daughter's abilities. To a therapist this may appear as over-protectiveness, lack of commitment to intervention programmes, or being unrealistic about an individual's abilities due to denial of his or her difficulties (Larson, 1996). These opposing perspectives must be shared and thoroughly examined if the tensions and stresses of working in opposing directions are to be removed from the therapeutic relationship.

In order to avoid this conflict between clinician and client, whether the carer or the person with the learning disability, it is important for the clinician to be able to empathize with the experiences of the client. There are various ways in which this can happen. When clients experience difficulty they may not always be able to clarify exactly what the problems are and it is important for the clinician to spend time with them to develop an understanding of their perspective. During the assessment process a story will be pieced together and, with the client, the clinician will clarify the key issues. The interviews at this early assessment stage provide a chance to clarify roles, identify and evaluate strategies currently in use and develop collaborative spirit (Crais, 1996). In this way, more attainable goals may be set, for as Fairbrother (1983) points out, goals set without consultation may lead to a lack of confidence on the part of carers and lack of achievement by the individual concerned.

The use of language is important at this stage; key phrases used by clients may be adopted by the clinician to demonstrate a willingness to understand their experiences. Semi-structured discussion allows clients the opportunity to raise issues spontaneously, while providing the clinician with a framework on which to hand the necessary information. The clinician takes the role of an active listener, reflecting back and allowing clients the opportunity to confirm or correct their interpretations. Selective questioning based on the clinician's past experience can be used to help clients expand on particular issues that relate to the problem (Hasselkus, 1990).

The use of a reflective contract facilitates shared knowledge and ownership of the problem and joint responsibility for the outcome of any intervention. Hasselkuss (1989) describes the use of reflection as a way of minimizing tension and facilitating shared ethical decision making. Spending time with a person, listening, observing and participating in his or her everyday life is similar to the ethnographic style of working and has been described as a style of assessment by Hasselkuss (1990) and

Crais (1996). This process enables the clinician to piece together the story with a client and is described by Mattingly and Fleming (1994) as story making or narrative thinking.

A number of methods based on these approaches have been developed to facilitate people with learning disabilities in a life-planning process. Richardson (1997) describes professionals developing a working alliance with people with learning disabilities using shared action planning (Brechin and Swain, 1989) and futures planning (O'Brien, 1987) to identify disabling barriers and set enabling goals and actions.

In addition, the practitioner has a range of clinical tools available, which include assessment packages, use of video and written contracts. There are several formal assessment processes especially designed for use with clients and carers that provide a framework for gathering relevant information. The Personal Communication Plan (Hitchings and Spence, 1991) contains a series of structured questions on the different areas of communication. These are completed by the therapist, the carer and the individual with a learning disability if appropriate. As the interview progresses, key issues become apparent and the last section provides an opportunity for shared action planning. This along with other packages (e.g. ENABLE, Hurst-Brown and Keens, 1990) provides an opportunity for staff, carers and clinicians to share perceptions of their clients (Money, 1997).

The use of video as a reflective tool has also been documented. It provides an objective way in which both clinicians and carers may observe and evaluate each other's skills on an equal basis, as well as capturing the 'transient experience of interaction' (Cummins and Hulme, 1997). Video recordings may feature as a key element in the training of care staff, to provide examples of strategies and feedback on their own techniques. They can also be useful when sharing details of behaviours or strategies with families.

The drawing up of written contracts in conjunction with the client at each stage of involvement (assessment, intervention or staff training) is another way in which therapists can ensure a clear understanding of roles and responsibilities (van der Gaag and Dormandy, 1993). They may also serve as a format for the clinician to identify and monitor precise aims and objectives throughout the process of assessment, intervention and evaluation.

Before the start of intervention it is important to understand how the family lives its story and how therapy approaches can integrate with this (Robinson, 1993). When working with paid carers, issues such as staff management and supervision structures will form part of the story. Whether carers are paid or unpaid, the clinician should try to identify both those routines or systems which are valued and essential and those which are open to change. Mattingly and Fleming (1994) describe the process as creating a therapeutic story to invent a new future.

In the case of paid care staff, some additional methods may be employed which would not always be considered when working with families. The provision of staff training is one way in which clinicians aim to influence the social and physical environment of a whole organization (such as a day centre or residential unit), rather than working purely on individual one-to-one relationships within it. This is a very necessary element of intervention for, as Cullen (1988) points out, in order to change the behaviour of people with learning disabilities one needs first to change the behaviour of staff. There is growing agreement that the traditional approach to training, in the form of occasional educational days, has little effect on working practice on its own (Cullen, 1987; van der Gaag and Dormandy, 1993). Instead, a combination of the theoretical and the practical is suggested for maximum efficacy (Money, 1997).

The practical element follows a needs-led approach to training (offering staff the opportunity to decide on topics), using staff as facilitators wherever possible, keeping groups small with high participant involvement relating to the workplace and led by local personnel. All training should ideally be combined with more direct assessment and intervention (Crawford, 1990; van der Gaag and Dormandy, 1993; Money, 1997), and workshops should include an opportunity for people to examine their own beliefs and values as well as to reflect on experience. The key to this area of work is the use of feedback techniques (verbal, written or video) to enable staff to link theory to practice with support from the clinician. In terms of evaluation, Money (1997) stresses a need for evaluating training programmes, looking at changes in the learning disabled individuals, rather than traditional feedback forms. These forms may give trainers a measure of changes in staff awareness, morale and theoretical knowledge, but are less likely to capture details of any real change. A commitment to record keeping by staff may also serve as positive feedback during the implementation of new methods of interaction.

In addition to the methods described above which can be incorporated into everyday practice, it is also possible to apply the same approaches to project work. Examples of some innovative partnerships include involvement of people with learning disabilities in co-facilitating courses (Walmsley, 1991; Hooper and Bowler, 1988). In the area of research, March *et al.*, (1997) describe a collaborative study between a researcher and a group of people with learning disabilities, in which they plan and carry out a research project together.

In this section we have discussed a number of ways in which the clinican can work in partnership with people with learning disabilities and their informal and formal carers. However, the feasibility and effectiveness of this way of working rests on a number of factors.

Schön (1991) describes some of the factors that need to be considered when employing reflective practice. This approach entails changes in role, of expectations and responsibility both from the clinician's and client's points of view. The clinician gives up some authority and the client takes on more responsibility. In the reflective model the clinician, traditionally considered the expert, shares the uncertainties and difficulties of the situation, sharing the more vulnerable position as learner or 'inquirer' together with the client. In some situations, where either party is unable or not prepared to relinquish or adopt these responsibilities, it is necessary to retain the more traditional approach to intervention. Equally, there will be times when urgent action needs to be taken or the intervention required is relatively clear-cut and reflective practice would be unnecessarily time consuming and complex. In these situations, the more traditional approach, entailing professional assessment and intervention or recommendations for interventions, would be carried out.

Conclusion

This chapter has described some of the structural and organizational factors that promote partnership between the agencies within which clinicians work. Different types of partnership between practitioners and people with learning disabilities and their carers have also been discussed. Traditional approaches that entail a power imbalance between client and clinician are slowly being replaced by a range of methods that use reflective practice as the overarching theme.

References

Barnes, M. (1997) Families and empowerment. In Ramcharan, P. *et al.* (eds), *Empowerment in Everyday Life: Learning Disability*, Jessica Kingsley, London

Baumgart, D., Brown, L., Ford, D., Messina, R., Nisbet, J., Pumpian, I., Schroeder, J. and Sweet, M. (1982) Principle of partial participation and individualised adaptations in educational programs for severely handicapped students. *Journal of the Association for Persons with Severe Handicaps*, **7**, 17–27

Brandon, D. (1991) The implications of normalisation work for professional skills. In Ramon, S. (ed.), *Beyond Community Care*, Macmillan Education, London

Brechin, A. and Swain, J. (1989) Creating a 'working alliance' with people with learning difficulties. In Brechin, A. and Welmsley, J. (eds) *Making Connections*, Hodder and Stoughton, London

Bush, A., Morris, S. and Williams, J. (1980) An activity period for the mentally handicapped. *British Journal of Occupational Therapy*, **42**, 19–20

Churchill, J. (1992) Contracts or partnerships? In Thompson, T. and Mathias, P. (eds), *Standards and Mental Handicap*, Baillière Tindall, London

Crais, E.R. (1996) Pre-assessment planning with caregivers. *American Speech and Hearing Association*, **38**(1), 38–39

Crawford, J.V. (1990). Maintaining staff morale: the value of a staff training and support network. *Mental Handicap*, **18**, 48–51

Crepeau, E.B. (1991) Achieving intersubjective understanding: examples from an occupational therapy treatment session. *American Journal of Occupational Therapy*, **45**, 1016–1025

Cullen, C. (1987) Nurse training and institutional constraints. In Hogg, J. and Mittler, p. (eds), *Staff Training in Mental Handicap*, Croom Helm, London

Cullen, C. (1988) A review of staff training: the emperor's old clothes. *Irish Journal of Psychology*, **9**, 309–323

Cumming, J. (1992) It is possible: a process for teaching community living skills. *Australian Journal of Occupational Therapy*, **39**, 35–38

Cummins, K. and Hulme, S. (1997) Video – a reflective tool. *Speech and Language Therapy in Practice*, Autumn, 4–7

Fairbrother, P. (1983) Needs of parents of adults. In Mittler, P. and McConachie H. (eds), *Parents, Professionals and Mentally Handicapped People* Brookline Books, Cambridge, Mass.

Finkelstein, V. and French, S. (1993) Towards a psychology of disability. In Swain, J. *et al.* (eds), *Disabling Barriers – Enabling Environments*, Sage, London

Gitlin, L.N., Corcoran, M. and Leinmiller-Eckhart, S. (1995) Understanding the family perspective: an ethnographic framework for providing occupational therapy in the home. *American Journal of Occupational Therapy*, **49**(8), 802–809

Glendinning, C. (1986) *A Single Door: Social Work with the Families of Disabled Children*, Allen and Unwin, London

Hasselkuss, B.R. (1989) The meaning of daily activity in family care giving for the elderly. *American Journal of Occupational Therapy*, **43**, 649–655

Hasselkuss, B.R. (1990) Ethnographic interviewing: a tool for practice with family caregivers for the elderly. *Occupational Therapy in Practice*, **2**(1), 9–16

Hattersley, J. (1995) The survival of collaboration and cooperation. In Malin, N. (ed), *Services for People with Learning Difficulties*, Routledge, London

Hitchings, A. and Spence, R. (1991) *The Personal Communication Plan (PCP)*, NFER Nelson, Windsor

Hurst-Brown, L. and Keens, A. (1990) *ENABLE: Enabling a Natural and Better Life Experience*, Forum Consultancy, London

Holliday, I. (1995) *The NHS Transformed*, 2nd edn, Baseline Books, Manchester

Hooper, H. and Bowler, D. (1988) Peer-tutoring of manual signs by adults with mental handicaps. *Mental Handicap Research*, **4**, 207–215

Hughson, E.A. and Brown, R.I. (1992) Learning difficulties in the context of social change: a challenge for professional action. In Thompson, T. and Mathias, P. (eds), *Standards and Mental Handicap*, Baillière Tindall, London

Jerosch-Herold, C. (1996) Patient compliance: a desirable goal of patient education? *British Journal of Therapy and Rehabilitation*, **3**, 154–157

Jones, D. (1995) Learning disability: an alternative frame of reference. *British Journal of Occupational Therapy*, **58**, 423–426

Kemmis, B.L. and Dunn, W. (1996) Collaborative consultation: the efficacy of remedial and compensatory interventions in school contexts. *American Journal of Occupational Therapy*, **50**(9), 709–717

Larson, E. (1996) The story of Maricela and Miguel: a narrative analysis of dimensions of adaptation. *American Journal of Occupational Therapy*, **50**(4), 286–298

Maggs, C. and Laugharne, C. (1996) Relationship between elderly carers and the older adult with learning disabilities: an overview of the literature. *Journal of Advanced Nursing*, **23**, 243–251

Manthorpe, J. (1995) Services to families. In Malin, N. (ed.), *Services for People with Learning Difficulties*, Routledge, London

March, J., Justice, S., Steingold, B. with Mitchell, P. (1997) Follow the yellow brick road! People with learning difficulties as co-researchers. *British Journal of Learning Disabilities*, **25**, 77–80

Mattingly, C. and Fleming, M. (1994) *Clinical Reasoning: Forms of Enquiry in a Therapeutic Practise*, F.A. Davis, Philadelphia

Money, D. (1997) A comparison of three approaches to delivering a speech and language therapy service to people with learning disabilities. *European Journal of Disorders of Communication*, **32**, 449–466

Nocon, A. (1994) *Collaboration in Community Care in the 1990's*, Business Education Publishers, Sunderland

Nocon, A. and Pleace, N. (1997) Until disabled people get consulted: the role of occupational therapy in meeting housing needs. *British Journal of Occupational Therapy*, **60**, 115–122

O'Brien, J. (1987) A guide to personal futures planning. In Bellamy, G. and Wilcox, B. (eds) *A Comprehensive Guide to the Activities Catalogue: An Alternative*

Curriculum for Youth and Adults with Severe Disabilities Paul H. Brookes, Baltimore

Overtviet, J. (1985) *Organisational Issues in Multi-Disciplinary Teams*, Brunel Institute of Organization and Social Studies, Health Services Centre working paper, Brunel University, Uxbridge

Peloquin, S.M. (1993) The depersonalization of patients: a profile gleaned from narratives. *American Journal of Occupational Therapy*, **47**, 830–837

Pool, J. (1993) The CARE approach to enabling independence. *British Journal of Occupational Therapy*, **56**, 120–122

Richardson, M. (1997) Crossing barriers: disabled rights and the implications for nursing of the social construct of disability. *Journal of Advanced Nursing*, **25**, 1269–1275

Robinson, C. (1993) Managing life with a chronic condition: the story of normalisation. *Qualitative Health Research*, **3**(1), 6–28

RCSLT (1996) *Communicating Quality*, 2nd edn, Royal College of Speech and Language Therapists, London

Schön, D. (1991) *The reflective practitioner*. Basic Books Inc. London

Sines, D. (1992) Service Provision: Developments in the National Health Service. In Thompson, T. and Mathias, P. (eds), *Standards and Mental Handicap*, pp. 16–22, Bailliere Tindall, London.

Smith, B., Wun, W-L., & Cumella, S. (1996) Training for Staff Caring for People with Learning Disability. *British Journal of Learning Disabilities*, **24**, 20–25.

Swain, J., Finkelstein, V., French, S. and Oliver, M. (eds) (1993) *Disabling Barriers – Enabling Environments*, Sage, London

van der Gaag, A. and Dormandy, K. (1993) *Communication and Adults with Learning Disabilities*, Winslow Press, Bicester

Walmsley, J. (1991) Working together: a participative approach to learning. *Mental Handicap*, **19**, 92–95

Wolfensberger, W. (1972) *The Principle of Normalisation in Human Services*, National Institute on Mental Retardation, Toronto

Young, H. (1979) DOCTA: a project for the profoundly mentally handicapped. *British Journal of Occupational Therapy*, **42**, 19–20

The practice of working in partnership

Sue Standing

Introduction

At first glance it would seem that therapists are an obvious example of people who work in partnership. After all, therapy intervention involves, in the first instance, two people – a clinician and a patient or client – who have agreed aims and goals to achieve a specific outcome. Therapists also invariably work as part of a team developing professional partnerships.

Let us look more deeply at the partnership philosophy.

- Are we, as therapists, truly the partners of patients and clients with learning disabilities?
- Do we share and utilize their perspectives?
- Are we prepared to share the risks and profits involved in joint decisions?
- Is the relationship an enabling and empowering one for the patient or client?
- Are we prepared to be supporters and advocates?
- Do we truly listen, recognize and appreciate the needs of our patients and clients, or are we too wrapped up in what we have to offer, the outcomes we wish to achieve and our own concerns as service providers?
- Are we on the same side as the patients and clients?

The main aim of services for people with learning disabilities, including the therapy services, is to bring about appropriate and positive change in the lifestyles of service users. This should be the culmination of a shared process where the therapist, client and other members of the team work in partnership with one another. This philosophy is developing and must continue to be the thrust for students, clinicians, educators and clients.

Empowerment in therapy practice

The concept of empowerment is difficult to define. Part of the difficulty of definition is that it takes different forms for different people and within different contexts (Rappaport, 1984). It is unique to the individual or group having a different meaning (e.g. for a poor, ill-educated Black woman, from that of a middle-aged business man or an elderly woman with learning disabilities). According to Dunst *et al.* (1992): 'Empowerment has no agreed upon definition. . . . Rather the term has been used loosely, to capture a family of somewhat related meanings.' Rappaport, whose work has been within mental health and self-help groups, suggests, however, that empowerment is:

> A sense of control over one's life in personality, cognition and motivation. It expresses itself at the level of feelings, at the level of ideas about self worth, at the level of something more akin to the spiritual . . . it is something that must be taken not given. (1984:7)

Partnerships need to be examined within the concept of empowerment. This will involve important interpersonal characteristics, including open communication, mutual trust and respect, shared responsibility and cooperation (Dunst *et al.*, 1992). Empowerment is likely to be achieved in situations and within programmes where professionals are not the key actors. The cognitive, motivational and personality changes experienced by those who gain a sense of control are the essence of empowerment. It is useful for professionals to think in these terms, as the previous medical perspective created an iatrogenesis that increased stress and dependency while reducing individual choice and control (Illich, 1976). Brian Stoker talks about the disempowering effect of his 14-year stay in a mental handicap hospital:

> I had the confidence in me to speak up and take control over my life. But I was prevented from speaking up because of physical abuse from the nurses. Therefore, their behaviour disempowered me (stopped me saying what I want) and prevented me from living a 'normal' life. Staff shouldn't stop people speaking up for themselves. They should let users say what they want to be confident and take control over their life. I left the hospital and have been out in the community for twenty years. (People First, December 1997)

Staff from human services, and carers who really understand the ideology of empowerment, can create conditions where people with learning disabilities can be empowered. It is not just about workers listening and responding to users' requests. It is about working partnerships where the worker is actively engaged in sharing ideas and thoughts and ensuring that the individual or group has the benefit of different points of view. Brechin and Swain (1990) warn professionals that their access to exclusive and privileged knowledge about people with learning disabilities puts them in a dependent, disempowering role.

Partnership is not easy to achieve and in the view of the Disabled People's Movement, including the organization People First, has not gone far enough. The relationship between disabled people and professionals has been an unequal one, with professionals holding most of the power. Professionals have defined, planned and delivered services, whereas disabled people have had little opportunity to exercise control (French, 1994). Although therapists may appear to have a technical approach, more akin to the medical model, in practice they can provide opportunities for people to take responsibility, to master their own environment and to maintain health and wellbeing through activities of their choice. The role of the therapist can be one of enabler, allowing the client to take the lead. This is illustrated in the following case study cited in, and adapted from Auty:

> A young man about to transfer from long-stay hospital to a community setting was unable to walk the distance to the local shops. The therapist involved wanted to find a meaningful way to engage the young man in activities which increased his exercise tolerance, afforded him enjoyment and, if possible, provided him with a hobby. The actual programme involved progression from exercise in a gym to a one-mile hike, followed by a five-mile hike around a nature trail and finished with an outward bound activity week. The programme was considered unrealistic by many and yet through the process the young man was given realistic opportunities to make his own decisions, make new friends and to develop a hobby. In addition he earned respect by his determination and efforts to accomplish each task of the process. (1991: 40–43)

The therapist should be seen as a member of a multidisciplinary team, the aim of which is to help create and support a lifestyle of choice for each individual client. O'Brien (1987) viewed the quality of services in terms of five accomplishments: choice, community presence, competence, community participation and respect. All of these should be borne in mind when the therapist is involved with a client in planning a programme. This may be particularly challenging when the client has multiple impairments and/or comes from an ethnic minority group. The following case study demonstrates how a woman with a severe learning disability, who is also blind and from a cultural background where English is not her first language, can enjoy an environment where she is enabled to become increasingly empowered and involved in her own life:

> Reeta is a young Bengali woman with cerebral palsy who is also blind. She cannot push her wheelchair and can only say a few words. She gets very frustrated if she is left to sit in her wheelchair. She starts to spit and rock her chair backwards violently and tries to scratch and pinch anyone within reach. Reeta loves to move, and when she goes swimming (she is able to swim without assistance) she greatly enjoys it.
>
> An assessment of Reeta was carried out by a physiotherapist and a speech and language therapist (with the help of an interpreter). The assessment also involved Reeta's family and a support worker at the day centre. It was discovered that Reeta understood very little spoken English and that this lack of communication was causing her frustration. Because she is blind it was not possible to use gesture, Makaton or Sign Along to facilitate her.
>
> A programme using a 'moulded signing' approach was devised. With this approach, objects and smells are used to communicate and to enable people to make a choice. For example, when Reeta is presented with a swimming costume she knows that she is being asked whether she wants to go swimming. Similarly before Reeta has a bath she smells

the soap and feels the face cloth. Reeta loves spicy food and at the day centre she enjoys shopping for the groceries, cooking (helped by her support worker) and then eating a good tasty curry. (The author would like to acknowledge Julie Waring, who provided this case study)

Therapeutic intervention – where to begin?

Assessment and planning an intervention

Assessment is the keystone to all therapy interventions, but in the case of the person with learning disabilities it may take many sessions to get to know the person, to win confidence and to establish rapport before a satisfactory assessment is achieved (Auty, 1991). This is illustrated in the following case study:

Angela is a woman in her twenties with Rett's syndrome. She has just moved into a new community home and has been referred to physiotherapy by the carer of the home, which she shares with three other people, because at bath time she refuses to cooperate. There have been two or three incidents where she has fallen during transfer into the bath.

Angela would rather not have a bath, she finds it distressing and is frightened of hurting herself again. The carer, on the other hand, is concerned that Angela needs to be washed but is also worried that she herself may get hurt through a back injury or by contact with Angela when she lashes out.

The physiotherapist, through an assessment, wants to identify the physical problems that prevent Angela from getting in and out of the bath so that she can devise a safer and more suitable method of doing so, or suggest, in consultation with the occupational therapist, the installation of a hoist, bath rails and other aids. She decides that a programme of activity in the hydrotherapy pool, where access and mobility can be observed in a wider context, may, in the first instance, be appropriate and that this will have the added advantage of assisting the decrease in mobility associated with Rett's syndrome. At every stage of assessment, ideas and possible interventions need to be discussed with Angela and other members of the team. (Case study supplied by the present author)

The assessment and interventions which follow may assist in turning a stressful situation into a positive experience. The intervention must be discussed with the client to achieve specific, measurable, achievable and timed objectives with appropriate parameters. The goals need to be divided into those which are short and long term. Quin Patton (1986) states that planning and evaluation should go hand in hand in order to ensure that the objectives set are met. Clear aims and objectives are a prerequisite of effective programmes to produce measurable outcomes. Outcome measures are nothing new to the therapist, but have been difficult to define, monitor and achieve within the field of learning disability. This does not mean they have not been addressed (Massie *et al.*, 1997; Standing, 1997). If the assessment and subsequent therapy programme delivered does not incorporate measurable outcomes to allow evaluation, it will not be possible to fully evaluate the effectiveness of therapy practice.

Therapy intervention

Traditional techniques and skills are not always appropriate when working with people with learning disabilities. This is illustrated in the following case study:

> Trevor is a 50-year-old man who has spent 20 years in a mental handicap hospital. He has no verbal skills but communicates using Makaton and facial gestures. He spent his days in the hospital walking around the large grounds greeting various members of staff, clients and visitors. He always returned to his villa for lunch and tea and never went out after tea. Trevor was relocated into a small terraced house in the city with two other men and several new staff. Despite a programme of resettlement he quickly became very agitated, depressed and aggressive, disrupting the other members of the household who began to live in fear of him.
>
> One of the staff members recognized that Trevor needed to get out of the house and that his behaviour resulted from fear, boredom, lack of stimulation and physical exercise and referred him to the physiotherapist as she felt she could not manage Trevor alone. The physiotherapist gradually introduced herself to Trevor and observed his behaviour on visits to the home, communicating with him using Makaton. She attempted to devise a physical programme to be carried out from the home, but this failed as Trevor refused to walk outside the house where there was only a small pavement between him and a very busy road.
>
> It was suggested that Trevor attended a hydrotherapy session. Initially he was interested but resistant to travelling in the car. When in the pool he quickly came to enjoy the activities and readily continued to attend. The staff member was amazed at what he could achieve and noted that his behaviour in the home began to change. She suggested that if the physiotherapist came along they could take Trevor to the local leisure pool together. This was discussed with Trevor who agreed, although he was apprehensive. The first two or three visits were met with resistance, but the activity rapidly became a happy event and staff were willing to accompany Trevor twice a week without the physiotherapist. During this time, Trevor gradually became more adventurous in leaving the house with staff to attend other venues. As he grew familiar with his surroundings, engaged in stimulating activities and gained confidence, Trevor became less depressed and agitated and his violent behaviour ceased. (Case study supplied by the present author)

Conclusion

People with learning disabilities have been labelled, stigmatized and disempowered, and it is only now that any coordinated attempt has been made to improve their situation. Working in partnership with people with learning disabilities demands of therapists far more than learning new techniques of treatment; it involves a willingness and capacity to respond imaginatively to every person as a unique individual and to help and support each person in the achievement of his or her own aspirations and desired lifestyle.

(The author would like to acknowledge Julie Waring for providing case study material.)

References

Auty, P. (1991) *Physiotherapy for People with Learning Difficulties*, Woodhead-Faulkner, London

Brechin, A. and Swain, J. (1990) Professional/client relationships: creating a 'working alliance' with people with learning difficulties. In Brechin, A. and Walmsley, J. (eds), *Making Connections: Reflecting on the Lives of and Experiences of People with Learning Difficulties*, Hodder and Stoughton, London

Dunst, C.J., Trivette, C.M. and La Pointe, N. (1992) Towards clarification of the meaning and key elements of empowerment. *Family Science Review*, **5**(12), 111–130

French, S. (1994) Uneasy alliances. *Therapy Weekly*, **21**(14), 4

Illich, J. (1976) *Medical Nemesis: The Exploration of Health*, Pantheon Books, New York

Massie, S., McCleod, M. and Chessman, R. (1997) Use of outcome measures in therapy departments in Scotland. *Physiotherapy*, **82**(12), 673–679

O'Brien, J. (1987) *Principles of Normalisation: A Foundation for Effective Services*, Campaign for People with Mental Handicap, London

Quin Patton, M. (1986) *Utilisation – Focused Evaluation*, Sage, London

Rappaport, J. (1984) The power of empowerment language. *Social Policy*, **3**, 19–21

Standing, S. (1997) *Magical, Mythical, Measurable*. A survey of outcome measures as understood and used by physiotherapists who work with people with learning disabilities, Portsmouth University

Stoker, B. (1997) People First Conference, December, London

Multidisciplinary teams

Sally French

Introduction

Though few objective evaluations have been taken of the effectiveness of teamwork over individual care (Pritchard and Pritchard, 1992), there is a widespread belief that people achieve more when working collectively than they do when working alone. Teams work by pooling knowledge, skills and resources; each individual has his or her specific role, but the team has common interests and objectives. Each member shares responsibility for the decisions made within the team, the overall functioning of the team and the quality of its output. Teamwork also allows a broader base of attitudes and values to be brought into decision making.

Multidisciplinary teams involved with people with learning difficulties include, first and foremost, the people with learning difficulties themselves as well as their relatives and those who assist them. It may also include a large number of professional and non-professional workers, including physiotherapists, occupational therapists, psychologists and care assistants. It will be argued in this chapter that the most central person in the team, that is, the person who should have most control, is the person with learning difficulties him or herself, although this is not always easy to achieve. A large team of professional workers can be intimidating to people with learning difficulties as well as their families and younger, less experienced members of the team.

This chapter will examine some of the factors which enhance the effectiveness of teamwork and ways of ensuring that people with learning difficulties maintain a central position of control within the team. It concludes with a discussion of generic versus specialist teams for people with learning difficulties.

Effective teamwork

Working with others is not always easy; we have probably all experienced teams that were fraught with conflict or which simply failed to gel. Effective teamwork is not, however, entirely a matter of chance, but involves skills that can be learned. Pritchard and Pritchard (1992) present four major facets of effective teamwork:

1 Team members need to understand the goals of the team and the tasks they will perform as individuals. It is important that team members are given some degree of autonomy so that they do not have to refer

constantly to others. It is vital, however, that a strong channel of communication exists between each member of the team and the person with learning difficulties as well as his or her family or assistants.

2 Teams work most effectively if members understand and value one another's roles.

3 Agreed procedures for carrying out tasks and evaluating them need to be negotiated.

4 Teams work most effectively if interpersonal relationships are good. Unresolved conflicts are likely to threaten seriously the effectiveness of the team.

These four facets interact; there are less likely to be problems with interpersonal relationships, for example, if goals, roles and procedures are clear.

It is very important that teams which work with people with learning difficulties do not become overpowering, controlling or oppressive, and that they do not allow their procedures and work patterns to become rigid. The purpose of such teams is to enhance the lives of people with learning difficulties according to their own goals and aspirations.

The realization of such principles can, however, be fraught with difficulties, particularly in ensuring the control of people with learning difficulties in decisions about themselves and their lives. The central dilemma is the possibility that the processes and procedures of multidisciplinary teamwork, while enhancing the effectiveness of professionals working together, disempowers the client about whom decisions are being made. Given that the client/professional relationship is an unequal one, a team of professionals can, of course, be so much more powerful than an individual professional. The ideal of teamwork, envisaged in this chapter, is that the work of professionals is coordinated and effective in realizing the goals and aspirations of the person with learning difficulties.

The importance of setting goals

The negotiation of goals is a cornerstone of teamwork. It is also crucial in ensuring the control of people with learning difficulties. This involves the recognition that people with learning difficulties may have problems in defining and/or communicating their goals, and that professionals may not be in the best position to enable clients to explore their aspirations (Brechin and Swain, 1987). Sometimes the team needs to include someone who can advocate for the person with learning difficulties (Macadam and Rodgers, 1997).

Goals may be challenging, but need to be within the team's capacity and reflect the aspirations and desires of the clients. Goals can be stated in terms of process (how things will proceed) and in terms of outcome (what will be achieved). A process goal, for example, might specify ways in which a group of clients can be helped to communicate their wishes more openly, whereas an outcome goal might specify how that improvement will be demonstrated or measured.

Understanding one another's roles

It is important that team members understand and value one another's roles. This is not always easy, as roles are constantly changing and role boundaries are rarely clear. This situation can, in itself, lead to uncertainty and lack of confidence and can raise, rather than reduce, inter-professional boundaries (Macadam and Rodgers, 1997). It can also cause confusion among clients and those who assist them. It is impossible to utilize the skills and experience of team members, including people with learning difficulties themselves, if their roles and abilities are not understood and valued, but it is also undesirable, from the client's point of view, for roles to be rigid and prescribed.

Roles are rarely static and will depend on the unique composition of the team. Roles may also be shared. The physiotherapist and occupational therapist, for example, may share the task of providing advice about orthotics and wheelchairs. Tasks such as counselling and health education may also be shared. Role negotiation is very important, especially when a new member joins the team. People from the same profession or occupation rarely have a matching set of skills. Flexibility and willingness to learn new skills are essential characteristics of multidisciplinary teamwork (Pritchard and Pritchard, 1992).

Relationships within the team

Harmonious, trusting relationships within teams are essential to effective teamwork (Hattersley, 1995). Team members need to support and encourage one another and provide sufficient time to discuss feelings and problems. This having been said, conflict within teams is inevitable; not only are team members likely to have different values and beliefs, but the management structures and legal frameworks under which they work may differ. It is not always best to avoid conflict if, as a result, problems are driven underground, leading to resentment, lack of trust and ineffective work. The development of trust, respect and friendship is best developed in small working groups where people, including those with learning difficulties and their assistants, can exchange ideas in an informal atmosphere.

Conflict can become debilitating, but in moderation it is healthy; as with all relationships it can deepen mutual understanding and respect, and can be diverted into creative activity and solutions. If, for example, a physiotherapist and an occupational therapist are in conflict over the appropriate way to reduce 'challenging behaviour' in a client, they may manage to reach a creative compromise that is superior to either of their original ideas. This, in turn, may give them confidence to deal with future conflicts and deepen their trust in each other. A team which speaks entirely 'with one voice' can be oppressive, rather than supportive, to clients and members with minority views.

An important barrier to the effective functioning of multidisciplinary teams is a hierarchical structure which has, until very recent times, typified such teams. This type of structure leads to an authoritarian style of leadership and management where decisions are made from 'above', with little on no consultation or discussion with colleagues and least of all with the clients themselves. A consultative style, in contrast, is characterized by discussion and negotiation. In view of the range of skills required and the diversity of multidisciplinary teams in this field of work, it is probably best for different people to lead different aspects of the team, always keeping the views and goals of people with learning difficulties centrally in mind. This will also serve to minimize the need for large team meetings which can be formidable and do little to foster interpersonal understanding.

Specialist versus generic teams

Health and social services for adults with learning difficulties are commonly provided through specialized community teams. These teams are multidisciplinary and multi-agency and comprise many professional and non-professional workers. This model of health and social care has existed for nearly 20 years and has expanded since the closure of institutions. It is responsible for direct services (e.g. occupational therapy and physiotherapy) and for liaising with other professionals and agencies (Macadam and Rodgers, 1997). The philosophy is to provide a holistic service in accord with the client's individual requirements and wishes. Children with learning difficulties frequently receive services (e.g. therapy) from professionals who work within their schools. Others receive services from more generalized paediatric community teams.

The most central members of the team are, of course, people with learning difficulties themselves and those who assist them. It is essential to understand and respect their aspirations and goals and to seek their views in order to evaluate the service provided. An anti-racist and multicultural perspective is also vital. It is important, for example, to observe and respect cultural practices and to provide equal services to people whose first language is not English by, for example, employing sufficient interpreters. Stereotypical views about ethnic minorities 'looking after their own' also need to be dispelled (French and Vernon, 1997).

Teams which are specific to people with learning difficulties have the potential to provide their clients with a high-quality service delivered by people who understand their needs (Bannerman and Lindsay, 1993). Health care and health education are not very accessible to people with learning difficulties because their needs and rights have not been taken into account. Health professionals may, for example, lack the necessary skills to communicate with a person with severe learning difficulties, health education literature may not be in a suitable format, and the pace at which information is given may be too fast (Howells, 1997).

The existence of a specialized team for people with learning difficulties may, however, segregate people unnecessarily and maintain the status quo. Mainstream professional workers may not feel the need to become knowledgeable or involved with people with learning difficulties if a specialist team is in place (Sperlinger, 1997). In addition, the existence of specialist services has the potential to create feelings of inadequacy and deficiency in other workers (Sperlinger, 1997)

There are some advantages to having a specialized team. The staff involved are likely to have specific knowledge of people with learning difficulties and to be interested in providing a service of quality – though additional training is not routine. In reality, however, it is a 'Cinderella' service with low status and shortages of therapists and other staff, particularly in adult services (Auty, 1991). Therapists may possess important skills of communication, or of coping with 'challenging behaviour', but lack specific skills that other therapists may have. Should they be treating a person who has had a stroke, for example, when therapists in the nearby general hospital have specialized in this field? It can be argued that every therapist, whatever his or her speciality, should be sufficiently competent and confident to work with people with learning difficulties. In reality, however, it is an area of work rarely seen in the curriculum of student therapists and the existence of a specialized team has the potential to inhibit the acquisition of such knowledge among therapists who work in other areas. Birchenall *et al.* (1997) speaks of these dilemmas in relation to nursing.

Macadam and Rodgers (1997) believe that adults with learning difficulties require both specialist and general health and social services. There is nothing inherent in specialist teams for people with learning difficulties which prevents this from occurring. One of their functions is to liaise with other agencies and to cross institutional and management boundaries, however difficult this may be, if it is in the best interest of the client (Barnes *et al.*, 1989). The NHS and Community Care Act 1990 encourages the use of statutory, voluntary and private providers when drawing up 'packages of care' for individual clients; the client's key worker or care manager (who may be a therapist) is an important advocate in this regard. The introduction of competition among providers, following the implementation of the above mentioned Act, tends, however, to lessen cooperation between them. There are also financial repercussions when calling upon the services of professionals employed by other organizations. A further barrier is the different ideologies and cultures among organizations which make joint working difficult and time consuming (Macadam and Rodgers, 1997).

An advantage of a specialized service for people with learning difficulties is that they may have swifter access to services and receive more time and attention. This does, however, have the potential to create dependency on specialized medical and social services which, in some instances, could be provided in more inclusive and creative ways.

In an unpublished questionnaire study (French, 1997), which gathered the opinions of 40 carers and key workers regarding the physiotherapy service for adults with learning difficulties in an area of London, physiotherapy was thought to have various wide-ranging benefits. Twenty-seven (67%) of the respondents said it helped to keep the client moving, 22 (55%) said that physiotherapy added to the client's enjoyment of life, and seven (17%) said that physiotherapy improved the client's social skills. It is likely, however, that such benefits could be obtained in more inclusive and less medical settings.

There is an ever-present danger of medicalizing the lives of people with learning difficulties, particularly in the context of a disabling society where people with learning difficulties may lack access to mainstream services and where they may not be welcomed. Medicalization can serve the interests of professionals far more than those of clients, by providing professionals with work and a valued role. The issue of whether people with learning difficulties require a specialized or a generic service is still contentious (Walmsley, 1997).

Conclusion

At the present time, many of the health and social needs of people with learning difficulties are provided by multidisciplinary teams. The challenge for multidisciplinary teams is to provide a relevant and effective service for people with learning difficulties without medicalizing or controlling their lives or creating unnecessary dependency. This will only be achieved if people with learning difficulties and those who assist them in everyday life are central to the decision-making processes of the team.

References

Auty, P.O. (1991) *Physiotherapy for People with Learning Difficulties*, Woodhead-Faulkner, London

Bannerman, M. and Linsay, M. (1993) Evolution of services. In Shanley, E. and Starrs, T.A. (eds), *Learning Disabilities: A Handbook of Care*, 2nd ed, Churchill Livingstone, Edinburgh

Barnes, J., Dennis, C., Barrell, A. and Jenkins, J. (1989) *Standards for Good Practice in Physiotherapy Services for People with Learning Disabilities*, leaflet 1, Association of Chartered Physiotherapists for People with Learning Disabilities, London

Birchenall, M., Baldwin, S. and Morris, J. (1997) *Learning Disability and the Social Context of Caring*, The Open Learning Foundation/Churchill Livingstone, Edinburgh

Brechin, A. and Swain, J. (1987) *Changing Relationships: Shared Action Planning with People with a Mental Handicap*, Harper and Row, London

French S. (1997) A survey of carers' opinions of a physiotherapy service for adult clients with learning disabilities. Unpublished questionnaire study

French, S. and Vernon, A. (1997) Health Care for people from ethnic minority groups. In French, S. (ed) *Physiotherapy: A Psycholsocial Approach*, Butterworth-Heinemann, Oxford

Hattersley, J. (1995) The survival of collaboration and cooperation. In Malin, N. (ed.), *Services for People with Learning Difficulties*, Routledge, London

Howells, G. (1997) A general practice perspective. In O'Hara, J. and Sperlinger, A. (eds), *Adults with Learning Disabilities: A Practical Approach for Health Professionals*, Wiley, Chichester

Macadam, M. and Rodgers, J. (1997) A multi-disciplinary, multi-agency approach. In O'Hara, J. and Sperlinger, A. (eds), *Adults with Learning Disabilities: A Practical Approach for Health Professionals*, Wiley, Chichester

Pritchard, P. and Pritchard, J. (1992) *Developing Team Work in Primary Healthcare: A Practical Workbook*, Oxford Medical Publications, Oxford

Sperlinger, A. (1997) Introduction. In O'Hara, J and Sperlinger, A. (eds), *Adults with Learning Disabilities: A Practical Approach for Health Professionals*, Wiley, Chichester

Walmsley, J. (1997) Learning difficulties: changing roles for physiotherapists. In French, S. (ed.), *Physiotherapy: A Psychosocial Approach*, 2nd edn, Butterworth-Heinemann, Oxford

Ethical decision making

Sally French

What is ethical decision making?

Physiotherapists and occupational therapists, whatever their field of work, frequently find themselves in situations where ethical decisions need to be made – indeed, ethical questions and dilemmas permeate the entire process of therapy. Homan (1991) describes ethics as 'the science of morality' and Sim defines health care ethics as '... the application of moral reasoning in the context of health care' (1997a:323). He points out that there is no such thing as 'health care ethics' as the ethical principles applied within therapy are universal. 'Morality' and 'ethics' are words which are used interchangeably, but 'ethics' has a more specific meaning – the systematic study of assumptions of what is right and wrong.

Ethics is a branch of philosophy which rests upon various fundamental principles. The principle of non-maleficence, for example, demands that we do not inflict harm on others, whereas the principle of beneficence demands that we strive to confer benefits on others (Sim, 1997b). The utilitarian principle, in contrast, stipulates that that which is right is that which satisfies the largest number of people (Shanley and Starrs, 1993). These fundamental ethical principles frequently conflict. Respect for a person's autonomy, for example, would promote self-determination, but this may conflict with the principle of beneficence if the person's chosen action is not considered to be in his or her own best interests. Therapists do, therefore, find themselves in situations of moral conflict.

The therapy professions have their own codes of conduct to guide the behaviour of their members. For example, in the publication *Rules of Professional Conduct* by the Chartered Society of Physiotherapy it is stated that 'Chartered physiotherapists shall respect the rights, dignity and individual sensibilities of every patient' (1995:2). Some of the principles espoused in these codes are, however, more to do with etiquette and protection of the profession than with morality. In the same publication it is stated that 'Chartered physiotherapists shall adhere at all times to personal and professional standards that reflect credit on the profession' (1995:2). Physiotherapists are also warned to avoid public criticism of colleagues except in a court of law.

The ethical principles given within such guidelines tend, inevitably, to be global rather than specific which may lead therapists to become unreflective and to view situations in stereotyped ways. Plummer (1983) believes that ethical guidelines can lead to 'dogmatic sterility', and Homan states '... ethical principles are established on the basis of a considerable measure of professional self-interest' (1991:3). Ethical values change over time and across cultures and there are, therefore, no absolute right and wrong answers. The ultimate responsibility for ethically acceptable therapy thus lies with individual therapists. Ethical guidelines can be helpful, but may serve to absolve therapists from the necessity of making ethical decisions.

In this short chapter some ethical principles relating to respect, informed consent, confidentiality and the avoidance of exploitation will be examined and applied to the work of physiotherapists and occupational therapists. Some wider ethical issues will also be discussed.

Ethical dilemmas in therapy

Sarah, who has severe learning difficulties, has recently been involved in a road traffic accident and, as a consequence, has a stiff and painful knee. Although she is keen on swimming, horse riding and other sports, Sarah will not cooperate with Jackie, the physiotherapist, to bend her knee and become more mobile. Jackie is reluctant to force or coerce her and yet she is aware that Sarah derives a great deal of satisfaction, self-esteem and dignity from her sporting activities.

The principle of beneficence dictates that Jackie should carry out the treatment on Sarah's knee as this is for Sarah's own good. This, however, conflicts with the principle of respect for autonomy which dictates that people have the right to choose for themselves even if they make unwise choices. Ethical decisions must, however, be justified in terms of ethical reasoning and in the light of the particular case. The decision must be based on an accurate assessment of the facts. Jackie would need to be sure, for example, that Sarah's unwillingness to cooperate is not simply an expression of fear or a lack of understanding of the outcome. She also needs to be sure that Sarah is still interested in sport, that she is not unduly depressed or anxious and that her judgement is not being distorted by pain or distress.

By checking out these factors Jackie is demonstrating respect for Sarah's autonomy far more than she would be by simply withdrawing treatment. If Sarah's behaviour is significantly influenced by any of these factors, basing action on the 'respect for autonomy' principle would be flawed. It could be considered unethical to allow Sarah to make the decision to refuse treatment without attempting to encourage her and give her information. The dividing line between persuasion and coercion is fine, however, especially in the context of an unequal relationship. Ethical decision making is not, therefore, 'a matter of common sense' but a rigorous process of deduction.

It is essential for therapists to have a clear and ongoing dialogue with their clients in order to make ethical decisions. As Sim says, 'It is hard to respect the interests and preferences of the patient if one hasn't made the necessary effort to find out what they are' (1997a:334). This may be particularly difficult with people who have severe learning difficulties where conventional means of communication are not possible and where understanding may be limited. It may be necessary, in this situation, to confer with carers and advocates, but every effort should be made to communicate with the person himself or herself. The person's wishes should also be monitored carefully in case they change over time.

Some ethicists have stressed that to make ethical decisions people need particular personality characteristics, for example courage, generosity and compassion. Ethical decision making can, however, be learned. Professional qualities and expertise do not automatically carry with them expertise in ethical decision making; indeed, ethical and clinical judgements frequently conflict. As Sim states:

> What may seem an appropriate decision on clinical grounds may be morally objectionable, and, conversely, what may seem a dubious decision purely in terms of clinical judgement, may have much to recommend it as a moral course of action. (1997a:323)

Questions of ethics

Respect

The welfare of clients should always be at the front of the therapist's mind. Until very recent times, people with learning difficulties were frequently treated as objects rather than people with feelings, needs and rights. It is essential that therapists respect the wishes of people with learning difficulties and adapt any help they give to suit the chosen lifestyle of the person concerned. Respect can be measured, to a large extent, by how much people are able to exercise control over their own lives. The greater the control, the less likely therapists are to infringe the person's rights.

Informed consent

If consent is to be valid, sufficient information must be given and the person receiving the information must comprehend its meaning (Sim, 1986). Consent should not be given under coercion or pressure although, as noted above, the boundary between persuasion and coercion is rarely distinct. In order to give informed consent, the person must also be competent to make a rational decision (Sim, 1997b).

Until recently, people with learning difficulties were deemed incapable of making decisions about their own lives, including decisions relating to their rehabilitation and medical treatment. Although the help of carers and advocates may be needed when people have severe learning difficulties, every effort should be made to communicate directly with the people themselves using every available means and taking sufficient time. It is very easy to assume that people with learning difficulties are automatically incapable of understanding information and are unable to give their informed consent, but such beliefs do little more than promote stereotyping.

The issue of informed consent, particularly with people with learning difficulties, is, however, deeply problematic. The amount and complexity of information that can be assimilated and comprehended by someone with a severe learning difficulty may be limited and, as Walmsley (1993) points out, 'explaining is an interactive process' involving negotiation and a sharing of perspectives, not merely a process of passing on information. Furthermore, subtle pressure (often unintended) may be placed on clients to comply (Swain *et al.*, 1998).

Confidentiality

All therapists are required by their professional codes of conduct to respect privileged information that they acquire about their clients. In a multidisciplinary team it is generally thought legitimate and beneficial, to the client and the team, for members to share information, but unethical to divulge such information to an outside party without the consent of the client. The information gathered in case notes has, however, come under criticism for being useful only to professionals and to 'objectify, pathologize and label' people with learning difficulties (Gillman *et al.*, 1997).

The principle of confidentiality is not absolute and may come into conflict with other ethical principles. An example of this is illustrated in the following fictitious case study:

> Mary, a woman with learning difficulties, is being treated by an occupational therapist for a shoulder dislocation. During one of the treatment sessions she becomes distressed and discloses to the therapist that her shoulder was dislocated by her partner during a heated row. She insists, however, that this has never happened before and that she does not want the information to go any further.

There is a conflict here between the duty to preserve confidentiality and the duty (based on the principle of beneficence) to protect Mary from further danger. Depending on the details of the particular case, the therapist may decide to reveal the information to others but this, as Sim (1997b) points out, can destroy the very essence of the therapist – client relationship. The client may, however, be referred to a professional counsellor who will be bound by the principle of confidentiality for as long as the client wishes.

Therapists and counsellors do, on occasions, come under extreme pressure to reveal information, for example by parents. They may also be legally obliged to give information about their clients or, alternatively, to break the law. In organizations such as The Samaritans, the duty of confidentiality is so crucial that workers have faced the consequences of breaking the law in order to uphold the principle of confidentiality.

Exploitation

The relationship between the therapist and the client is an unequal one, with the therapist having more power and more knowledge of the treatment procedures and how they will be used. Therapists are, therefore, in a position to exploit clients in ways which may be overt but also so subtle that they are barely noticeable. Therapists may, for example, make it difficult for people with learning difficulties to refuse treatment, or embarrassing for them to withdraw from treatment. People with learning difficulties may comply against their wishes because they mistakenly view the therapist as a person who has the power to bring about favourable changes to their situation, or a fear that the valued social contact with the therapist may be withdrawn.

Although therapists may sometimes be exploited by clients, for example by being sexually harassed (Swain, 1995), vulnerable people, such as people with learning difficulties, are particularly susceptible to exploitation. An ethical dilemma always arises when permission to involve people with learning difficulties as clients is granted by someone in authority, especially when the client concerned is in an institution or is, in some other way, 'captive'. In this situation, people are often dependent on the same people for their physical, social and emotional needs, so to go against their wishes may have huge personal repercussions. People with learning difficulties need to be able to make as informed a choice as possible and their rights should be carefully safeguarded. It is helpful, when attempting to make an ethical decision, to acknowledge that the motivations and vested interests of therapists may be different from those of their clients. It is easy for the agendas of professionals to dominate those of the clients.

Wider ethical issues

There are many wider ethical issues with regard to people with learning difficulties which, although they may not impinge directly or frequently on the day-to-day work of therapists, are nevertheless of great concern. Where allocation of health care resources is scarce, for example, therapists may use their power to ensure that people with learning difficulties receive a fair share and are not marginalized or neglected because of disablist attitudes and assumptions about their worth or quality of life.

Therapists may also become involved in decisions concerning the right of people with learning difficulties to marry, live independently, have sexual relationships and become parents. In situations such as these there are, understandably, fears that the person may not understand the implications of his or her actions, or may have insufficient skills and insight to cope practically, socially or emotionally. A stringent demand that people with learning difficulties should demonstrate competence and understanding can, however, be oppressive. Few people know themselves well enough or understand the complexities of situations or relationships sufficiently to guarantee their own happiness or success. It is important that people with learning difficulties, like other people, are allowed to take risks and make mistakes and that standards are not applied to them that we would not apply to others. Shanley and Starr remark '... if we do not allow for errors no one is ever competent' (1993:301) and Manthorpe and colleagues state that '... risk is a barometer of ordinary living and is as much to do with opportunities as threats' (1997:80).

Bioethics is an area where therapists may, at a political level, choose to become involved. There is much criticism by disabled people, for example, of prenatal screening, genetic testing and euthanasia (Disability

Awareness in Action, 1997). Underlying these measures is a frequently erroneous assumption that disabled people are incapable of happiness because of their impairments, and are unable to lead productive lives (Swain and French, 1997).

Conclusion

Every aspect of a therapist's work involves ethical decision making. This is reflected in many topics within this book including bereavement, sexuality, and challenging behaviour. The key to making ethically sound decisions is the willingness to give control to people with learning difficulties, to help them lead the lives they choose and to help build their potential in order to reach their own self-defined goals.

References

Chartered Society of Physiotherapy (1995) *Rules of Professional Conduct*, London

Disability Awareness in Action (1997) *Life, Death and Rights*, London

Gillman, M., Swain, J. and Heyman, B. (1997) Life history or 'case' history: the objectification of people with learning difficulties through the tyranny of professional discourses. *Disability and Society*, **12**(5), 675–694

Homan, R. (1991) *The Ethics of Social Research*, Longman, London

Manthorpe, J. and Walsh, M. with Alaszewski, A. and Harrison, L. (1997) Issues of risk practice and welfare in learning disability services. *Disability and Society*, **12**(1), 69–82

Plummer, K. (1993) *Documents of Life*, Allen and Unwin, London

Shanley, E. and Starrs, T.A. (eds) (1993) *Learning Disabilities: A Handbook of Care*, 2nd ed, Churchill Livingstone, Edinburgh

Sim, J. (1986) Informed consent: ethical implications for physiotherapists. *Physiotherapy*, **72**, 584–587

Sim, J. (1997a) Ethics and moral decision making. In French, S. (ed.), *Physiotherapy: A Psychosocial Approach*, 2nd ed, Butterworth-Heinemann, Oxford

Sim, J. (1997b) *Ethical Decision Making in Therapy Practice*, Butterworth-Heinemann, Oxford

Swain, J. (1995) *The Use of Counselling Skills: A Guide For Therapists*, Butterworth-Heinemann, Oxford

Swain, J. and French, S. (1997) Whose tragedy? *Therapy Weekly*, **24**(13), 7

Swain, J., Heyman, B. and Gillman, M. (1998) Public research, private concerns: ethical issues in the use of open-ended interviews with people who have learning difficulties. *Disability and Society*, **13**(1), 21–36

Walmsley, J. (1993) Explaining. In Shakespeare, P., Atkinson, A. and French, S. (eds), *Reflecting on Research Practice: issues in Health and social welfare*, Open University Press, Buckingham

Institutional discrimination: people with learning difficulties from Black and ethnic minority communities

John Swain

Introduction

There are three possible interrelated themes in an exploration of institutional discrimination, each raising issues for the provision and practice of therapy with people with learning difficulties. The first is the nature of institutional discrimination: the unfair or unequal treatment of individuals or groups which is built into institutional organizations, policies and practices at personal, environmental and structural levels (Swain *et al.*, 1998). People with learning difficulties face institutional discrimination in a social and physical world that is geared by, for and to non-disabled people. Essentially, to understand discrimination as being 'institutional' is to eschew individualized, or victim-blaming, explanations of unjust treatment. This includes psychological models of attitudes that give no account to the historical and social context of prejudice. To see discrimination as institutional is to recognize that inequalities are woven into the very structure and fabric of British society and organizations. Discrimination is constructed at different levels within social divisions, hierarchies and inequalities, between people with learning difficulties and non-disabled people and the power relations that maintain the marginalization of people with learning difficulties.

The second theme is one of connections and commonalities. People with learning difficulties are by no means the only group within our society to face institutional discrimination. It is a way of understanding that applies to, and connects, the experiences of people with learning difficulties with those of other disabled people, Black and ethnic minority groups, gays and lesbians, old people and women. The commonalities in issues of racism, sexism, homophobia and disablism can be explored through themes such as prejudicial attitudes and discriminatory language (Thompson, 1997). From this point of view it is perhaps particularly significant that the struggles of people with learning difficulties, against discrimination, are aligned with those of other disabled people and the Disabled People's Movement.

The third theme highlights differences in the forms of discrimination faced by different groups, particularly groups whose day-to-day experiences involve simultaneous or multiple discrimination. Thus, as argued by Stuart, Black disabled people are subjected to a unique form of institutional discrimination which is different from the sum of racism experienced as a Black person and disablism experienced as a disabled person. Their experiences 'isolate black disabled people and place them at the margins of the ethnic minority and disabled populations' (1993: 95).

The particular focus for the chapter is the provision of therapy for Black and ethnic minority people with learning difficulties. In 1991, Mildrette Hill drew attention to the extremes of oppression faced by Black disabled people. She stated that the cumulative effect of discrimination is such that Black disabled people are 'the most socially, economically and educationally deprived and oppressed members of society' (1991: 6). This chapter aims to provide a framework for therapists to reflect on the experiences of people with learning difficulties from Black and ethnic minorities as a foundation for formulating principles and strategies of anti-discriminatory practice.

What is institutional discrimination?

The notion of institutional discrimination has played an important role in the development of theories of disability (Barnes, 1991) generating from a social model and developed by disabled people. People with learning difficulties are disabled by institutional barriers that prevent their full participative citizenship in society, and access to and participation in organizations. Figure 22B.1 depicts these barriers as the bricks in a wall of institutional discrimination. The wall (rather than more usual concentric circles) graphically illustrates the marginalization of disabled people. In this model of institutional discrimination, attitudinal barriers are constructed on environmental barriers, which are themselves constructed on structural barriers. No graphics can depict the interlinking and interaction between the three levels, although, as discussed below, ideology plays a key role in the articulation and interreliance between each layer.

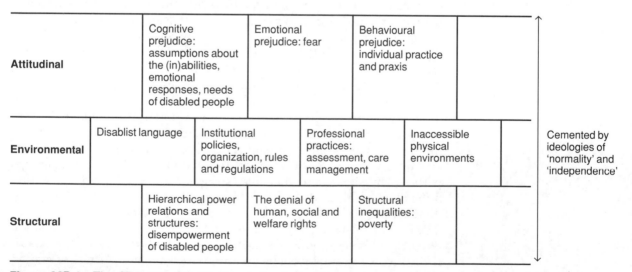

Attitudinal	Cognitive prejudice: assumptions about the (in)abilities, emotional responses, needs of disabled people	Emotional prejudice: fear	Behavioural prejudice: individual practice and praxis		Cemented by ideologies of 'normality' and 'independence'
Environmental	Disablist language	Institutional policies, organization, rules and regulations	Professional practices: assessment, care management	Inaccessible physical environments	
Structural	Hierarchical power relations and structures: disempowerment of disabled people	The denial of human, social and welfare rights	Structural inequalities: poverty		

Figure 22B.1 The SEAwall of institutional discrimination

The foundations of the wall are built at the Structural level. Institutional discrimination is founded on the social divisions in society and, in particular, hierarchical power relations between groups (e.g. disabled and non-disabled people). Inequalities in the distribution of resources, particularly economic, underpin hierarchical power relations, with people with learning difficulties being marginalized from open employment and condemned to poverty. People with learning difficulties, as a group, are denied political, social and human rights that non-disabled people take for granted.

The Environmental level of barriers is constructed, on these foundations, in the interaction between the individual and the social and physical environment. These, then, are the barriers confronted by people with learning difficulties in relation to rules, procedures, patterns of behaviour, shared understandings, timetables and so on (i.e. social organization), that are geared to the needs and norms of the non-disabled majority. The barriers are also created by aids that are geared to the needs and norms of non-disabled people (steps, taps, cars, buses, etc.), the needs of disabled people being marginalized to 'special' aids.

The third layer, Attitudinal, which is built on the previous two, is constructed in the direct interactions between disabled and non-disabled people, as individuals or in groups. These barriers are manifest in the attitudes and personal prejudices of non-disabled people, their expectations and actions. This includes the beliefs, feelings and practices of individual professionals. These relate to, but can differ substantially from, the collective professional practice, including training, ideology and organizational structures, which is conceived at the environmental level in this model. Thus, our analysis acknowledges that, despite the constraints, individual professionals can and do support the struggle of people with learning difficulties against institutional discrimination, even though the general practice of their profession contributes to this SEAwall of barriers.

The cement of normality and independence

If each brick in this wall of institutional discrimination was separable from all the others, the wall could be dismantled brick by brick. However, as the Disabled People's Movement has recognized, piecemeal approaches are ultimately ineffective in dismantling institutional discrimination, and it needs to be recognized that all these barriers are closely bound and interrelated. Part of the dynamic of this interlinking is through ideology.

Thompson (1997) refers to ideology as the 'glue' that binds together the levels in his model of institutionalized discrimination. In doing so, a dominant ideology operates in a number of ways:

- legitimizing social inequalities, power relations and structures;
- establishing 'what is "normal" and therefore, by extension, what is "abnormal" ' (Thompson, 1997: 25);
- defining cultural values and desirable goals;
- being 'naturalized, taken for granted and almost all-embracing' (Barnes, 1996: 48).

There are a number of dimensions to the ideological basis of institutionalized discrimination faced by people with learning difficulties:

(a) The individual model: in which disability is seen as a problem, and the problem is located in the impaired individual.
(b) The medical model: which is a form of the individual model and strengthens the legitimization of inequality based on biology.
(c) Stereotypes of people with learning difficulties.
(d) Societal values of 'normality–abnormality' and 'dependency–independency'.

These values not only define people with learning difficulties as 'abnormal', but also as needing care, cure and control to become, if not normal and independent, then as nearly so as possible. Such ambitions are rarely those of disabled people themselves (Swain and French, 1998).

Simultaneous discrimination: people with learning difficulties from Black and ethnic minorities

The simultaneous discrimination faced by people with learning difficulties from Black and ethnic minority communities manifests itself in many ways in day-to-day living. Though the evidence relating to this particular group is sparse, it points to major barriers at all three levels of the SEAwall of institutional discrimination. Two studies of the families of Asian people with learning difficulties (ADAPT, 1993; Azmi et al., 1996), for instance, provided evidence of high levels of poverty, with 69 per cent of families having no full-time wage earner and half of the families being on income support. Significant language barriers were found in the same studies. Ninety-five per cent of carers had been born outside of Britain and only a minority could speak or write English (Nadirshaw, 1997).

However, there are dangers in such statistics. First, they can feed presumptions and stereotyping which belie diversity. In her study of Asian parents, for instance, Shah found that 'the majority of parents had a good command of English and, for some, English was their first language' (1998: 186). She also cites language barriers as an example of preconceived notions of discrimination experienced by Asian families. Secondly, there is a danger of oversimplifying language barriers. As the Black Perspectives Sub-group points out, language is 'about freedom of expression, release of emotion, cultural identity and shared values' (1998: 97) and a common language is no guarantee of shared understanding. At the attitudinal level of institutional discrimination, 'there is a lack of understanding among the majority population concerning the life style, social customs and religious practices of people from ethnic minority groups' (French and Vernon, 1997: 62)

Discrimination within the provision of services has received particular attention as a major brick in the SEAwall of institutional discrimination experienced by people with learning difficulties from Black and ethnic minority communities and their families, and they can receive little or no appropriate services. Yet discrimination has been denied and rationalized through myths that, for instance, Black families prefer 'to look after their own' (Baxter, 1995). As Nadirshaw (1997) points out, parents' expectations and use of services depends on a number of factors, including the way in which they learn about their child's learning difficulties. Baxter and colleagues suggest that if the family is from a Black or ethnic minority community, good standards in 'breaking the news' are less likely to be met. They provide an example:

> One Asian mother told us: 'When my baby was born, there were no professional staff who could speak my language. Eventually staff identified a cleaner who could speak to me working on the ward. The cleaner was asked to break the news to me. (1990: 33)

Institutional discrimination is manifest in many ways in the provision, policy and practice of services. Three related themes recur in the literature: normalization, assessment and individual programme planning. The ideologies of normality and independence pervade the provision of services and professional practice, with little or no account being taken of the wider social, political and economic issues of institutional discrimination. The dominant rhetoric of meeting individual needs and normalization underlies the failure of services to recognize and address the effects of racism and disablism on both clients and providers of services. For instance, the section on *normalisation* in a workbook for nurses working with people with learning difficulties acknowledges that 'the idea of normality as a constant needs to be challenged' (Birchenall *et al.*, 1997: 48), but there is no reference to racism or disablism as an integral part of the culture of white non-disabled society.

Though the literature documenting the views of Black disabled people is sparse, it consistently speaks to experiences of segregation and marginalization within services. In Vernon's research, disabled Black and ethnic minority women felt that, in many ways, they had not had access to equal education. The following is an illustrative example:

> Momta, who came to Britain at the age of 12 from Uganda, found that her education suffered because of a focus on medical and rehabilitation needs. 'At the top of everybody's priorities was the physical side. You know, get you on your feet and get you moving was the most important thing in special school. Like swimming and physio was more important than the actual study side. There was a lot of disappointment as far as I was concerned.' (1996: 55)

Therapy and institutional discrimination

It is not the aim of this chapter to provide detailed practical advice for therapists, and indeed to do so would be in danger of compromising the principle of diversity that is central to the analysis presented here. Some general implications are, however, evident.

Provision of race and disability equality training for therapists

Both forms of training espouse, in general terms, the institutional discrimination perspective outlined above. French and Vernon, advocating race equality training, state:

> 'Race' equality training, when skillfully carried out by people from ethnic minority groups, can help people to become aware of their attitudes and behaviour in a relaxed and non-threatening environment. (1997: 66)

The same can be said in relation to disability equality training which has the following characteristics:

- it is about discrimination rather than impairment;
- it is about challenging understanding of 'disability', and changing practices, rather than about improving general attitudes towards people with learning difficulties;
- it is seen as part of the wider struggle for equality of opportunity in policy and practice (for women, Black and ethnic minority communities, lesbians and gays);
- it is devised and delivered by disabled people (Swain and Lawrence, 1994)

Listening and consultation

Therapists are predominantly white and non-disabled, and have no direct personal experience of the institutional discrimination faced by people with learning difficulties from Black and ethnic minority communities. Whatever their working knowledge of cultural diversity, it is essential that the 'voice' of clients directs the provision of appropriate and culturally-sensitive services. This applies through listening to individual clients whose daily experiences are likely to be fundamentally different from the experiences of therapists. It also applies through the consultation of organizations of people with learning difficulties and people from Black and ethnic minority communities at every stage of service planning and implementation.

Facilitation of communication

There is a continuing need for trained interpreters, carefully matched to the client and his or her family, and independent of the particular organization. There is a need too for the provision of information about services in languages and forms accessible to all clients, potential clients and their families.

Employment of disabled, Black and ethnic minority staff

As Nadirshaw (1997) points out, Black and ethnic minority staff can communicate with clients in their own languages and can contribute to the evaluation of the adequacy of services, though it is important that such staff do not become restricted, in their role, to 'race experts'.

Conclusion

From the viewpoint of institutional discrimination, meeting the particular needs of this group of clients is not a matter of simply confronting racism in the provision of services. As Begum states:

> The very nature of simultaneous oppression means that as Black Disabled men and women, and Black Disabled lesbians and gay men we cannot identify a single source of oppression to reflect the reality of our lives. No meaningful analysis of multiple oppression can take place without an acknowledgement that Black Disabled people are subject to simultaneous oppression and as a consequence of this we cannot simply prioritize one aspect of our oppression to the exclusion of others.
> (1994: 35)

Jackie who is a woman, a Black person and a person with learning difficulties expressed a similar view: 'My view is that I can't separate them. This is me. I relate to them all in different ways' (Walmsley and Downer, 1997: 45).

The issues are much broader and, as Stuart says, go well beyond the reductionist view that 'racist processes are the only primary cause of all the unequal outcomes and exclusions which black people experience' (1996: 96). Indeed, it is questionable whether Black and ethnic minority people with learning difficulties can or should be considered as a heterogeneous group. The central challenge to the policies and practices of therapy addresses diversity as well as commonality of need. As Williams (1992) points out, the task is to relate the diversity and differences between different forms of discrimination to the need for an anti-discriminatory alliance and for anti-discriminatory practice.

References

ADAPT (1993) *Asian and Disabled: A Study into the Needs of Asian People with Disabilities in the Bradford Area*, Asian Disability Advisory Project Team, The Spastics Society and Barnardos, West Yorkshire

Azmi, S., Emerson, E., Caine, A. and Hatton, C. (1996) *Improving Services for Asian People with Learning Difficulties and their Families*, Hester Adrian Research Centre/The Mental Health Foundation, Manchester

Barnes, C. (1991) *Disabled People in Britain: A Case for Anti-discrimination Legislation*, Hurst, London

Barnes, C. (1996) Theories of disability and the origins of the oppression of disabled people in western society. In Barton, L. (ed.), *Disability and Society: Emerging Issues and Insights*, Longman, London

Baxter, C. (1995) Confronting colour blindness: developing better services for people with learning difficulties from Black and ethnic minority communities. In Philpot, T. and Ward, L. (eds), *Values and Visions: Changing Ideas in Services for People with Learning Difficulties*, Butterworth-Heinemann, Oxford

Baxter, C., Poonia, K., Ward, L. and Nadirshaw, Z. (1990) *Double Discrimination: Issues and Services for People with Learning Difficulties from Black and Ethnic Minority Communities*, King's Fund Centre, London

Begum, N. (1994) Mirror, mirror on the wall. In Begum, N., Hill, M. and Stevens, A. (eds), *Reflections: Views of Black Disabled People on their Lives and Community Care*, Central Council for Education and Training in Social Work, London

Birchenall, M., Baldwin, S. and Morris, J. (1997) *Learning Disability and the Social Context of Caring*, Churchill Livingstone, Edinburgh

Black Perspectives Sub-group (1998) Black perspectives on residential care. In Allott, M. and Robb, M. (eds), *Understanding Health and Social Care: An Introductory Reader*, Sage, London

French, S. and Vernon, A. (1997) Health care for people from ethnic minority groups. In French, S. (ed.), *Physiotherapy: A Psychosocial Approach*, 2nd edn, Butterworth-Heinemann, Oxford

Hill, M. (1991) Race and disability. In *Disability – Identity, Sexuality and Relationships: Readings*, K665Y course, The Open University, Milton Keynes

Nadirshaw, Z. (1997) Cultural Issues. In O'Hara, J. and Sperlinger, A. (eds), *Adults with Learning Difficulties*, John Wiley and Sons, London

Shah, R. (1998) 'He's our child and we shall always love him' – mental handicap: the parents' response. In Allott, M. and Robb, M. (eds), *Understanding Health and Social Care: An Introductory Reader*, Sage, London

Stuart, O. (1993) Double oppression: an appropriate starting-point? In Swain, J. *et al.* (eds), *Disabling Barriers – Enabling Environments*, Sage, London

Stuart, O. (1996) 'Yes, we mean black disabled people too': thoughts on community care and disabled people from black and minority ethnic communities. In Ahmad, W. I.U. and Atkin, K. (eds), *'Race' And Community Care*, Open University Press, Buckingham

Swain, J. and French, S. (1998) Measuring up to normality: the foundations of disabling care. In Brechin, A. *et al.* (eds), *Care Matters: Concepts, Practice and Research*, London, Sage

Swain, J., Gillman, M. and French, S. (1998) *Confronting Disabling Barriers: Towards Making Organisations Accessible*, Venture Press, Birmingham

Swain, J. and Lawrence, P. (1994) Learning about disability: changing attitudes or challenging understanding? In French, S. (ed.), *On Equal Terms: Working with Disabled People*, Butterworth-Heinemann, Oxford

Thompson, N. (1997) *Anti-Discriminatory Practice*, 2nd edn, Macmillan Press, Basingstoke

Vernon, A. (1996) A Stranger in many camps: the experiences of disabled black and ethnic minority women. In Morris, J. (ed.), *Encounters with Strangers: Feminism and Disability*, The Women's Press, London

Walmsley, J. and Downer, J. (1997) Shouting the loudest: self-advocacy, power and diversity. In Ramcharan, P. *et al.* (eds), *Empowerment in Everyday Life: Learning Disability*, Jessica Kingsley, London

Williams, F. (1992) Somewhere over the rainbow: universality and diversity in social policy. In Manning, N. and Page, N. (eds), *Social Policy Review*, Social Policy Association, London

The human relations of therapy: power over or power with?

Phyllis Jones

Introduction

The relations between humans are fundamental to the quality and effectiveness of all aspects of life. The quality of the relationships that grow between therapists and people with learning difficulties can be the key to the type of partnership developed. It can open the door to a true partnership – one which enables both parties to share and contribute in a context of mutual respect and value. Conversely, it can open the door to a relationship that is hierarchical and characterized by dominance and compliance. Human relations are very powerful and need to be handled with care and sensitivity. Swain defines human relations within the context of therapy as 'a social interaction involving: self-awareness and awareness of others, including experiences, actions and feelings; the personal relationships between those involved' (1995:17).

Intrinsic to the quality and equality of human relations is the notion of power. From this comes the concept of empowerment. This chapter will consider these concepts in the context of the human relations that develop between therapists and people with learning difficulties.

The term 'empowerment' has become something of a cliché in the context of disability and therapy. To explore the essence of the concept, it is necessary to consider the concept of power. Neath and Schriner (1998) identify three forms of power:

- 'Personal power', which relates to the power of an individual to influence his or her environment. This could be, for example, choosing to change the channel on the television when watching it alone.
- 'Power over', which relates to authoritarian and hierarchical power, for example, a parent choosing to switch off the television at the watershed time when youngsters are in the room.
- 'Power with', which is egalitarian social power, referring to people acting together, for example, a group of people deciding to change the channel on the television to watch another programme.

These three forms of power are evident all the time throughout society, although it is true to say that most Western institutions, no matter how benevolent, are based on the 'power over' form of power. This type of power permeates through all organizations to some extent and has a major influence on all the people working within them. This influence can be constraining for all concerned.

An occupational therapist told the story of an incident that occurred in a community wing of a long-stay hospital for people with learning difficulties. The story highlights the influential and disabling role of 'power over' within the community hospital. An explicit aim of the occupational therapy work was to try to enable personal choice and advocacy for the young people. The occupational therapy rooms were open to residents at various times throughout the week. A young man with Down's syndrome had been assigned, through discussion, to activities and tasks in the garden. The young man continuously left his place of work throughout the day to go to the occupational therapy rooms on the first floor. He appeared to be particularly happy there. However, he was not allowed to stay in the suite of rooms. It was either 'not his time', or it was 'staff meeting time' where it was deemed inappropriate for him to stay.

A problem was thus created. There followed a period of trying to dissuade the young man from staying. This often led to physical interventions by staff to remove him. The situation was stressful for the young man and for the staff on duty. The occupation therapist telling the story said she would not have minded if he had stayed, but explained that the routines within the hospital did not allow for this. This is an example of the limiting implications and consequences of 'power over'.

Considering the concept of empowerment in the context of relations between therapists and people with learning difficulties raises the issue of where power lies in the relationship and the extent to which the power structures of the organization encourage or discourage the movement of power within the context of therapy. It involves the perceptions professionals hold relating to the role of power. Some may feel threatened by the notion of empowering people with learning difficulties and see it as a disempowerment of themselves. The concept of empowerment will now be explored by examining three main questions concerned with the 'Why?', 'What?' and 'How?' of human relations and the role of power within these.

The 'Why?'

It is important to be aware of the driving force that impels people to want to relate to one another: the 'Why?' question in human relations. With this question the notion of power emerges. The work of Maslow (1954) offers one illustration of the perceived hierarchy of human needs that appears to drive human relations. Figure 22C.1 illustrates this model.

According to Maslow it is necessary to satisfy the needs at the bottom of the hierarchy before the 'higher' needs can be satisfied. Self-actualization cannot, therefore, be achieved until all four proceeding levels of need in the hierarchy have been satisfied. Immediately one can envisage circumstances where this hierarchy of needs may not be correct. For example, a person who is in a great deal of pain may develop, nevertheless, higher level needs. An issue that occurs with some people

+---+
| Self-actualization (full potential) |
| Self-esteem |
| Love and belonging |
| Safety |
| Physiological |
+---+

Figure 22C.1 The hierarchy of human needs (after Maslow, 1954)

who have difficulty communicating is enabling them to express their feelings and needs. A brief explanation of the levels proposed by Maslow (1954) reveals some of the dilemmas that relate to human relations and the concept of empowerment.

Physiological

These are life-sustaining needs. They relate to basic needs, such as alleviation from hunger and thirst, but also refer to medical considerations. For example, a child with cystic fibrosis will need physiotherapy as a basic human need to free the mucus from his or her lungs. Until this level of need is met, it is difficult for the child to experience other levels of need positively. The question of who perceives the physiological need reveals a dilemma. Is it the child with cystic fibrosis or is it the therapist?

Safety

This need refers both to physical and psychological safety: the need to feel secure. For example, a man with learning difficulties who has recently experienced major changes within his life, such as the loss of a parent, will need to regain his sense of security before moving on to another level. It can be very difficult and even dangerous to quantify and judge the psychological needs of others. People with learning difficulties have psychological needs that they can express and deal with themselves, often without the intervention of professionals. While supporting people with learning difficulties, it is important not to 'medicalize' or 'professionalize' their lives.

Love and belonging

This refers to the need to love, to be loved and to have a sense of belonging. Brammer and Macdonald (1996) suggest that the personal aspect of being loved, and feeling wanted and accepted, is a precursor to being able to love and value others. For example, an adolescent with challenging behaviour may need to feel loved and wanted before he or she feels secure enough to reciprocate.

Self-esteem

Self-esteem refers to the need to feel good about oneself. Swain explains self-esteem as 'the value or worth that people put upon themselves or single aspects of their self images' (1995:20). It is important not to make assumptions about the level of self-esteem of others. Situations are always viewed from a deeply personal perspective. It is important to be sensitive and open and not to make judgements from a personal perspective in order to enable people with learning difficulties to express how they feel about themselves. For example, when relating to a young woman who has a severe physical impairment, a therapist may perceive the situation as tragic from a personal perspective, thinking that he or she would never cope in a similar situation. This can lead to wrong assumptions being made. The young woman will be living her life as she knows it, and therefore her viewpoint may be entirely different from that of the therapist.

Self-actualization

This refers to the need to strive for self-development, autonomy, individuality, personal identity and challenge. Self-actualization involves reaching one's full potential and becoming everything one is capable of becoming. It includes concepts of self-advocacy and personal power. It is in enabling these needs to be met that institutional power and the role of the therapist may be threatened. It is at this stage that true empowerment can take place.

For everyone, depending on personal and environmental circumstances, striving to meet varying levels of need in the hierarchy may be operating at any one time. Even those who have developed a high level of self-actualization must, at the same time, satisfy at least some of the lower level needs for any quality of life to continue (Minardi, 1997).

The 'What?'

The 'What?' question is concerned with relationships. Nelson-Jones offers a clear definition of relationships as 'the connections that we make with others' (1996: 21). Connections between ourselves and others can take any form. They can be of any length, depth or strength. Relationships involve something happening or passing among two or more people. They are interactive processes that are dynamic. Any relationship is a process of coming together from different perspectives to create a single and united interaction. The nature of relationships may be seen to be shaped by the interplay of power between the people involved. Bulmer (1987) (cited in Bayley, 1997) developed a model that represents the range of relationships needed in order to fulfil cognitive and emotional needs. Figure 22C.2 sets out this model. It represents a typology of relationships and does not illustrate a hierarchy. However, the quality of relationships and the balance of power may be enhanced or adversely affected through experiences in the various types of relationships. In relationships that involve attachment and intimacy, feelings can be expressed freely in a secure and supported context; for example, with a close friend or parent. Some relationships enable social integration and encourage participants to share concerns, interests and goals; for example, those found in a social support group. Relationships that offer opportunities for nurture encourage the sense of being needed and valued; for example, that of looking after a child or pet animal. Relationships that encourage reassurance of worth, assist in developing

Attachment and intimacy
Social integration
Nurturance
Reassurance of worth
Reliable assistance
Obtaining guidance

Figure 22C.2   The range of relationships, after Bulmer (1987)

and demonstrating individual competence within a role; for example, that of the cook within a group of friends living together. Relationships which provide reliable assistance create support networks; for example, a neighbour who always buys the milk.

The last type of relationship in the model is based upon obtaining guidance. Such guidance may be obtained from a priest, a physiotherapist, an occupational therapist or someone who is deemed to have knowledge and experience. This does not, of course, necessarily have to be a professional.

It is worth remembering the negative elements that can also develop in any of these types of relationship. For example, the cook, while receiving positive feedback on his or her role as cook, may also feel taken for granted because he or she always has to do the cooking! The first four types of relationship appear to support the development of self and self-worth, whereas the last two types offer external support and guidance. Pertinent questions may be 'Which type or types of relationships do therapists encourage and practise within the therapy context?', and 'Which types of relationships do people with learning difficulties encourage within the therapy context?'.

The 'How?'

How, then, does power manifest itself within society? One way is through the roles that are adopted by people and the way in which these roles are perceived by others. The roles people adopt and the interplay of these within a relationship can be overt or subtle, but are always complex. Does this have implications for the professional role adopted by the therapist within the context of the therapy? The role of the therapist is perceived as a professional one. A therapist can contribute a professional knowledge base of skills and experience to the therapy which naturally carries status and power. Therapists can be said to enter the therapy context with a perceived powerful role. The power of this role will be greater than the perceived power of a person with learning difficulties. The therapist is the expert, the professional, and may be perceived to hold 'power over' power because of his or her role. However, people with learning difficulties live constantly with their particular abilities and disabilities. Within the context of the therapy, they are the natural experts and have much to contribute.

Lovett develops the theme of 'power over' within institutions for people with learning difficulties. He states:

In the world of people with learning disabilities, compliance is often the chiefest of virtues. In this world, being controlled by others is the norm and to break with that standard exacts punishments from one's controllers. (1996: 159)

Lovett offers some disturbing examples of how extreme punishment has been administered over the years in the name of behaviour modification to people whose very behaviour challenges the 'power over' form of power. He goes on to comment on the effect that this 'power over' role has on staff who work the closest with people with learning difficulties. They too are ruled, rewarded and punished because of their clients' behaviour – the needs of the institution clearly coming before the needs of the individual. Although the staff acknowledge the danger of hierarchical power, they too may be powerless to influence or impact upon it (Wardhaugh and Wilding, 1998).

Neath and Schriner illustrate the positive interrelationship that can occur between the three forms of power:

Personal power enables people to work together, exercising 'power with' and challenging social structures based on 'power over'. (1998:218)

There needs to be a level of 'personal power', made stronger in the context of sharing of 'power with', to enable the status quo of 'power over' to be challenged. A recent research project by Melton (1998), concerned with the role of an occupational therapist with a group of young people with mild learning difficulties, showed that the occupational therapist was perceived by the young people in a very positive way. She was seen by them as helping to develop their autonomy and encouraging them to take responsibility for their choices. Another study by Cattermole *et al.* (1988) carried out some detailed research with people who had significant learning difficulties and who were about to move out of the mental handicap hospital where they had lived for many years. The findings of the study demonstrated that the people that they interviewed held very strong opinions about their circumstances and the standard of service they received.

To enable empowerment to take place, there needs to be a shift in the perceived balance of power away from the therapist as expert towards the therapist and person with learning difficulties sharing the power. This is similar to the 'power with' form of power described by Neath and Schriner (1998). However, it is important to enable and support the development of 'personal power' with the person with learning difficulties. This, in turn, will help to create the ambience and context for the 'power with' form of power to be developed and sustained. This has major repercussions for the role and style of working adopted by the therapist.

The therapist can enable this to happen by adopting the role of collaborator and facilitator. Within the research carried out by Melton

(1998), the role of the occupational therapist was seen by the young people as a flexible and changing one. They used terms that referred to her as 'teacher', 'facilitator' and 'supporter'. Are there skills that can be learned to enable the therapist and people with learning difficulties to improve their roles within the relationship? Minardi (1997) offers an example where mental health nurses were given direct teaching in relation to identifying emotions through non-verbal communication. The study showed that direct teaching could enhance the communication skills employed by the nurses. Another example of similar work was carried out by Ware (1994). This study highlighted the tendency of some professionals, in this case a group of teachers in a special school for pupils with severe and profound learning difficulties, to intervene too quickly in the interaction. The research revealed the teachers were very committed to encouraging active responses from their pupils, but in practice did not allow enough time for the pupils to respond before they intervened again within the communication. The research showed greater incidence of pupil initiation and responses within the communication dialogue after the in-service training of their teachers.

These two pieces of research show that communication skills can be taught. However, effective communication involves more complex processes than skills and strategies, and there is a school of thought that the promotion of counselling skills with professionals can be dangerous. Counselling skills can be very powerful. They can be utilized to empower people with learning difficulties. However, within institutions dominated by 'power over' forms of power, counselling skills may strengthen the power of the therapist. The work of Swain (1995) highlights principles for human relations within a helping context. These principles relate to the relationships formed between therapists and people with learning difficulties. Exploring principles rather than skills and strategies can be helpful when examining the purpose and nature of the relationship. Table 22C.1 sets out these principles.

Table 22C.1   Principles for relationships between therapists and people with learning difficulties (after Swain, 1995)

---

1 Promotion of prediction and control over decision making
2 Development of understanding concerning important issues central to therapy
3 Promotion of mutual understanding
4 Development of awareness of others' preferences, wishes and needs
5 Promotion of self-understanding
6 Promotion of people's struggles against oppression regarding equal opportunities and full participation
7 Development of self-awareness, self-motivation and self-monitoring
8 Questioning of power relations and structures

---

288 Therapy and Learning Difficulties

When examining the principles it becomes clear that they apply equally well to the relationships between therapists and people with learning difficulties. They are helpful in that they represent a philosophy that encourages shared partnership and makes positive moves towards empowerment. They can also be seen as a challenge to the 'power over' form of power which is common in many institutions (Lovett, 1996). Whatever communication skills therapists develop, the above principles will affect why and how the specific skills and strategies are employed. There is a range of skills and strategies that come from counselling that could help the therapist fulfil these principles (Swain, 1995).

Conclusion

This chapter has explored the three questions set out at the beginning relating to the 'Why?', 'What?' and 'How?' of human relationships. The complex role that power plays can never be understated. In exploring these issues, more questions and dilemmas have been raised that need further exploration and development. The continual pressure and presence of the 'power over' type of power, typical of organizations, continues to have a strong influence on the potential response of therapists and people with learning difficulties.

The notion of 'power with' replacing 'power over' suggests one possible way forward in the pursuit of a more balanced and equal distribution of power within the relationship. This may be seen as a diminution in the role of the therapist and may create a personal dilemma, but it can also be viewed as an empowerment for both parties as it may strengthen the quality of the human relations and the subsequent power of the relationship that develops from this. This, in turn, will lead to a richer outcome of the therapy and may be a powerful force that can begin to present a challenge to the institutional power. (For further information on the concept of empowerment, the reader is referred to Chapters 21A–C.)

References

Bayley, M. (1997) Empowering and relationships. In Ramcharan, P. *et al.*, (eds) *Empowerment in Everyday Life: Learning Disability*, Jessica Kingsley, London

Brammer, J. and Macdonald, G. (1996) *The Helping Relationship: Process and Skills*, Schuster, London

Bulmer, M. (1987) The Social Basis of Community Care, Allen and Unwin, London

Cattermole, M., Johoda, A. and Markova, L. (1988) Life in a mental handicap hospital. *Journal of the British Institute of Mental Handicap*, **16**, 136–139

Lovett, H. (1996) *Learning to Listen: Positive Approaches and People with Difficult Behaviour*, Jessica Kingsley, London

Maslow, A. (1954) *Motivation and Personality*, Harper, New York

Melton, J. (1998) How do clients with learning disabilities evaluate their experience of cooking with the occupational therapist? *British Journal of Occupational Therapy*, **61**(3), 106–110

Minardi, H. (1997) *Communications in Health Care: A Skills-based Approach*, Butterworth-Heinemann, Oxford

Neath, J. and Schriner, K. (1998) Power to people with disabilities: empowerment issues in employment programming. *Disability and Society*, **13**(2), 217–228

Nelson-Jones, R. (1996) *Relating Skills*, Cassell, London

Swain, J. (1995) *The Use of Counselling Skills: A Guide for Therapists*, Butterworth-Heinemann, Oxford

Wardhaugh, J. and Wilding, P. (1998) Towards an explanation of the corruption of care. In Abbott, M. and Robb, M. (eds), *Understanding Health and Social Care: An Introductory Reader*, Sage, London

Ware, J. (1994) *Educating Children with Profound and Multiple Learning Difficulties*, Fulton, London

22D	# Vulnerable to abuse

Hilary Brown

Introduction

This chapter explores responsibilities in relation to abuse and mistreatment of children and adults with learning disabilities, and examines different ideas about how such abuse comes about and what is currently considered best practice in responding to it. It is illustrated by quotes from a group of service users who were survivors of sexual abuse and who met together in late 1995 to make tapes about sexual abuse for service users and for staff (Brown and Stein, 1996; Stein and Brown, 1996).

The day-to-day involvement and advice of therapists may serve to prevent abuse from happening in the first place and to increase the confidence of staff in positive interventions. Social services take the lead in cases involving child protection and usually it will be their responsibility (or that of the inspection unit) to act on any specific concerns or allegations concerning vulnerable adults.

The role of health-related professionals certainly extends to being alert to risks and sensitive to hints or cues which might indicate that someone might have been abused. Independent practitioners, moving in and out of family and service settings, are in a relatively powerful position to pass on concerns: care staff, for example, might be afraid of losing their jobs if they were to 'blow the whistle' about standards of care within their agency. Also in the course of consultations they may notice bruises, injuries, signs of neglect, problems with medication, and changes in daily activities and confidence.

Therapists may also be on the receiving end of disclosures and 'confidences' which they must deal with in the framework of local multiagency policies and procedures and not as an individual making decisions 'on the hoof' in an unaccountable way. For example, it may not be the best course of action for a therapist to take a person's stated wish that they do nothing about abuse which they have disclosed at face value when they may have been intimidated and/or other people may be at risk – this is the kind of decision about which all practitioners are expected to consult.

This chapter recommends a proactive stance to abuse and vulnerability; in other words it urges an *appropriate* level of suspicion on behalf of clients/patients. This does not mean that practitioners should over-react by seeing abuse everywhere or assuming malicious motives behind every situation in which care is less than perfect. But it does mean keeping that possibility in the back of one's mind when working with individuals who give rise to concern, or care agencies and their managers or proprietors who seem to be failing service users or to be overly excluding or defensive.

An important place to start is to acknowledge that people with learning disabilities are not alone in having to recognize their vulnerability to personal violence, bullying or sexual assault: these are issues faced to some extent by *all* children, women and men in their neighbourhoods, families and relationships. However, research suggests that children and adults with learning disabilities may be more at risk because of their own difficulties in understanding or communicating, but also because of the way they receive services and the fact that they may be actively targeted or taken advantage of. Moreover, risk is increased by

- the congregated and isolated settings in which people with learning disabilities live and work – in group homes and day centres;
- their needs for support and assistance – often provided by people who do not know them well or stay long in their lives;
- the fact that all too often they lack independent advocacy.

But despite the fact that people with learning disabilities are likely to be more vulnerable, they are afforded less protection and more restricted access to justice or redress than other citizens.

Children with learning disabilities are included within statutory child protection procedures (although these do not always work well for them) and increasingly abuse of vulnerable adults is being addressed through explicit policies and procedures that formalize some aspects of the decision-making process. Sometimes these policies are generic in that they refer to abuse of other adult 'client groups', or they may be specific to people with learning disabilities or to particular issues or settings. The ADSS (Association of Directors of Social Services) has mandated all social service departments (in their role as lead agency for community care) to develop overarching policies or a set of interlocking and consistent statements to cover all types of abuse, of all client groups in all settings, and that these should be multi-agency wherever possible. This may seem cumbersome or bureaucratic and it certainly limits discretion to act alone, as do child protection procedures which mandate the sharing of information and set out agreed decision-making structures and processes. For example, therapists are probably required to report concerns even if they have been told them in confidence. But there are very good reasons for doing so and for occasionally overriding the usual tenets of good practice around confidentiality and risk taking, especially if there is a risk of repeated abuse to an individual or to other vulnerable adults which justifies such caution.

What do we mean by the term 'abuse'?

'Abuse' is a rather loose term that has been criticized from opposing points of view. Williams (1993) has argued that it minimizes the impact of incidents that are often serious criminal offences, such as theft, assault or rape. Others have argued that it is too heavy-handed. Often the word is only applied to harm caused or sustained within an ongoing relationship marked by dependency and other inequalities. This focus on family, or other 'carer' relationships, draws attention away from the abuse and exploitation which vulnerable adults experience in day and residential services or in their neighbourhoods and communities (Flynn, 1987), including assaults from other service users or mistreatment by staff.

Consensus is beginning to emerge in relation to which *categories* of abuse should be covered within adult protection procedures, but practitioners usually say that it is not the *category* but the *threshold of seriousness* (the point at which they should report their concerns) that they find difficult to pinpoint. Policies usually cover

- physical
- sexual
- psychological (sometimes called emotional, or social abuse)
- financial
- neglect (Brown and Stein, 1998).

If we take each of these types of abuse in turn we can see that there are some special issues which arise for people with learning disabilities in relation to each category of abuse and some potential omissions from this list.

Physical abuse

This form of abuse includes hitting and rough handling and manifests itself as bruising, finger marking and so on. It is more likely to occur in settings where carers, whether family members or paid staff, have little understanding of challenging behaviours, or assume that any difficulties are directed at them personally. Although it is important to treat adults distinctly from children, training in recognizing non-accidental injury in children or in older people does to some extent translate into situations involving adults with learning disabilities and alert people to signals for concern. Any evidence of such injuries, however minor, should be acted upon, so that it can be followed up in an appropriate multidisciplinary forum. Over-medication or misuse of medical procedures might also fall within this category, for example the use of enemas without sound medical reasons or safeguards in their administration.

Sexual abuse

Any sexual behaviours, whether they involve direct contact or not, can be abusive in the absence of valid consent or in the presence of force or intimidation. Even non-contact abuse such as voyeurism, involvement in pornography, indecent exposure, harassment, serious teasing or innuendo, can be experienced as seriously abusive, especially if they take place in a threatening atmosphere. The act(s) might have happened once only or be part of an ongoing sexual relationship. Consent issues are dealt with in full by Murphy and Clare (1995), but as a shorthand formulation there are three issues (Brown and Turk 1992):

- Whether the person *did* give their consent because if they did not they have been raped or assaulted like any other woman or man.
- Whether the person *could* give their consent, that is if they understood enough about sexual behaviour and knew what was happening: at law people with severe learning disabilities are deemed not to be able to give consent to sexual acts.
- A judgement has to be made as to whether the person with learning disabilities was *under undue pressure* in this particular situation, for example due to an authority or care-giving relationship, such as might be the case if sex is initiated by a staff or family member, or where force, trickery or exploitation are used. Physical force or the threat of violence or reprisals also cut across any meaningful consent.

You can be in an environment where you can't bloody well say no.

The law specifies a distinction between people with severe intellectual impairments and those with milder degrees of disability. It is important that services undertake, or draw on, clear assessments of the capacity of individual service users who are engaging in sexual activities. When people with severe learning disabilities are sexually active the service should enquire what evidence there is that they have mutual or reciprocal relationships. When supporting people with mild learning difficulties, judgements hinge upon whether the relationships appear to have exploitative or threatening elements.

For people with learning disabilities, sexual abuses often take place against a background of negative expectations about sex. People may have little in the way of credible or reliable sex education, have few opportunities to make friends or be private and always be swimming against the tide if they wish to establish an independent sexual life. Unfortunately, this kind of protective veneer does not keep people safe, merely ignorant. It means that they are often ill-equipped to make a complaint, to appreciate when they might be putting themselves at risk or to have their problems picked up through routine health checks. Because people often assume that people with learning disabilities are asexual, their sexual health needs tend not to be routinely addressed. They may not be offered smear tests, ordinary help with menstruation (as opposed to more drastic measures like hysterectomy) or safer-sex education. But there are many instances of excellent practice on the part of health visitors, psychologists and other professionals (e.g. Baum, 1994; Carlson *et al.*, 1994; Flynn *et al.*, 1996; Cambridge and Brown, 1997).

Psychological abuse   This type of abuse is often involved in the situations outlined above but is obscured because the mental health needs of people with learning disabilities are overlooked. Signs of mental distress tend to be explained away as part of the person's condition rather than as a valid emotional response to life events. A recent research study on 'elder abuse' defined this term to mean mainly verbal assault, threats and insults, including humiliation in relation to bodily functions such as incontinence and threats to abandon the vulnerable person (see Pillemer and Finkelhor, 1988: 53, who term this 'chronic verbal aggression').

Financial, or material, abuse

This form of abuse is also an issue for people with learning disabilities, although one which is not often reported within the framework of abuse policies. Practitioners are often aware that people with learning disabilities have very restricted access to money and property. It is, however, striking that this does not lead to reports under the policies in the way that more tangible or fraudulent transactions involving older people do (Brown and Stein, 1998). Families may subsume benefits into the family income, and irregularities in managing personal moneys in residential services are also commonplace (Davis *et al.*, 1995). Professionals need to satisfy themselves about whether transactions of gifts are valid and uncoerced. Consent needs to be considered carefully, as it does in relation to sexual interactions. Occasionally, formal measures are taken where individuals lack capacity, but more often people make informal arrangements which are condoned by those around as long as they seem to work in the interests of the person concerned. Health professionals may be aware of these arrangements and should be alert to problems, especially when the care provided is in other ways inadequate, or bordering on neglect, in which case financial motivation may be at the root of a particular care arrangement, or an unwillingness to 'allow' a learning disabled adult to leave home.

Neglect

This includes those situations within which an individual's basic physical, social and health care needs are not being met; for example, failure to

● access proper medical or dental care
● give prescribed medication or pain relief reliably
● enable someone to use services such as a day centre or leisure group.

Sometimes negligence is also included, implying a more active failure to take risks into account.

In practice, the types of abuse outlined in the above text often overlap. In a recent study of cases reported in two authorities over one year, multiple abuses were documented in at least one-fifth of cases (Brown and Stein, 1998).

Complex dynamics, abusive regimes and double standards

The various definitions given above are not exhaustive but they do provide a framework within which risks can be addressed. An important part of any definition is the extent to which the harm was intentionally caused, but where abuse is perpetrated by another service user it should not be assumed to be less serious or to have less of an impact on the individual. Nor should the status of the perpetrator confuse or cut across the right of a *victim* to receive help. Accessing help for victim *and* perpetrator in such situations is an important measure of good practice.

Moreover, when abuse takes place within a service it is important to be alert to the nature of the whole regime, rather than just the behaviour of an individual abuser. If the abuse is the act of a lone worker, the management should deal with it openly and summarily. But it could also reflect more widespread negligence on the part of management, resulting in lack of knowledge, support and resources for direct care staff. Workers in abusive regimes are often underpaid, untrained and insecure. They may be afraid of the proprietor, management or union and be unable to 'blow the whistle' (Wardaugh and Wilding, 1993; Pilgrim, 1995). A further dynamic to take into account in both institutional and informal settings is the distortion of behavioural programmes or sanctions. Occasionally, serious assaults are carried out under the guise of punishment or control.

Independent practitioners have to make a judgement about whether a service has done enough to seek outside expertise or if they have been negligent in tackling aspects of their work, such as dealing with challenging behaviour, difficulties in communication or feeding. Where there are concerns that practice is well outside standards commonly agreed within the professional community, there is a duty to alert social services or the inspection unit, in addition to the usual role of designing and monitoring relevant interventions.

Indicators of abuse

We have seen that there are social as well as medical/physical indicators of abuse which independent practitioners should be alert to. By their very nature, it is often the case that such abusive incidents do not come to light. They 'leak' out, sometimes through the distressed, angry or sexualized behaviour of a victim or the sexualized, authoritarian or persecutory behaviour of the perpetrator. Many text book lists alert practitioners to *sudden* changes of mood or behaviour, but even this can be misleading since abuse is often long-standing and/or introduced gradually: nevertheless such changes, along with newly sexualized language or dislike for particular individuals or activities, should always be taken seriously. Cycles of weight loss or gain, gagging and, more dramatically, elective mutism are among the disguised ways in which some people communicate their distress (Vizard, 1989; Flynn and Brown, 1997). One woman attending a workshop for survivors of sexual abuse (Brown and Stein, 1996) swallowed a needle so that she could be taken to hospital, after being sexually assaulted by a member of her family. Otherwise practitioners should be alert to agencies which are characterized by closed systems and rigid hierarchies (Wardhaugh and Wilding, 1993).

However, by far the most common route for discovery is disclosure or partial disclosure (Turk and Brown, 1993). Practitioners are often reluctant to listen or to ask (Rose *et al.*, 1991), where acknowledgement that one is willing to hear, and take seriously, a disclosure of abuse would allow someone to say what is happening to them. It is important to acknowledge how difficult it can be for someone to disclose abuse when they are afraid: they may wait a long time before trusting someone enough.

'I didn't know it was wrong. ... I was told not to tell anyone, because it was all my fault. ...'

Where practitioners are working with someone who discloses abuse, they should follow the guidance set out in the Memorandum of Good Practice (Home Office/DoH 1992)[1]:

- listen rather than directly question;
- don't stop someone who is freely recalling important events, they may not tell you again;
- at the first opportunity make a note of exactly what they said, in their own words wherever possible, noting especially details about the time, setting and any witnesses who might have seen what happened;
- date and sign the record.

This allows the initial disclosure to be followed up with a more formal and evidentially sound interview as soon as practicable.

'It's not good for you to bottle it in ... which I found out ... this is the first proper year that I'm sort of starting [to sort it out].'

If individuals are abused or exploited, the legacy for them can be very long-standing and this may affect their service needs over a long period. Practitioners may also have a role in accessing immediate or longer-term support from other agencies such as rape crisis, women's refuges or specialist counselling services.

'It stops you from getting all tight up and I think I can sleep better you know ... because it still goes through your mind doesn't it when you are still sleeping ... as though it is still happening you know when you are asleep. I mean he was coming, I was thinking he was coming into my bedroom, you know, standing there ... and giving me horrible looks ... I was staying awake the whole time and that's why counselling is a good thing.'

Conclusion

People with learning disabilities are vulnerable to a range of exploitative and abusive experiences and need professionals to act for them by building proper safeguards and by keeping alert to signs of distress or to

---

[1] The guidance in this document is specific to *child* protection, but a similar standard in relation to vulnerable adults is recommended for those cases in which disclosure may eventually lead to prosecution.

their attempts to tell someone that something is wrong. Working within the framework of adult protection policies allows all practitioners to be part of a safety network and not a weak link in the chain. A commitment to empowerment has to include supporting people who have been exploited or abused and helping them to recover.

'Since I've been with the women's group they've helped me get a lot better and they've got me stronger and stronger.'

Acknowledgements

The quotes are taken from a group of service users who were survivors of sexual abuse and who met together in late 1995 to make two tapes about sexual abuse for service users and for staff. I should like to thank them and the people who facilitated the workshop with them, especially June Stein, Margaret Flynn, Michelle McCarthy, David Thompson and Paul Cambridge.

References

Baum, S. (1994) Interventions with a pregnant woman with severe learning disabilities: a case example. In Craft, A. (ed.) *Practice Issues in Sexuality and Learning Disabilities*, Routledge, London

Brown, H. and Stein, J. (eds) (1996) *But now they've got a voice* (a tape about sexual abuse for services users made by service users), Pavilion Publishing, Brighton

Brown, H. and Stein, J. (1998) Implementing adult protection policies in Kent and East Sussex. *Journal of Social Policy*, **27**(3), 371–396

Brown, H. and Turk, V. (1992) Defining sexual abuse as it affects adults with learning disabilities. *Mental Handicap*, **20**, 44–55

Cambridge, P. and Brown, H. (eds) (1997) *HIV and Learning Disabilities*, BILD, Kidderminster

Carlson, G. Taylor, M., Wilson, J. and Griffin, J. (1994) Menstrual management and fertility management for women who have intellectual disability and high support needs: an analysis of Australian policy. Department of Social Work and Social Policy, University of Queensland, Australia

Davis, A., Eley, R., Flynn, M., Flynn, P. and Roberts, G. (1995) To have and have not: addressing issues of poverty. In Philpot, T. and Ward, L. (eds), *Values and Visions: Changing Ideas in Services for People with Learning Difficulties*, Butterworth-Heinemann, Oxford

Flynn, M. (1987) Independent living arrangements for adults who are mentally handicapped. In Malin, N. (ed.), *Reassessing Community Care*, Croom Helm, London

Flynn, M. and Brown, H. (1997) The responsibilities of commissioners, purchasers and providers. In Churchill, J. *et al.*, (eds), *There Are No Easy Answers: Working with Service Users Who Sexually Abuse*, ARC/NAPSAC, Chesterfield

Flynn, M., Howard, J. and Pursey, A. (1996) *GP Fundholding and the Health Care of People with Learning Disabilities*, NDT, Manchester

Home Office in conjunction with the Department of Health (1992) *Memorandum of good practice* (video-recorded interviews with child witnesses for criminal proceedings), HMSO, London

Murphy, G. and Clare, I. (1995) Adults' capacity to make decisions affecting the person. In Bull, R. and Carson, D. (eds), *Handbook of Psychology in Legal Contexts*, Wiley, Chichester

Pilgrim, D. (1995) Explaining abuse and inadequate care. In Hunt, G. (ed.) *Whistleblowing in the Health Service: Accountability, Law and Professional Practice*, Edward Arnold, London

Pillemer, K. and Finkelhor, D. (1988) The prevalence of elder abuse: a random sample survey. *The Gerontologist*, **28**(1), 51–57

Rose, S., Peabody, C. and Stratigeas, B. (1991) Undetected abuse amongst intensive case management clients. *Hospital and Community Psychiatry*, **42**(5), 499–503

Stein, J. and Brown, H. (eds) (1996) *A nightmare . . . that I thought would never end*, (a tape about sexual abuse for staff made by service users), Pavilion Publishing, Brighton

Turk, V. and Brown, H. (1993) The sexual abuse of adults with learning disabilities: results of a two year incidence survey. *Mental Handicap Research*, **6**(3), 193–216

Vizard, E. (1989) Child sexual abuse and mental handicap: a child psychiatrist's perspective. In Brown, H. and Craft, A. (eds) *Thinking the 'Unthinkable': Papers on Sexual Abuse and People with Learning Difficulties*, FPA, London

Wardhaugh, J. and Wilding, P. (1993) Towards an explanation of the corruption of care. *Critical Social Policy*, Summer, 4–31

Williams, C (1993) Vulnerable victims? A current awareness of the victimisation of people with learning disabilities. *Disability, Handicap and Society*, **8**(2), 161–172

23 Enhancing communication with people with severe and profound learning difficulties

Caroline Downs

Introduction

Enabling clients to communicate their feelings and needs, thoughts and interests, likes and dislikes is possibly the most important aspect of a therapist's work. Nowadays, most settings in which people with learning difficulties live, work and learn ascribe to a philosophy of empowerment and self-advocacy or advocacy. The implementation of this requires that carers and professionals develop ways of supporting service users to make and express choices, however they may do this. Workers therefore need to be able to understand and, where self-expression is unconventional, interpret service users' communications. They must also be competent to engage, interact and communicate with each person in the most appropriate way, and have the knowledge and skills to provide the necessary environment and means to support such communication.

The greater the level of difficulty in communication experienced by the client, the more difficult both of these tasks become; comprehending or interpreting the often highly idiosyncratic and ambiguous communications of many of our service users is a great responsibility and requires specific skills. Similarly, fostering and promoting clients' different means of communication becomes correspondingly more complex, demanding, in addition to a good understanding of and empathy with the person concerned, specialized interests and skills as well as knowledge of different methods of communication. While it is, of course, vital that clients experience the motivation to communicate, it is not sufficient, when working with people with very severe learning difficulties, simply to provide a rich environment and trust that intentional communication, which others may come to understand, will develop. For these reasons and because an increasing proportion of the people with whom we work have very severe, complex and profound learning difficulties (Male, 1995), emphasis in this chapter will be on enabling and developing communication with this particular client group.

Ten years ago a widespread study of children in what were then named 'Special Care Units' was conducted in schools in England and Wales (Evans and Ware, 1987). Over 80 per cent of the 800 children involved in the survey were described by their teachers and therapists as 'non-communicating'. Since that time our understanding of communication has become more sophisticated and it is unlikely that such a term would be used nowadays. Indeed, definitions of communication which inform and underpin contemporary practice include 'pre-intentional communication', i.e. information decoded by care givers from the behaviour of people who are not yet intentionally sending messages (Goldbart *et al.*, 1994).

Not only is it widely accepted nowadays that all behaviour is communicative or potentially communicative, strategies for helping clients to develop intentionality in their communication are both written about and practised. Jean Ware (1994) stresses that it is only by a carer or member of staff providing a 'responsive environment', responding to a person's actions *as if* they were acts of communication, that the client has the opportunity to perceive that their actions can convey a purpose and have an effect on the world; both of these factors are known to be prerequisites for intentional communication (Schweigert, 1989). While recognizing that all people are different and, as such, express themselves differently and have different needs, Helen Bradley offers guidelines to help us to create a responsive environment for clients communicating in a variety of different ways (Bradley, 1994). She recommends, for example, that where a person seems to react to internal feelings rather than trying to communicate or to change the situation, it is helpful to respond by establishing a close relationship with him or her, to have clear, consistent routines and to respond quickly to any overt demonstrations of happiness or distress.

Where a client does not yet respond intentionally but tries to affect or alter a situation, e.g. by pushing someone or something away, Bradley suggests responding to this as if intentional; as: 'Go away!' or 'I do not like this!' Opportunities should be created wherever and whenever possible for the client to act on the environment. So, for example, rather than routinely clearing a client's cup away after a drink, the therapist or carer should allow time and the opportunity for him or her to push it away. Bradley also suggests introducing, at this stage, objects of reference as indicators of what is to happen next. This is explored in detail below.

Once the client recognizes that she or he can affect the world, Bradley suggests that constant opportunities be given for him or her to influence carers and to make choices. Responses should be given quickly so that the association between the gesture or vocalization and the outcome is strengthened. While responding to gestures, it is helpful if carers model a more sophisticated form of communication, e.g. introduce the sign or a symbol for drink in addition to responding in the usual way.

Where an individual uses a conventional form of communication, whether symbols, signs or words, it is important that all carers should both understand and respond to the system and use it themselves, encouraging and extending its use. The range of symbols used with clients to open up channels of communication is discussed below.

It is likely that the increase in knowledge and skill among therapists and teachers in the use of alternative augmentative communication

(AAC) will have resulted in a substantially higher percentage of service users today using signs or symbols than the 2.6 per cent of children noted in the Evans and Ware study (Goldbart, 1995). Practitioners seem to be more skilled now at recognizing and cultivating potential communication than they were 10 years ago, when it was demonstrated that more than half of the communication and potential communication of a group of children with profound and multiple learning difficulties were either misinterpreted (as judged by the principal carer/mother) or were missed altogether (Brown and Lehr, 1989). It appears that we have succeeded in developing the willingness, the sensitivity and the skills, advocated by McLean and Snyder McLean (1987), to recognize and to assign communicative significance to actions which previously may have been disregarded or may have passed unnoticed. However, as we shall explore below, despite having apparently enhanced our practice quite substantially over the past 10 years, scope remains for improvement in the development and quality of communication between carers and clients, particularly in relation to interpreting the more idiosyncratic or ambiguous communications of clients with very severe disabilities.

The 'How?', 'What?' and 'Why?' of communication

Before proceeding to examine some of the factors which may increase the quality of communication between therapist and client, and some of the strategies we might introduce to support an individual's communication, it is useful to explore, as Jones (1990) suggests, the 'How?', 'What?' and 'Why?' of communication.

The content of our communication or *what* we communicate will depend on context and individuals' experiences and interests. It includes all imaginable topics and ideas, from exploring the meaning of life to discussing the previous evening's episode of Coronation Street; from examining the implications of feudalism to stating that the dog has been sick.

The purpose of communication or *why* we communicate will depend on our immediate, or long-term, aims or intentions: for example, to gain attention; to stop or prolong an interaction or activity; to express wishes; to fulfil needs; to make contact with others; to obtain shared attention; to give or acquire information; to explore issues and ideas. It is helpful to remember the possible range of intentions a client may have, otherwise it becomes easy to misinterpret, for example, an invitation to share attention, assuming it to be a request. Park (1997) suggests that it is an all too frequent assumption that any communication will be a request; a misunderstanding of purpose leads to a different, and an inappropriate, response, resulting in feelings of frustration and powerlessness for the client.

If we look at *how* we communicate, this can clearly encompass a wide range of methods; for example, abstract means such as writing, speaking, Morse code, braille, communication aids, sign language (other than iconic signs), finger spelling, and some symbols. Iconic signs, mimicking the object or action they represent, (e.g. ball, table, house) are more concrete and therefore easier to learn and remember than other signs. How we communicate also includes less abstract representation of people, items, feelings and so on; for example, iconic signs, many symbols, pictures and picture boards, drawings, photographs, and objects of reference. Other methods of communication include informal, intentional, concrete gestures like pointing and reaching, grabbing, hitting out, some vocalizations and facial expression. Lastly there are the generally unintentional or pre-intentional acts; for example, body posture and movement towards or away from someone or something, involuntary and spontaneous actions which may include laughing, crying, smiling, self-injurious behaviour, throwing objects, rhythmic or repetitive acts, and seeking or avoiding attention. While several of those in the last category may sometimes be used intentionally, they may also be, and often are, simple reflex actions, unlike communication in the other three categories, in which the communicator inevitably engages with a purpose.

From the viewpoint of people with learning difficulties

The aim of many therapies and, indeed, other methods of intervention is a better understanding of a person's life, experiences and insight into the world from his or her point of view. Prevezer (1991), for example, discusses the notion of 'tuning in' to the perspective of the client with whom she is working, in order that she may become 'micro-responsive' to any signals given out. She sees her role as a therapist to support and facilitate any interaction, interpreting and reacting to every contribution offered by the client.

Several methods currently favoured by other practitioners also stress the importance of endeavouring to understand the world view of the communicator, offering warmth, solidarity and reciprocity within the interaction. This may be viewed as 'behaviourism at its best' (Jones, 1990) or as a 'posture' and methodology based on parent – child type bonding between care givers or therapists and the client with a learning difficulty (McGee et al., 1987); Gentle Teaching exemplifies such an approach.

The widely used method of Intensive Interaction (Nind and Hewett, 1994), with its predecessor Augmented Mothering (Ephraim, 1986), share this value system and consciously draw on and imitate the early parent – infant interaction, (see, e.g., Lewis and Coates, 1980; Harding, 1983; Scoville, 1984). For many years, unquestioning adherence to a misinterpretation of age-appropriateness caused practitioners working with people with learning difficulties to eschew practices or equipment designed for infants or young children, often despite parents' and carers' requests to the contrary, arguing that to offer non-age-appropriate materials or activities is disrespectful to the person with learning difficulties. However, it is now generally recognized that age-appropriateness is more concerned with the image of people with learning difficulties than with the individual himself or herself (Szivos and Griffiths, 1990; Emerson, 1992) indeed, respect for a person demands that we use approaches which might begin to meet his or her needs, irrespective of the prejudices and norms of society, which can oppress people with learning difficulties (Corbett, 1994). As Chappell demonstrates, if we deny clients access to learning opportunities, simply because they are not age-appropriate, then 'the onus is on changing them to make them more like "normal" people, rather than on unconditional acceptance' (1992:43). This view has liberated practitioners to draw on useful theory and practice around the development of communication.

Structuring and organizing

Intensive Interaction requires that any form of expression is given a response: a sound, a movement, something on which the client is focusing, or a phrase, with the therapist using the client's mode of expression creatively in order to draw attention to the outside world. Caldwell (1996) discusses the importance of the therapist recognizing what is significant to the client and using his or her 'language' in order to develop a conversation between equals; the therapist offers back to the client a balance between the familiar, i.e. the same mode of expression as the client, and an element of surprise, in order both to affirm his or her means of expression and to engage his or her interest in the outside. She quotes David Stern's suggestion that if the therapist responds in the same mode, he or she is conveying to the client: 'I know what you are thinking.' If the response given is in a different mode, for example a client rocking is responded to in the same rhythm, through sound, he or she is saying to the client: 'I know what you are feeling.'

A prerequisite for communication to develop is an enjoyment of the other person in the interaction or at least a willingness to participate in a world outside, to share personal space and an understanding of the turn-taking inherent in communication. It is also necessary to ensure that clients want to notice and communicate about the things and people around them. Cirrin and Rowland (1985), cited in Goldbart (1995), state that clients may not use or demonstrate all the communication skills they have at their disposal unless the context encourages their use. Such encouragement will include a range of structured experiences on which to comment, and stimuli using different senses: attractive things to look at, to feel; different sounds – music, voices; a variety of tastes; different feelings or emotional responses to activities and sensations. Responses may be verbal, or may be communicated through sign, symbols, by pointing or other gestures; they may be facial or body movements or a range of behaviours indicating pleasure, fear, excitement, or anger.

As communication develops, many clients with learning difficulties, in addition to requiring help and structured opportunities, also require strategies to organize their experiences. For example, encouragement in focusing and in selective attention – comparing people and objects and noticing their features is helpful; so too are systems for categorizing, sorting and classifying into: things I like/do not like; what I can/cannot eat; what I wear when it is hot/cold; how I behave in this/that situation. Clients also often need help with category inclusion and exclusion, to aid their comprehension of the boundaries between one concept and another. Just as toddlers may pass through a stage of calling all men 'Daddy', or disbelieving that any breed other than their own may be classified as a 'dog', so too may clients use a label, whether a word or a sign or symbol, with a different meaning from the one we immediately assume. One young woman with a severe learning difficulty caused both excitement and consternation by informing her parents and key worker that she wanted to get married. Further questions revealed that what she really wanted was a big party, with all her friends and lots of presents.

Clients also frequently need help to notice cause-and-effect reasoning, whether at the more sophisticated level of 'I have no money, therefore I cannot buy a video' to 'I press this switch and music goes on' to, at the more concrete level, 'I make this gesture with my hand and I get a drink'. As we noted earlier, without recognizing one's effect on the world, intentional communication does not develop and it is possible that the outcome of successive lack of response for the client is a feeling of learned helplessness (Seligman, 1975).

Interpreting

To establish or confirm for a client the association between a certain gesture and an outcome, it is of course necessary to ensure consistency of response from all those working or interacting with him or her. This involves members of a staff team feeling confident to agree on an interpretation of the person's possible or actual communicative intent or meaning. While many familiar adults do feel confident in their interpretations of client's unconventional responses to an experience (Goldbart, 1995), many do not and, in fact, report feeling concerned that they may frequently be 'getting it wrong' (Downs and Craft, 1997). Indeed, staff are justified in not always trusting their 'gut level' interpretations of unconventional communication; an assumed rejection of food may simply be a tongue thrust outside of a person's control. In addition, customary expressions of pleasure, fear, anger, sadness and so on are frequently distorted for people with poor muscular control, and communications which are generally assumed to be responses to an external event may, in fact, be reactions to discomfort due to, for example poor positioning or constipation (Withers, 1991; Hogg *et al.*, 1995; Downs and Craft, 1997; Bunning *et al.*, in press; Goldbart, 1995).

Furthermore, staff members' perceptions of people's communications are frequently distorted by their own feelings, needs, wishes and beliefs, which result in the lack of agreement between communication partners as to meaning or intention of a specific piece of communication. This was shown in a recent national project (Downs and Craft, 1997; Downs, in press). As we saw earlier, even familiar adults were judged, by the principal carer/mother, to misinterpret or miss more than half of a group of children's attempts to communicate (Brown and Lehr, 1989).

The inevitable subjectivity inherent in interpreting communication, and therefore the likelihood of differences of view regarding meaning, has been further recognized as a cause for concern since Facilitated Communication was introduced as a method for working with children and adults who have very limited expressive communication. When working in this way, the communication partner or facilitator gives the client physical support to enable him or her to point to a symbol, picture or object or to spell out words. Although the method has been found to be useful for some clients, successive experiments designed to test the authenticity of the method, in which a client and the communication partner are asked different questions, have shown that the answer given has generally been a response to the question posed to the partner (Intellectual Disability Review Panel, 1989; Eberlin *et al.*, 1993; Felce, 1994; Moore *et al.*, 1993). Such findings lend weight to the contention that messages generated through Facilitated Communication, purported to come from the client, actually originate in the unconscious mind of the facilitator (Von Tetzschner, 1996).

One method devised to increase the confidence and competence of staff to interpret more accurately clients' communications, explores the distortion of interpretations, referred to above, which result from individual personal feelings, beliefs and motives. It has been demonstrated that enhanced awareness of these influencing factors results in increased agreement within staff teams as to the meaning of a specific, ambiguous communication (Downs and Craft, 1997). It is acknowledged that it is possible, in theory at least, for all members of a staff team to misinterpret a piece of communication; that is, the validity or accuracy of the interpretation is not confirmed by unanimity. Furthermore, it is recognized that the culture of a setting can influence a staff team to perceive a client or a certain behaviour in a common way and peer pressure can lead a therapist to acquiesce to the majority view. Nevertheless, Downs and Craft (1997) argue that it is reasonable to assume that a high level of agreement among several self-aware communication partners, who claim a feeling of empathy with their client, increases the reliability of the interpretation; accuracy is a matter of degree and therefore substantiating the interpretations of a behaviour is successfully worked towards only by questioning and checking out evidence from a range of sources. Another method devised to help staff to interpret their service users' communications is a set of guidelines shortly to be published (Bunning *et al.*, in press).

A further, and frequently used, strategy for checking out interpretations of ambiguous or unconventional communication is the Affective Communication Assessment (ACA) (Coupe *et al.*, 1985). This offers a detailed observation sheet to list responses to a range of stimuli and an identification sheet which highlights consistencies in patterns of response. Tentative interpretations which emerge from this may then be checked out and the information gained may be used as a basis for individual communication indices for clients. A communication index lists, for example, categories of statements the individual is believed to communicate; for example, 'I like that!'; 'Come here!'; 'I'm angry!'; 'Go away!'. Beside each of these will be detailed the way in which these meanings are thought to be conveyed, either intentionally by the individual or by means of gestures which have been identified as potentially communicative. Finally, the response which all carers will give is agreed and written onto the sheet, in order to ensure consistency of experience for the client.

For service users who have developed clear, intentional communication and who express themselves through speech, sign or symbols clearly and unambiguously, other assessment profiles are useful (van der Gaag and Dormandy, 1993). The Personal Communication Plan (Hitchens and Spence, 1991) is used widely in individual action plans and involves all those in the care, education and therapy of the client. Similarly, the Communication Assessment Profile (CASP) (van der Gaag, 1988) involves all key staff and carers in the communication assessment and explores not only the client's skills in language comprehension and expression but also the 'communicative demands' placed on him or her in everyday life.

Signs and symbols

As we have noted above, for many clients with severe and profound learning difficulties, using signs and/or symbols can open up otherwise very restricted channels of communication. These may be used by the communication partner or therapist to augment spoken language and be introduced as a means of communication for clients. For many service users, sign can provide a bridge as a means of expression, more concrete than words.

When working with people with additional impairments, for example people with visual impairment, signs will inevitably need to be adapted (Kohl, 1981; McInnes and Treffry, 1982; Freeman, 1985; Gallagher and Lewis, 1987). Clark (1988) suggests that clients with visual impairment have particular difficulty in learning signs that: are produced in open space; require sophisticated hand positions to start or complete the sign; comprise a very small movement; or contain ambiguous tactile information which make them very similar to other signs.

When adapting signs, it is important to keep certain principles in mind. It is useful, first, to remember that while many clients will have sufficient vision to read signs visually, the visual field may be very narrow and care must be taken that signs are not presented, or are not allowed to move outside of, the field of vision. Signing must be consigned to a small area within the frame of vision and must be at the optimum distance. The orientation of some signs may need to be changed; for example, a sign which generally involves movement towards the client may not be perceived, whereas if this is changed through 90 degrees, it may be more easily read.

Signs must be clear and precise, and the significant movements and aspects of the hands must be emphasized. Irrelevant factors and sloppiness must be minimized. 'Air' signs formed in space are more difficult for all clients to learn, whether or not they have additional visual impairment; tactile and kinaesthetic feedback is an important aid to memory. For this reason, Clark (1988) recommends that the sign for 'apple' be formed with the right hand touching the chin and 'home' with hands touching the chest. Where it is difficult to adapt a sign to involve the body, it may be possible to have the hands touching in the production of a sign. For example, in 'play' they may either touch little finger to little finger or be placed one on top of the other before making a circular movement in the vertical–parallel plane.

Where a sign is formed using one hand, the passive hand may be introduced to give support to, or be used as a reference point for, the active hand. For example, the active hand may be supported and held at the wrist by the passive hand in its forward circular action to form the sign 'train', or the active hand may meet the reference hand held in front of it at the end of each circular movement.

As was noted earlier, iconic signs, which mimic the object or action they represent, are learned more quickly than more abstract signs. However, it is easy to make the mistake of assuming that what comprises iconicity for one person, does for another, for people who drink unaided or who are helped to lift a cup to their lips, the sign for 'drink' will be iconic; for those for whom the experience of a drink is to feel the spout of a feeding cup brush their lips, the iconic carries no such association. When deciding on a sign – or symbol – for a client to learn, it is important, therefore, to try to see the world as he or she experiences it and to examine the relevance for the individual. Is the notion of 'chair' portrayed meaningfully by the conventional sign of two horizontal arms, held in space, moving downwards as if resting on the arms of a chair, for example, or might it be better represented for that person by a picture or drawing or symbol of a chair? Or can the experience be better conveyed by the fabric with which the chair is covered? Or by the sensation of hard surface being brought to touch the bottom?

Symbols and signs are not only used as a means of communication; they can also develop understanding and thinking skills and help memory. When choosing a symbol system appropriate for an individual, it is helpful to select the most abstract one which a person can comprehend. If pictures, rebuses or line drawings are meaningful for a client, these should be used and provide a useful means of communication in themselves and a focus for discussion when an array of such symbols are presented in a book or on a communication board. For many people, however, abstract symbols of this type carry little or no meaning and a more concrete way of representing experiences has to be found. Objects of reference can be used in a variety of different ways and are being used increasingly with clients with severe and profound learning disabilities as well with deaf-blind clients with whom this method has been in use for many years (Grove and Park, 1996).

At their most 'concrete', the same objects may be used as the focus of communication as those which are used in the event. For example, a client may be given a spoon to indicate that it is lunchtime; the client holds onto the spoon and then uses it to eat his or her lunch. Once the association between the spoon and food has built up, a spoon may become a symbol for food. A spoon mounted onto card, in order to indicate that it is different from the actual spoon to be used, is given to the client to indicate that it is lunchtime. Similarly, the client is encouraged to point to or hand the mounted spoon to someone to communicate 'I am hungry'.

However, to have a 'vocabulary' of many such objects is unwieldy and, where possible, clients are encouraged to move on to use smaller, more manageable objects of reference, either those which have a shared feature with the object it represents or are a miniature version of it. So, for example, a small piece of fabric may come to signify a chair or mother, and may be gradually cut in size so that it can be contained in a small communication book which the client carries with him or her on all occasions. Doll's house furniture is useful for some clients, although for many it does not carry the necessary associations.

Where signs and objects are both used with a client, it is helpful for them to resemble one another. Park (1997) gives the example of a client for whom the conventional sign for car, formed in space, was inappropriate. Rather than adapting the sign so that the two hands made contact, which was an option, it was decided to introduce a body-referenced sign, tracing the line of the seat belt, which resembled the object already in use, in this case a 'seat belt mate' (a 35 cm piece of sheepskin wrapped around the car safety belt).

Other criteria to be considered when selecting an appropriate object as an aid to communication for an individual, as we have seen above, are: the significance or meaningfulness for that individual; the possibility and/or desirability of having shared objects of reference for a group of clients; the pertinence or relevance for the person. Clients are most highly motivated to communicate about people and events which are familiar, liked and occur frequently in their lives; it is more useful to introduce an object for mealtime, as this occurs three times a day, than for a trip to the shops if this only takes place once a week.

Conclusion

Helping a client to communicate requires an understanding of her or his lived experience, derived from close, non-judgemental observation and the ability to distinguish the client's perspective or motives from one's own. As has been seen above, the latter requires insight into one's own feelings and beliefs, without which perceptions and interpretations of the client's communications are inevitably distorted. Furthermore, it is useful for therapists to have an understanding of how communication develops and how typical interactions between carers and infants which effect this development may be adapted for use with clients. Finally, it is important for therapists to be acquainted with the range of alternative augmentative communication systems and be skilled in their use.

Useful contacts and organizations for further information about communication methods and resources described in the chapter:

The Makaton Vocabulary Development Project
31 Firwood Drive
Camberley
Surrey GU15 3QD.   (tel: 01276 61390)

Signalong Communication and Language Centre
All Saints Hospital
Chatham
Kent ME4 5NG   (tel: 01634 407311)

References

Bradley, H. (1994) *Encouraging and Developing Early Communication Skills in Adults with Multiple Disabilities*, Focus factsheet, RNIB Publications, London

Brown, F. and Lehr, D.H. (1989) *Persons with Profound Disabilities: Issues and Practice*. Paul H. Brooks, Baltimore

Bunning, K., Downs, C., Emerson, A., *et al.* (in press) *See What I Mean: Guidelines to Aid the Understanding of Communication by People with Severe and Profound Learning Difficulties*, MENCAP, London

Caldwell, P. (1996) *Getting in Touch*: Ways of Working with People with Severe Learning Disabilities and Extensive Support Needs, Pavilion Publishing, Brighton

Chappell, A.L. (1992) Towards a sociological critique of the normalisation principle. *Disability, Handicap and Society*, **7**, 35–51

Clark, P. (1988) Adapting signs for deaf-blind children. *Talking Sense*, Spring, 16–17

Corbett, I. (1994) A proud label: exploring the relationship between disability politics and gay pride. *Disability and Society*, **9**, 343–358

Coupe, J., Barton, L., Barbef, M., Collins, L. Levy, D. and Murphy, D. (1985) *Affective Communication Assessment*, MEC, Manchester (available from Melland School, Holmcroft Road, Gorton, Manchester M19 7NG)

Downs, C. (forthcoming) Sexuality: challenges and dilemmas. In Lacey, P. and Ouvry, C. (eds), *Interdisciplinary Work with People with Profound and Multiple Learning Disabilities: A Collaborative Approach to Meeting Needs*, David Fulton, London

Downs, C. and Craft, A. (1997) *Sex in Context: A Personal and Social Development Programme for Children and Adults with Profound and Multiple Impairments: Staff Development and Working with Parents and Carers*, Pavilion Publishing, Brighton

Eberlin, M., McConnachie, C.J., Ibel, S. and Volpe, L. (1993) Facilitated communication: a failure to replicate the phenomenon. *Journal of Autism and Developmental Disorders*, **23**, 507–530

Emerson, G. (1992) What is normalisation? In Brown, H. and Smith, H. (eds), *Normalization: A Reader for the Nineties*, Tavistock/Routledge, London

Ephraim, G. (1986) *A Brief Introduction to Augmented Mothering*. Playtrac (available from the Horizon Trust, Harperbury, Harper Lane, Radlett, Herts. WD7 9HQ)

Evans, P. and Ware, J. (1987) *'Special Care' Provision: The Education of Children with Profound and Multiple Learning Difficulties*, NFER-Nelson, Windsor

Felce, D. (1994) Facilitated communication: results from a number of recently published evaluations. *British Journal of Learning Disabilities*, **22**, 122–126

Freeman, P. (1985) *The Deaf-Blind Baby: A Programme of Care*, Heinemann Medical Books, London

Gallagher, P and Lewis, C. (1987) Sign communication. *Talking Sense*, **33**(1), 15–16

Goldbart, J. (1995) *Interdisciplinary Work with People with Profound and Multiple Learning Disabilities: Communication*, University of Birmingham

Goldbart, J., Warner, J. and Mount, S. (1994) *The Development of Early Communication and Feeding for People Who Have Profound and Multiple Disabilities*. Mencap/PIMD, London

Grove, N. and Park, K. (1996) Life quilts for people with severe and profound learning disabilities: a journey into the unknown *PMLD Link*, **24**, 10–12

Harding, C. (1983) Development of the intention to communicate. *Human Development*, **25**, 140–151

Hitchens, A. and Spence, R. (1991) *The Personal Communication Plan*, NFER-Nelson, Windsor

Hogg, J., Reeves, D., Mudford, O. and Roberts, J. (1995) The development of observational techniques to assess behaviour states and affective behaviour in adults with profound and multiple intellectual disabilities. Unpublished paper, White Top Research Centre, University of Dundee

Intellectual Disability Review Panel (1989) *Report to the Director General on the Validity and Reliability of Assisted Communication*, Melbourne, Victoria, Australia

Jones, S. (1990) *Intecom* (a package designed to integrate carers into assessing and developing the communication skills of people with learning difficulties), NFER-Nelson, Windsor

Kohl, F.L. (1981) Effects of motoric requirements on the acquisition of manual sign responses by severely handicapped students. *American Journal of Mental Deficiency*, **85**, 396–403

Lewis, M. and Coates, D.L. (1980) Mother–infant interactions and cognitive development in 12-week-old infants. *Infant Behaviour and Development*, **3**, 95–105

Male, D. (1995) Who goes to SLD schools? *Journal of Applied Research in Intellectual Disabilities*, **9**(4), 307–323

McGee, J.J., Menolascino, F.J., Hobbs, D.D. and Menousek, P.E. (1987) *Gentle Teaching: A Non-aversive Approach to Helping Persons with Mental Retardation*, Human Sciences Press, New York

McInnes, J.M. and Treffry, J. (1982) *Deaf-Blind Infants and Children*, Open University Press, Milton Keynes

McLean, J. and Snyder-McLean, L. (1987) Form and function of communicative behaviour among persons with severe developmental disabilities. *Australia and New Zealand Journal of Developmental Disabilities*, **13**, 83–98

Moore, S., Donovan, B. and Hudson, A. (1993) Brief report: facilitator-suggested conversational evaluation of facilitated communication. *Journal of Autism and Developmental Disorders*, **23**, 541–552

Nind, M. and Hewett, D. (1994) *Access to Communication: Developing the Basics of Communication with People with Severe Learning Difficulties through Intensive Interaction*, David Fulton, London

Park, K. (1997) A Communication continuum. In Downs, C. and Craft, A. (eds), *Sex in Context: A Personal and Social Development Programme for Children and Adults with Profound and Multiple Impairments: Strategies for Devising a Programme and Recommendations for Teaching and Learning*, Pavilion Publishing, Brighton

Prevezer, W. (1991) Musical Interaction: some ideas to help your child enjoy communication and develop basic conversational skills. *I Can Speech and Language Disorders Newsletter*, Summer

Schweigert, P. (1989) Use of the microswitch technology to facilitate social contingency awareness as a basis for early communication skills. *Augmentative and Alternative Communication*, **5**, 192–198

Scoville, R. (1984) The development of the intention to communicate: the eye of the beholder. In Fegens, L. *et al.* (eds), *The Origins and Growth of Communication*, Ablex, New Jersey

Seligman, M.E.P. (1975) *Learned Helplessness*, Freeman, San Francisco

Szives, S.E. and Griffiths, E. (1990) Effects of infant sociability and the caretaking environment on the infant cognitive performance. *Child Development*, **50**, 340–349

van der Gaag, A. (1988) *The Communication Assessment Profile (CASP)*, Speech Profiles, London van der Gaag, A. and Dormandy, K. (1993) *Communication and Adults with Learning Disabilities*, Whurr, London

Von Tetzchner, S. (1996) Strategies for validating facilitated communication techniques: the use of a research paradigm for practice. Paper presented at conference: *Interpreting the Communication of People Who Are Non-verbal*, May, Institute of Education, London University

Ware, J. (1994) *Educating Children with Profound and Multiple Learning Difficulties*, David Fulton, London

Withers, P. (1991) Assessing the response of adults with profound learning difficulties to various forms of stimulation. Unpublished BPS Diploma in Clinical Psychology, Bolton, Lancs

24

Creative arts activities and therapies

Frances Reynolds

Introduction

A woman with profound learning disabilities and sensory impairment is engrossed in applying paint thickly around the edges of her paper (Rees, 1995). A lonely man, who regularly keeps most people at bay by screaming, listens with cautious interest to a piano being played. It has taken the therapist 18 months to help him cope with his anxieties and achieve this state of attentiveness (Ritchie, 1993). A habitually withdrawn woman who lacks speech presents a very different aspect of herself in drama, playing the role of a fearsome giant, clashing cymbals with sweeping gestures (James, 1996a). A young woman commonly described by staff as disruptive and 'attention-seeking' learns self-acceptance and body awareness through seven months of dance movement therapy and ultimately engages collaboratively in a group (MacDonald, 1992). A group of adults with learning disabilities experience the achievement of running their own poetry group (Simons, 1995). These and other published case examples indicate that adults with a wide range of learning disabilities gain experience of personal development and change through creative therapies. Such examples indicate that participation in the arts is more than 'simply' recreational.

The term 'creative arts' embraces a multiplicity of experiences. In the confines of a single chapter, discussion will focus more on the shared rather than unique features of different art forms. The chapter draws both on published work and also interviews with seven practitioners, in order to explore current issues. The views of four arts therapists, two occupational therapists and a nurse, all with substantial experience of creative work with adults who have learning disabilities, have helped to identify issues for discussion, although the material selected remains the decision of the author.

Creative activities are viewed by some as examples of 'complementary therapies'. Sensory integration, aromatherapy and massage, for example, share certain features with the creative therapies in offering clients with learning disabilities a variety of stimulation and a supportive therapeutic relationship. Such experiences may help to reduce self-injurious behaviour and increase relaxation and awareness (Reisman, 1993). Nevertheless, this chapter focuses specifically on creative activities and therapies because they share an emphasis on active rather than passive participation. Furthermore, many arts therapists resist the notion that their work is 'simply' complementary or adjunctive.

The chapter will examine therapists' views of the potential value of both creative activities and therapies. The particular issues and needs of adults with learning disabilities that are thought to be addressed through creative therapies will be discussed. The effects of creative experiences are interpreted in the light of some key foundational theories. As most research has been carried out in institutional settings, interviews with practitioners shed light on the current issues for those working in the community with adults with learning disabilities.

The creative arts as recreation, remediation and therapy

Creative activities include art, music, drama, dance and the construction of stories and poems (Atkinson and Williams, 1990; Payne, 1993; Gilroy and Lee, 1995). 'Creative' is a term with multiple meanings, but it tends to be applied to processes which incorporate active participation in sensing, intuiting and problem solving. Such processes often involve novelty and hence sustain attention. Although awareness of social norms is not completely suspended during creative activity, the person may feel a welcome degree of personal freedom to move beyond the normal confines of social roles.

It is clear that participation in creative activities can serve many purposes for all people, regardless of cognitive abilities. Schalkwijk (1994) distinguishes among recreational, remedial and therapeutic activities in his own field of music, and these categories can be usefully applied to other creative arts work (although the distinctions are ones of emphasis rather than being absolute).

Creative experiences may be engaged in primarily as 'recreational' or leisure activities, with the prime purpose of gaining enjoyment and enhanced quality of life. Leisure participation in the arts can be passive (e.g. as audience for drama or art exhibitions) or active (e.g. engaging in writing poetry, painting or dance). Recreational arts activities may help to stimulate thinking, heighten sensory awareness and increase self-esteem. They are hence much more than 'time fillers'.

Performance artists and adult education tutors in community settings offer a variety of creative activities as leisure opportunities. Activities with an apparently recreational purpose may also be facilitated by health professionals such as occupational therapists in day centres and hospital settings. However, patient–therapist roles then risk distorting the activity away from genuinely self-chosen 'recreation'. People with learning disabilities may themselves set up or take on the running of groups, and some arts workers empower their groups to do so if possible (James, 1996a).

'Remedial' arts activities may be facilitated by occupational therapists, nurses and arts therapists. In remedial activity, the therapist plans the intervention to work towards specific learning objectives. Schwalkwijk (1994) argues that remedial activities can promote emotional growth and self-actualization, as well as facilitating the development of cognitive, motor and social skills. The 'success' of the activity may be assessed in terms of the creative product as well as the process. For example, the facilitator may encourage productive activity through setting up a theme or set of structured activities for the session, rather than expecting the client to initiate the focus.

Recreational and remedial activities tend to focus on stimulating positive emotion and personal growth. Arts therapists more clearly offer psychotherapy, and commonly apply psychodynamic concepts to understand the therapeutic process occurring between client and therapist (Read Johnson, 1998). The therapeutic experience facilitates expression of positive emotion, but also offers a therapeutic channel for exploring negative, possibly repressed feelings. Indeed, arts therapists are open to working with mixed or ambivalent emotions. For example, an art therapist explained: 'A client may draw a happy memory but yet feels the sadness of time passing.'

In common with psychotherapists who work with verbal interactions, specialist arts therapists regard the therapeutic relationship with the client as catalytic of growth and change (Payne, 1992; Gilroy and Lee, 1995). The client may find it easier to build a trusting relationship with the therapist through the mediation of the art object, whether it is a painting, improvised music or dance (Case and Dalley, 1992).

Creative arts therapists are more likely to work in one-to-one relationships with adults who have learning difficulties, although there are also published accounts of effective groupwork (e.g. Strand, 1990). Many therapists, in accordance with client-centred values, argue that the therapeutic relationship is based on the therapist's empathy with the client's perspective and experience, unconditional regard or respect for the client as a person and genuineness in the relationship (Silverstone, 1997). For many people with learning disabilities, the experience of being in a collaborative, respectful relationship, where time and space are given to express personal feelings, may be highly unusual and much needed (James, 1996b). While skilful occupational therapists and nurses work to develop a sound therapeutic relationship with clients, specialist arts practitioners are more likely to interpret aspects of that relationship in psychodynamic terms, attempting to interpret clients' behaviour (however 'bizarre') as meaningful communication. An art therapist described this process:

> [The patient] would come in and constantly lick her hands and wipe her face, especially around the eyes. I couldn't figure out why she was doing this. Most people, of course, would think that she's just being odd, but then it suddenly clicked. It was as if she was washing her face, like you do when you get up in the morning. . . . She was trying to wake herself up, to keep herself conscious because she tended to cut off, or distance herself if she felt herself threatened. I fed this back to her and this seemed to work. . . . After that session she would enter the Art Therapy room saying 'I'm asleep now' or 'I'm awake now'. Gradually she became more able to stay awake, or conscious, in my presence.

Because clients are more likely to confront disturbing feelings in therapy (rather than in remedial activities), arts therapists pay very careful attention to the client's sense of safety by establishing firm therapeutic boundaries (including a predictable context, regular timing of sessions and a known place for safe storage for all art products such as paintings). Permission is given for 'being' as well as 'doing' and so periods of silence and stillness are regarded as equally therapeutic as activity (Chesner, 1995).

What needs do adults with learning disabilities bring to arts activities and therapies?

Coping with chaos

For some people with learning difficulties, the experience of meaning and order in the external environment may be further confused by sensory impairments. Difficulties in gaining sensory information may also fragment the body image. Sensory impairments may also result in a craving for stimulation that leads to repetitive self-injury.

Coping with feelings of loss, rejection or failure

Psychological and medical interventions for adults with learning disabilities have been dominated by a preoccupation with the irreversibility of cognitive impairment, and a focus on the intellectual domain to the exclusion of other aspects of the person (Brechin and Swain, 1989). This may communicate to people with learning disabilities a strong sense of failure. Other life experiences also leave some adults with learning disabilities with much more than cognitive impairment to overcome. In many cases, the individual has experienced serial losses and also possible abuse in childhood (Sinason, 1992). In an interview, a dance movement therapist suggested:

> I think the learning disability is an eighth of what we're dealing with. . . . What we're really working with are all those feelings of loss and rejection and difference.

Coping with social stigma and secondary disabilities

The experience of self and agency may be further compromised for people whose early parenting was impersonal or actively rejecting. Poor-quality institutional care, with restrictive choices, and emphasis on the need for compliance may induce child-like behaviour and 'secondary handicaps'. Sinason (1992) writes about people with learning disabilities smiling constantly and inoffensively to appease carers, thereby smothering perceptions of their own feelings and increasing their experience of powerlessness. Some discover that exaggerated cognitive and behavioural difficulties provoke extra attention. Such strategies may be adaptive within an institution, yet increase ostracism and other difficulties for those living in the community.

Coping with excessive demands for 'normal' behaviour

In addition to experiencing emotional hurt, some adults with learning disabilities have experienced lives marked by numerous restrictions. While drives towards 'normalization' supported by intensive education and training can usefully increase social and independence skills, people with learning disabilities may perpetually feel themselves to be 'learners' (Brechin and Swain, 1989). Their dominant experience is one of always having to comply with others' goals and agendas rather than expressing individual needs and views. Extensive time spent in training, and carers' demands for 'adult' behaviour, may also have the effect of limiting life's usual opportunities for exploration, curiosity and play throughout childhood and into later years. A dance movement therapist in interview suggested:

> A lot of learning disabled people and physically disabled people have an experience (of) being mollycoddled. 'We'd better not let him go and do that, because if he fell down or whatever' . . . which I think is why a lot of learning disabled people in their movements walk very stiffly and find it really hard to sit down on the floor or roll around. That's one of the things I do a lot of . . . just exploring crawling and rolling and stretching on the floor and it's very releasing but it can be very scary to them.

How do creative activities enhance well-being and promote functioning of people with learning disabilities?

Creative arts activities and therapies are holistic, acknowledging that a person's emotional life and self-image need to be respected and fostered, regardless of intellectual ability. Although socially useful skills may also be acquired, their primary aim is to help clients experience their own abilities, needs and viewpoint, rather than imposing compliance with external standards Numerous theories, including psychoanalytic and humanistic perspectives, explain the therapeutic effects of arts activities and there is space here only for a brief, selective review.

Whether set up for recreational, remedial or therapeutic purposes, creative activities may be potent catalysts of change on a number of levels. For all people, regardless of cognitive functioning, practitioners (Case and Dalley, 1992; Payne, 1993; Oldfield and Adams, 1995) commonly describe such activities as:

- engaging attention and motivation
- developing sensory and motor skills
- facilitating non-verbal channels of communication
- permitting emotional expression
- providing a safe space or container for emotions
- heightening self-awareness, integration and self-esteem
- enhancing the experience of play
- developing social skills.

Engaging attention and motivation

For people with marked cognitive and sensory difficulties, behavioural problems such as head banging and self-mutilation may reflect a craving for stimulation of any sort (Reisman, 1993). Such behavioural problems may also be expressions of high levels of frustration. Some practitioners note that arts activities can reduce such self-harm by their power to engage attention and channel negative emotion (e.g. wielding a heavy paintbrush or playing a tuned percussion instrument loudly).

Developing sensory and motor skills

For people with more profound learning disabilities associated with sensory or physical impairments, remedial creative activities may develop sensory and motor skills and thereby share goals similar to occupational therapy and physiotherapy interventions. A dance movement therapist may work with a client who has profound learning disabilities to develop increased coordination, for example by tapping a hand or foot to a rhythm. In art therapy, the physical grip of the brush may be problematic and need to be practised. Improved physical control over the body also brings about an enhanced perception of stability in the environment, so reducing anxiety (MacDonald, 1992).

Facilitating awareness and expression of emotions and needs

Perhaps most importantly, all arts activities and therapies facilitate communication, particularly about emotions. Musical improvisation, art work, dramatic role-play and dance all open up non-verbal channels of expression, and so may be helpful whether or not the client has the use of speech. Writing of dance movement therapy, MacDonald (1992:203) argues: 'The smallest movement, even if it is assisted, affords each individual a window, however small, into their own feelings.'

In arts therapies (although not always in recreational or remedial arts work), the client's own pace is respected, with therapists providing an attentive space rather than overt training in skills. Adults with learning disabilities who have rarely had the experience of being listened to, may feel a range of negative emotions, including high levels of frustration or anxiety. Emotional release (e.g. through painting of images, stamping in a circle dance or striking percussion instruments in a music therapy session) may in itself be an effective form of therapy, promoting relaxation of mind and body. Practitioners also describe creative arts work as not only helping to release psychological pain but also fostering the experience of positive emotion:

> It is important not to undervalue **joy**. Joy is more than fun, more than just having a good time. There is something transcendent about the purity of joy, something that relates to an original realization of one's full humanness . . . joy in discovering self-expression or in achieving musical creation with a therapist can be momentous. (Robbins, 1993: 15)

Arts activities facilitate dialogue between client and practitioner and may even improve relationships with other health professionals. For example, once a client has been 'listened to', general care arrangements may be changed in line with expressed needs and preferences, as noted by a dance movement therapist in interview:

> I was working with one particular chap who was really causing quite of lot of headaches on the ward and would attack quite a lot, or was very lethargic, but he came along to my sessions and I never saw any of that. From Day One, he never made any attempt to attack, he just smiled and

> beamed and showed that he really enjoyed both the music. . . . He would say 'up, up', the only word he'd say, and he just wanted to be dancing, moving and be active. . . . I went into one of the ward rounds and . . . I said it seemed to me that this man did not like being inactive, he's very overweight and he's very drugged, but he loves activity. And they looked at me – 'are you talking about the same person?'. I said in his movements all I see is this 'upness', he wants to get going, and all his words are about moving.

She described how these insights led to a varied programme of activities which ultimately facilitated the man's transfer into the community.

Some arts therapists, particularly those influenced by Jung's theory, view creative activities as not only releasing personal feelings but enabling contact with the deeper human issues that we all share, through the vehicle of symbols, metaphor or myth. In drama, for example, the playing out of roles – and exploring the nurturant, threatening or aggressive characters of folktales – may help clients find their own voice and power (James, 1996a, 1996b). Psychotherapists used to regard people with learning disabilities as unable to respond to symbolic meanings, but sensitive case studies suggest that, for some, intellectual impairments are no barrier to symbolic expression. For example, Hughes (1988) described a woman with learning disabilities who retained a fantasy that she would one day be able to return to the idealized family that she had left many years previously. Her preoccupation with waiting for this reunion seemed to resonate with her repetitive drawings of clocks.

Most forms of art work can be viewed as a bridge between the conscious and the unconscious (Case and Dalley, 1992; Dekker, 1996), giving the individual freedom of expression but also some protection from confronting the full force of inner feelings. There is simultaneously an engagement in the product (I made that) and a detachment (that is not me). The art medium (as well as the therapeutic relationship) may provide a sense of containment and safety. In art, the frame is sometimes regarded both as the boundary of the image and the container of symbolized feelings (Schaverien, 1989; Rees, 1995). Of drama therapy, Jennings (1987:15) wrote: 'Drama is both the container of chaos and the means of exploring it.'

Where practitioners are not sensitive to hidden meanings in the art work, the client with learning disabilities may find that feelings are casually invalidated. In an interview, an art therapist described the following experience:

> I remember . . . a woman with learning disabilities in a residential home, where someone was employed to do art activities. It was noticed that the woman would draw a picture and then she would totally cover it in black crayon. The person running the art activity didn't like this and so removed the black crayons, without thinking about what the black meant to the client.

The art therapist regarded the woman as attempting to work through feelings about a bereavement, but this deeper meaning had not been perceived by those facilitating the activity.

Some therapists regard non-verbal emotional expression as therapeutic in itself, whereas others believe that the client's understanding is increased through the therapist's feedback. Some are careful never to interpret, respecting clients needs to express emotions obliquely (Aldridge, 1996; Pearson, 1996). They argue that direct interpretation of unconscious issues may be too painful for the client to bear. Some therapists communicate their growing understanding non-verbally. For example, in music therapy, the therapist may reflect the client's apparent feelings via improvised musical responses. If a client appears unable to proceed in an art therapy session, the therapist may also sit for a while with blank paper to convey that it is indeed 'acceptable' for people sometimes to feel unsure how to proceed.

Explicit verbalizations may also prematurely fix interpretations of a process that is continuing to evolve (Schaverien, 1989). However, some therapists move beyond the non-verbal, carefully verbalizing the meanings that the client's behaviour seems to embody in order to increase conscious awareness of underlying feelings (Tipple, 1994). For instance, the therapist may tentatively suggest that they understand the client's destructive behaviour reflects frustration. Ritchie (1993) describes reflecting back both musically and verbally the deeper meanings of a man's continuous screaming in a music therapy session. Once the client felt understood and accepted, the motivation for his 'challenging' behaviour appeared to fade.

In practical terms though, the therapist requires great sensitivity to the client's needs to offer such interpretations back to the client. Many layers of implicit meaning may be contained even within single images or actions. The client may feel judged rather than understood and the therapist has to be aware of his/her powerful position of influence and the risk of error. The therapists' emotional sensitivity generally requires lengthy periods of contact with the client and considerable reflection in clinical supervision. Groupwork can also offer clients opportunities for mutual understanding and support of peers (Strand, 1990).

Facilitating self-image and self-esteem

Creative activities and therapies offer not only the opportunity of expressing feelings but becoming 'whole' (Aldridge, 1996). An adequate self-image is considered vital to well-being and to the capacity to form relationships with others. The self may be constructed from many sources of information, including sensory and emotional feedback from the body, as well as the responses of others.

Sensory feedback may be very limited for people with more profound learning difficulties and may restrict awareness and recognition of body parts and the boundaries of the body. Creative activities – whether recreational, remedial or therapeutic – permit participants to try out new skills and roles, and to experience some power (over the body and over events) and so develop a stronger sense of self (Chesner, 1995).

Many theorists argue that self-awareness is also shaped by social experiences. Winnicott (1965) regarded the early mother–baby relationship as crucial to the child's growing understanding of the boundaries of self, with the small ways in which the mother fails to respond exactly to the baby's demands as helping the baby to distinguish self from non-self. However, marked failures to respond to the baby's communications may create an overwhelming sense of helplessness and worthlessness. People with learning disabilities who have experienced confused and perhaps rejecting responses from carers, may have difficulty in understanding their own needs, because they have not previously been adequately interpreted and attended to by others.

Others' reactions may also provide the foundations of self-esteem. People with learning disabilities may be vulnerable to low self-esteem if they have lacked praise from others and/or acquired a 'false self' in order to be socially accepted.

Creative experiences may strengthen the boundaries of the self in many ways. For example, the mutual improvisation in a music session may incorporate elements of the turn-taking of the early mother–child relationship, helping the person to make up for missed experiences of reciprocal interaction. Painting or other art work helps individuals to 'make their mark' on the world, leaving a visible record of their presence in the room. In interview, an art therapist suggested:

> I find that art therapy is very useful when people have a poor sense of themselves, and fragile egos. They may not know who they are or if they are real and often this can be reflected in their images of very weak and fragile figures. Drawing gives instant feedback, it confirms your existence and provides an opportunity to literally leave an impression on the world. The majority of my clients have a poor sense of self.

Dance movement activities increase awareness of the body and its sensations. The social dimensions of the therapy also clarify body boundaries. For example, turn-taking and mirroring of movements with the therapist may help to define 'me' and 'not-me'. Self-initiated movement may help the person to experience a greater sense of agency. In drama, experimentation with roles may help the person expand the sense of self, from exploring a wider repertoire of behaviours than is usual, and observing the effects of this new behaviour on others (Chesner, 1995).

Creative therapies offer many ways in which people can reject negative self-definitions that they have absorbed from others' prejudices. James (1996a) describes how role-play in drama may help the individual express and challenge inner criticisms which she terms the 'spoiling voice'. If experiences of negative labelling can be explored in role-play, the individual may be able to challenge and disown damaging labels and feel greater self-worth.

Enhancing the experience of play

Playful activities are spontaneous, active, pleasurable and basically self-affirmative. Some people with learning disabilities appear to have been given little opportunity to play – sometimes because of lack of resources, judgemental social attitudes or access to appropriate facilities.

The theories of Jung and Winnicott have had particular influences in the creative therapies, in their explanations of the human need for play.

Jung regarded creative acts as combining facets of the unconscious and conscious mind, contributing to a sense of wholeness (Noack, 1992; Tuby, 1996). Winnicott (1965) linked creativity to play and noted that even babies show an evident delight in play. However, in order to experiment and explore, the child needs a strong sense of safety, or being psychologically 'held' by the mother's presence. Children who feel insecure and anxious, clearly appear more restricted in their play activities and do not enjoy a physical and psychological 'play space' (Case and Dalley, 1992).

Winnicott's perspective helps to explain why arts therapists place such emphasis on the therapeutic relationship and boundaries for giving even adult clients a sense of safety and thereby 'permission' to play or explore. Some (e.g. James, 1996a) also emphasize that people with learning disabilities may need regular, explicit reminders that they have permission to initiate activities and explore because their usual care arrangements too often assume passive acceptance of others' decisions.

Facilitating social development

Social development is thought to be closely related to the capacity to conceptualize the self. Relationships are sometimes problematic for people with learning disabilities even when living in small community homes, for several reasons. Those with profound impairments may have an exceedingly narrow range of social relationships, tending to experience themselves only in a dependent cared-for role. Social roles, even for those with moderate learning disabilities, may be constrained by patronizing institutional care which perpetuates childlike behaviour, limiting choice and decision making. The person with learning disabilities may face further social difficulties in smaller group homes in the community, from having little choice about co-residents and limited opportunities for friendship outside the home (Howard and Spencer, 1997).

Even if not a primary goal, creative activities in a group setting clearly stimulate social interaction. Group activities, whether in music, drama or movement, encourage turn-taking, and observation of others' behaviour, in order to synchronize cooperative activity. Social development may be further promoted by giving increasing responsibility for the activity to the group. For example, in drama therapy the group may take on increasing decision making for the structure and themes of sessions, eventually enabling the group to function without the therapist (Steiner, 1992; James, 1996a).

The client, through building a trusting relationship with the therapist in the safe and non-pressurized environment of creative activity, may eventually gain confidence to enter other groups, expanding their social network. However, on the problematic side is the dependence that may be fostered by long-term work with clients. Practitioners need to work very carefully at the closure of therapy to ensure that the client has adequate access to alternative social support and can adequately express any feelings of loss or abandonment.

Discussion

Creative arts experiences for people with learning difficulties – whether recreational, remedial or therapeutic – may enrich lives, actualize potential and facilitate communication. They clearly stand in contrast to the medication, behaviour modification or 'warehousing' strategies that have dominated treatment regimes. However, the voices and opinions of people with learning disabilities about the value of creative pursuits are almost missing in the published literature.

A number of issues emerge as problematic in the literature on creative activities and therapies, particularly for people with learning disabilities who live in the community. Research evidence regarding effectiveness is limited, social prejudices may inflate estimates of how many people with learning disabilities need remedial and psychotherapeutic help, and funding processes may be undermining provision of creative therapies for those in need.

Regarding leisure and recreation, there is limited evidence suggesting that a wider range of recreational activity is available to people moving into small group homes from larger institutions (e.g. Howard and Spencer, 1997). However, access to adult education and community arts centres still seems to be limited, both by social attitudes, practical barriers such as transport, and by costs (Russell, 1995).

The evidence base for the remedial and therapeutic use of the creative arts is somewhat limited and needs to be developed as the National Health Service is increasingly linking funding to proven effectiveness. However, research in this area is difficult to conduct for a number of reasons. Arts tutors and therapists, by virtue of their initial interests and training in the performance arts, are often rather poorly equipped to carry out scientific research (Edwards, 1993). They may feel daunted by objective evaluation processes, believing that the processes of change which are observed are too subtle to be measurable. For example, an art therapist in interview said:

> It's the measuring that's the difficult bit, because (behaviour) does change but in very gradual and small ways. What I look for, in change, is a shift in the client from being very passive to being able to lead the session. It's a good sign when that happens. . . . There can be changes in the artwork, the strength of the marks or colours may get stronger. A client might start off with a tiny postage stamp sized drawing and then become bolder, or bigger, or use more space and bigger brushes. Of course their relationship with me will shift and change as it will with their artwork. Another thing to look out for is how the client invests themselves in their artwork, and how much they own it, as some people may just dismiss their artwork in the early stages.

Changes such as these seem clearly beneficial for the client, yet are difficult to measure objectively. People who have more profound learning disabilities may not be able to express their own evaluation. There are further difficulties about documenting whether or not changes achieved in therapy generalize to home settings.

The extent of provision of creative arts therapies (remedial and depth approaches) varies across regions. Although there are centres of excellence, some concern was expressed by practitioners in interviews about increasingly limited resources for community-based work. One dance movement therapist who was interviewed reflected on how difficult it was now to gain funds for working with vulnerable groups. She had recognized that Arts Council Funding, for example, could only be directed towards 'recreational' arts workshops, rather than therapy. This pattern suggests that at least some vulnerable people who would benefit from creative arts therapies are finding that it is not available.

Creative arts therapists emphasize the quality of the relationship between client and therapist. Traditionally, this has led to very long-term work in some instances. For example, Ritchie (1993) reports working with a client in an institution over four years. In the community, long-term psychotherapy is rarely funded by the health service, regardless of 'need'.

Creative therapies have had a long history within hospital settings. This form of therapy (as with other forms of psychotherapy) can stir up strong and unfamiliar feelings, possibly more manageable within the structured hospital setting than in the community. There is some recognition in the general psychotherapy literature that clients may have difficulties in 'holding' released emotions until the following week's therapy session. For people with learning disabilities who have limited social contacts, there may be risks in offering weekly sessions that contact deeply buried negative emotions. There is certainly a need to work with carers so that they can provide extra support if necessary.

However, to bring in carers is to risk breaking certain therapeutic boundaries. If the creative therapies are to stimulate meaningful exploration and communication, the client needs to engage voluntarily in the activity. Carers can create undue pressure to continue with activities, regardless of personal wishes. Conversely, the client's wishes to continue may be overruled by practical barriers such as lack of transport.

Furthermore, it is uncertain whether the novel rules within psychodynamically-based therapy sessions may be confusing to some clients. Free, expressive movements may be encouraged in dance, music or drama. The art therapy room may offer almost unlimited scope for exploration. While such activities provide a healthy antidote to the restrictions of 'normal' living, clients with more severe learning disabilities may become confused as to what is permitted in different situations. Generalization of newly-discovered behaviour into other everyday contexts – often the ultimate goal of therapy – may also be problematic if it conflicts with the ideas of 'normality' that prevail in the person's home. More research is needed to establish whether clients with learning disabilities find such 'rule changes' confusing.

While the provision of arts-based therapies may help people with learning disabilities to manage and resolve negative feelings, the models of disability that underpin therapy need to be carefully examined. Creative arts therapies tend to reflect 'individualistic' models of disability. However, some of the therapists interviewed were also aware that remedial and therapeutic sessions have limited value when the client returns to an unchanged environment, in which inclusion in community, work and leisure activities is still highly restricted. Any heightened awareness of negative feelings, stigma and inner potential that is gained through therapy simply exacerbates everyday frustration unless the person's 'eco-system' adapts to their new skills and aspirations.

Conclusion

Creative activities span a diverse set of experiences. There is relatively little evidence about how adults with learning difficulties prefer to pass their recreational and leisure time, although active involvement in creative pursuits may offer one route to enhancing quality of life and self-esteem. In terms of therapy, practitioners regard remedial and therapeutic arts work as facilitating non-verbal communication, and the growth of self-awareness and self-esteem, based upon the creative process itself, satisfaction with the creative product and trust in the relationship with the therapist. Remedial creative work tends to be based on humanistic (client-centred) principles and can provide multiple learning opportunities, helping to develop skills and potential, as well as promoting positive emotional experiences. Creative arts therapies overlap with remedial work, but may work in more depth and intensity, particularly in facilitating the expression and working through of conflicting emotions. A wide variety of humanistic and psychodynamic theoretical perspectives help the arts therapist to attempt communication and understanding of the client. There needs to be more research into the psychological and social effects of creative therapy, to test and substantiate theory. However, the benefits may be short term or elusive, unless the whole ecosystem of the person with learning disabilities is addressed.

Acknowledgements

The author would like to acknowledge the practitioners who were so generous of their time and whose views helped to clarify current practices and issues. The author would particularly like to thank Christine Lyle, Art Therapist, Psychological Services, Coventry Healthcare NHS Trust, not only for providing a valuable insight into her work during an interview, but also for her helpful comments on the chapter.

References

Aldridge, D. (1996) *Music Therapy Research and Practice in Medicine: From Out of the Silence*, Jessica Kingsley, London

Atkinson, D. and Williams, F. (eds) (1990) *Know Me As I Am: An Anthology of Prose, Poetry and Art by People with Learning Difficulties*, Hodder and Stoughton, London (in association with the Open University Press)

Brechin, A. and Swain, J. (1989) Creating a 'working alliance' with people with learning difficulties. In Brechin, A. and Walmsley, J. (eds), *Making Connections: Reflecting on the Lives and Experiences of People with Learning Difficulties*, Hodder and Stoughton, London

Case, C. and Dalley, T. (1992) *The Handbook of Art Therapy*, Routledge, London

Chesner, A. (1995) *Dramatherapy for people with Learning Disabilities*, Jessica Kingsley, London

Dekker, K. (1996) Why oblique and why Jung? In Pearson, J. (ed.), *Discovering the Self through Drama and Movement*, Jessica Kingsley, London

Edwards, D. (1993) Why don't arts therapists do research? In Payne, H. (ed.), *Handbook of Inquiry in the Arts Therapies: One River, Many Currents*, Jessica Kingsley, London

Gilroy, A. and Lee, C. (eds) (1995) *Art and Music Therapy and Research*, Routledge, London

Howard, S. and Spencer, A. (1997) Effects of resettlement on people with learning disabilities. *British Journal of Nursing*, **6**(8), 436–441

Hughes, R. (1998) Transitional phenomena and the potential space in art therapy with mentally handicapped people. *Inscape*, Summer, 4–8

James, J. (1996a) Dramatherapy with people with learning disabilities. In Mitchell, S. (ed.), *Dramatherapy: Clinical Studies*, Jessica Kingsley, London

James, J. (1996b). Poetry in motion: drama and movement therapy with people with learning disabilities. In Pearson, J. (ed.), *Discovering the Self through Drama and Movement*, Jessica Kingsley, London

Jennings, S. (1987) *Dramatherapy: Theory and Practice 1*. Routledge, London

MacDonald, J. (1992) Dance? Of course I can! Dance movement therapy for people with learning difficulties. In Payne, H. (ed.), *Dance Movement Therapy: Theory and Practice*, Routledge, London

Noack, A. (1992) On a Jungian approach to dance movement therapy. In Payne, H. (ed.), *Dance Movement Therapy: Theory and Practice*, Routledge, London

Oldfield, A. and Adams, M. (1995) The effects of music therapy on a group of adults with profound learning difficulties. In Gilroy, A. and Lee, C. (eds), *Art and Music Therapy and Research*, Routledge, London

Payne, H. (ed.) (1992) *Dance Movement Therapy: Theory and Practice*, Routledge, London

Payne, H. (1993). Introduction to inquiry in the arts therapies. In Payne, H., (ed.), *Handbook of Inquiry in the Arts Therapies: One River, Many Currents*, Jessica Kingsley, London

Pearson, J. (1996) Discovering the self. In Pearson, J. (ed.), *Discovering the Self through Drama and Movement*, Jessica Kingsley, London

Read Johnson, D. (1998) On the therapeutic action of the creative arts therapies: the psychodynamic model. *The Arts in Psychotherapy*, **25**(2), 85–99

Rees, M. (1995) Making sense of marking space: researching art therapy with people who have severe learning difficulties. In Gilroy, A. and Lee, C., (eds), *Art and Music Therapy and Research*, Routledge, London

Reisman, J. (1993) Using a sensory integrative approach to treat self-injurious behaviour in an adult with profound mental retardation. *American Journal of Occupational Therapy*, **47**(5), 403–411

Ritchie, F. (1993) The effects of music therapy with people who have severe learning difficulties and display challenging behaviour. In Heal, M. and Wigram, T. (eds), *Music Therapy in Health and Education*, Jessica Kingsley, London

Robbins, C. (1993) The creative processes are universal. In Heal, M. and Wigram, T. (eds), *Music Therapy in Health and Education*, Jessica Kingsley, London

Russell, J. (1995) Leisure and recreation services. In Malin, N. (ed.), *Services for People with Learning Disabilities*, Routledge, London

Schalkwijk, F. (1994) *Music and People with Developmental Disabilities: Music Therapy, Remedial Music Making and Musical Activities*, Jessica Kingsley, London

Schaverien, J. (1989). The picture within the frame. In Gilroy, A. and Dalley, T. (eds), *Pictures at an Exhibition: Selected Essays on Art and Art Therapy*, Routledge, London

Silverstone, L. (1997) *Art Therapy: The Person-Centred Way*, Jessica Kingsley, London

Simons, K. (1995) Empowerment and advocacy. In Malin, N. (ed.), *Services for People with Learning Disabilities*, Routledge, London

Sinason, V. (1992) *Mental Handicap and The Human Condition: New Approaches from the Tavistock*, Free Association Books, London

Steiner, M. (1992) Alternatives in psychiatry: dance movement therapy in the community. In Payne, H., (ed.), *Dance Movement Therapy: Theory and Practice*, Routledge, London

Strand, S. (1990). Counteracting isolation: group art therapy for people with learning difficulties. *Group Analysis*, **23**, 255–263

Tipple, R. (1994) Communication and interpretation in art therapy with people who have a learning disability. *Inscape*, **2**, 31–35

Tuby, M. (1996) Jung and the symbol: resolution of conflicting opposites. In Pearson, J. (ed.), *Discovering the Self through Drama and Movement*, Jessica Kingsley, London

Winnicott, D. (1965) *The Maturational Process and the Facilitating Environment*, Hogarth Press, London

25

Conclusion: Reflections on *Therapy and Learning Difficulties*

Sally French and John Swain

Introduction

Some edited books include a concluding chapter which is a critical review of the whole book either by the editors themselves or an invited commentator. We have followed the same general idea, but through a different approach. We asked three groups of commentators for their views on the book and the issues it covers: physiotherapists; occupational therapists; and people with learning difficulties.

We first wrote and audiotaped a summary of the book. This was a difficult task in itself, to reduce a 150 000-word text to a 2000-word précis which provides a fair reflection of the book. The summary consisted of an introduction to the book as a whole (including aims, intended audience and structure) and a brief overview of each chapter, consisting of a couple of sentences to convey the general topic being covered, and a very short quotation chosen to illustrate the essence of the overall argument within the chapter and as a catalyst for discussion.

We approached three groups inviting them to participate, and then sent them each a copy of the audiotaped summary and a blank audiotape. The following extract from the summary provided the participants with the instructions for the task:

> On this tape we shall summarize just a few of the things in the book. We would like to ask you to listen to the tape and then discuss what you have heard. You might pick out particular points that you think are important or interesting, or points that you disagree with, or things that you think are very important but might not have been said within the book. How does the book apply to you and your work? We are asking you to tape your discussion, to send us the tape, and we shall use what you have said for the concluding chapter in the book.

While listening to and transcribing the tapes, we were struck first and foremost by the contrasts between the views and concerns expressed by the three groups, not only between therapists and people with learning difficulties, but also between occupational therapists and physiotherapists. The groups tackled the task in different ways, despite having exactly the same materials and instructions. The groups of therapists listened to and then discussed the summaries of each section of the book, whereas the group of people with learning difficulties turned off the summary tape, and had a discussion after each separate chapter. The group of people with learning difficulties also tended to talk more about personal experiences and concerns than the therapists. Analysing the content of the discussions, we found differences not only in what was said about particular issues, but also which issues were seen as important.

Our original plan for this chapter was simply to include the transcripts of the discussions, with as little editing as possible. In the following analysis, we attempt to convey the participants' views through key quotations, but in a framework of themes which compares and contrasts the viewpoints of the different groups. Perhaps inevitably, given the nature of this exercise, the four themes are, first, the book as a whole and then the three major themes of the book: advocacy, participation and partnership.

The book

The first issue for two of the groups was the client group and how they are referred to. The group of people with learning difficulties did not like the label:

> *PLD* ... We don't like the word 'learning difficulties', we like to be called clients.

> *PLD* Nobody's got learning difficulties, everyone is clever.

> *PLD* I think to label people it discriminates them in different ways. In this chapter they shouldn't put about the labelling, it should be cut out all together, and it's really down to asking people like us to put on research.

The physiotherapists, on the other hand, had no problems with using labels, but their preferred label was 'learning disabilities':

> *P* My thought is, you talk about people with learning difficulties, in this area we talk about learning disabilities although in education I know they still talk about learning difficulties. That threw me a bit.

The physiotherapists had further concerns about the possible client group addressed by the book:

> *P* So is the book going to be inclusive of people with more profound learning disabilities as well as those who can say 'I'd like to get married' or 'I'd like to have a baby' or whatever? Because that is an enormous part of therapeutic work isn't it? Really the large proportion of people we work with are those who can't communicate because those are the ones who tend to have the greatest physical disability.

The same concerns did not arise in the occupational therapists' group. Indeed, they use the term 'learning difficulties' throughout their discussion, while the physiotherapists consistently referred to people with 'learning disabilities'.

In terms of audience, all three groups wondered whether people would be attracted to reading the book, but for quite different reasons. For people with learning difficulties, it was the repeated use of the term 'learning difficulties':

PLD It's using the word too much. It puts people off reading it.

For occupational therapists the problem was societal values and attitudes in general and professional attitudes in particular:

OT I don't know who would be reading this book, apart from professionals. I think other people who work with people with learning difficulties might benefit as well. I know with other occupational therapists, when you say you work in learning difficulties, they well, not recoil exactly, but they say 'Oh no, that's not something I could do'. They're very wary of the area without knowing why, it's the unknown really.

The physiotherapists also discussed possible lack of interest in working with people with learning difficulties, but for them the main concerns seemed to be professional status and job satisfaction.

P About the fact that people have always worked with these people to a certain degree, but that it is only fairly recently that the field of work has opened up and people actually appreciate how much can actually be achieved with a client group like this and that you do get job satisfaction from it as well, whereas it's always been a bit of a Cinderella service hasn't it?

Nevertheless, all three groups felt that the book should reach a wider audience than therapists, and the people with learning difficulties felt it should be in a format accessible to people with learning difficulties.

Another subject for some comment and discussion by the two groups of therapists was the general approach taken in the book. The physiotherapists like the broad social approach, though did think medical knowledge is useful:

P I think it's a good introduction to learning disabilities, not getting too bogged down in the medical conditions but looking at the people you're working with as a whole. That is the emphasis that it needs really.

P Obviously you need some background knowledge of the medical conditions they've got, but you need to see them as people and not clients don't you?

The occupational therapists seemed to put more emphasis on the social approach, referring particularly to human rights:

OT We like the way you look at things from more than one perspective, getting the views of people who have worked with people with learning difficulties as well as people with learning difficulties themselves. Giving a real insight into how people feel and what has happened to them.

> *OT*   The abuse of basic human rights was so entrenched in our society, only now are we beginning to address the balance and even so there are still areas where we can go a long way to improve.

The approach of the book was not directly discussed by the people with learning difficulties, though 'equal rights' was referred to in their discussions a number of times. Medical conditions received no mention whatsoever.

Advocacy

There was some discussion of advocacy by the three groups, but again there were clear differences in their viewpoints. Physiotherapists argued that most people with learning difficulties cannot advocate for themselves, and that they as professionals have a role as advocates:

> *P*   In the chapter where somebody said 'We're just expected to sit there and accept what's given to us' and they're not expected to participate or to disagree with it. To a certain extent that's how a lot of our clients have to be because they are unable to communicate their needs, or the means in which they can communicate have yet to be discovered. Having said that you can respond to, you know whether the client likes the music therapy, or if they like going in the water, you can sense what they like and dislike and obviously you don't continue with what they dislike.

> *P*   With many people with learning disabilities they can't be self-advocates, they haven't got the communicative ability to do that. So it needs something about people working with them being able to understand so they can be their advocates. We have to do it for them and for an awful lot of people that therapists work with that is the case.

The occupational therapists also discussed the difficulties that people can have when advocating for themselves, but they talked of possible barriers and included the work of professionals being a barrier:

> *OT*   People are very passive in a way and I think we encourage people to be that way. I'm not talking about us personally, I'm talking about therapists and the medical profession generally. If somebody says 'No' then we label them as non-compliant, or difficult or challenging, whereas if we actually put ourselves in their position we may well say 'No' as well.

> *OT*   People are expected to be grateful and toe the line. If you say 'You've got an appointment' they're expected to come.

> *OT*   Absolutely, it's very much going by our agenda rather than that of the person with learning difficulties. Let's face it, it's their life not ours.

> *OT*   There are plenty of meetings where the client is basically talked at, they're being told where to go and what to do. It's quite difficult to change the culture.

The group of people with learning difficulties referred to and discussed self-advocacy at a number of points in their discussion. Mainly they spoke of its importance in their lives:

> *PLD* It's all to do with having confidence, sticking up for yourself and telling them what you want to do. The tutors say you cannot do this for the reason they cannot tell us.

> *PLD* If there's something you don't want to do and there's someone telling you you've got to do it, why should you do it?

> *PLD* Yes, they can't force you to do anything if you don't want to. If someone at L says I've got to do lighting and I don't want to do it then I don't have to do it, and that's quite correct. No-one can't force you to do anything if you don't want to do it.

Doubts were raised, however, in relation to the idea of people with learning difficulties telling their stories, but these concerned painful memories and trusting professionals:

> *PLD* Well why shouldn't people lead their own lives? If they want to tell their own story they can.

> *PLD* Yer, I don't want to talk about what happened a long time ago, like my mother died, my father died. I don't want to bring the past up, that's horrible. I like to think about nice things.

> *PLD* Yer, that's what I think. You've got to be so careful who the person is that wants to know about you. Before that you should ask the person why they want to know your story and what's going to happen to the story, because you don't want people thinking, what's this person on about? Why are they saying it? And what will it do to that person? And why should they tell a story, and what's going to happen to the story?

Participation

The main themes in the discussion of the people with learning difficulties in relation to participation concerned their experiences of, first, segregation:

> *PLD* When you are a child ... I used to go to school, as you know, boarding school. I went to B.M., boarding school, I couldn't understand why. When I was at B.M. it was a boarding school, this was back in 1964, I was in a child's home by then. When I went to boarding school I thought you were being locked up for the rest of your life. Actually, I went to a lot of schools in Bristol and I was pushed from one school to other schools, and I ended up in B.M.

and, second, barriers that limit participation in inclusive settings, including expectations, lack of support, attitudes and prejudice:

> *PLD* I go to college and people say to me, 'Why do you want to do level 2?' I say to them, 'I want to get more qualifications'. Because if you do a higher job you get better pay.

PLD Well vocational at level 2. People have been saying to me 'You can't do that', and I say 'why not'. And they say 'I think you are going to get really tired', and I say 'I'm not'. That is what I want to do, that is what my aim is.
[So what sort of help do you think you need in schools and colleges?]

PLD Support. Like in vocation, what you want to do and why you want to do it. Anybody with learning disability needs support. You can't just go into a research group, like what we were talking about, without thinking what support do I need, when do I need it.

PLD I think that some people with learning disabilities, is that you get laughed at. Some people just laugh at you and think it is funny.
[And does that happen in college?]

PLD Yes it does a hell of a lot, especially with people who do a course and think he'd be no good for that.

PLD Abusing people is a very wrong thing I think, for their colour and their race. I think that should be stopped straight away.
[Abuse is something sometimes related to colour and race.]

Occupational therapists also discussed barriers to participation, concentrating on the denial of opportunities particularly in families:

OT People manage very well really. Saying that though one thing that I find quite a challenge is when somebody's referred to you and this person's got a lot more abilities than they've ever been allowed to use. That they could be a lot more independent, but they have this role in the family of being 'the child' and the parents do everything for them.

Whereas the people with learning difficulties talked of the difficulties of segregation, physiotherapists talked of the difficulties of integration:

P Inclusive schooling for those with a profound disability will need enormous funding in terms of having the right level of assistance in the classroom to enable that person to get the most out of their schooling. Even within policies at the moment of trying to integrate, quite rightly so, physical disability, they struggle. We know teachers who are really struggling with knowing what to do with the more profoundly disabled child because they haven't got enough staffing levels.

Partnership

The physiotherapists specifically discussed the notion of partnership in their work with clients with learning difficulties. Though they were generally in favour of negotiation in practice, they also wanted the notion of partnership to include others, and argued that there were limitations to partnerships:

P I'm hoping that chapter does highlight that often you're working in partnership with carers and other people involved with the client as well as the client themselves. It's interesting that they brought up the ethical issue of informed consent; much discussion has gone on here in terms of when you've got a child with a profound disability then it's quite easy to get informed consent from parents but once they are post-18 there are decisions that you feel the parents aren't making appropriately that you need a multidisciplinary team decision on it. That's an enormous issue particularly when you've got people who can't speak for themselves.

P Perhaps it's even more difficult when you've got a client who is capable of communicating but is not fully able to understand what they're dealing with. Perhaps our clients who are profoundly handicapped and can't have a voice for themselves are almost better off because they don't have to make a decision, whereas there are clients who fall between two stools, they can perhaps talk to you and hold a conversation but they might not necessarily be able to assimilate knowledge to make an adequate informed choice.

The occupational therapists also saw partnership as 'good practice' and an ideal that they promoted. Like the physiotherapists, they discussed the barriers to partnership, but from a different standpoint. Whereas for physiotherapists the main concerns seemed to lie with the limitations of the client, in terms of capacities to communicate and understand, the occupational therapists focused on the constraints they faced in realizing the ideal of partnership:

OT I know we have this philosophy but I do wonder how empowered we are to make some of these things work. It's lip service to a lot of things. You need to involve service managers. I was thinking about abuse. I mean people are abused all the time aren't they, by not giving them choice, not giving them time to do something they enjoy doing, making decisions, taking away their independence and doing things for them. People think that because people are out in the community things are much better but it's not good enough yet is it? I certainly get quite frustrated as an OT; you suggest something and people just won't take it on board.

OT I don't know about you but listening to this I think 'Yes, I try to be all these things' but I don't know how much I do because it's really, really difficult to empathize. We can think of what it might be like to have a severe learning disability and to be in a wheelchair, but there is a power struggle, we are the people 'doing' and they are the people being 'done to'. They don't get the chance to do enough.

The group of people with learning difficulties, however, had a broad discussion about their experiences, but they emphasized choices, rights and being listened to:

PLD   Yer, I got my own life to lead.
[Because most people do have a choice?]

PLD   It's my choice about who I want to live with. Well it is my choice.

PLD   But most people don't get what they want really. It depends.

PLD   But people with learning difficulties have their rights. People with learning difficulties yes, I think they should have their rights.

PLD   Depends who wants to listen to you. This block in this chapter, I think it's a great idea, people listening to you, and why they listen to you, for different reasons. It might be disability reasons, maybe for housing reasons, caring reason. They're there to listen to you, and care is a big thing in this.

Conclusion

We have written this chapter by juxtaposing the views of people with learning difficulties, physiotherapists and occupational therapists. We have done so, not to be obstructive, but in the belief that for therapists and people with learning difficulties to work together, recognition needs to be given to their different viewpoints and experiences. Certainly each group saw possibilities for positive changes as reflected, coincidentally, in the final statements on each of the tapes we received, and we think they provide an appropriate ending for this chapter.

The physiotherapists looked towards reflecting on their own practice as one possibility for change:

P   There certainly should be reflective practice. As therapists we're moving into a new place of doing that, we haven't done that enough in the past, in terms of looking at what we're doing and why we're doing it, and are we being successful? It's good that that's mentioned in the book.

The occupational therapists saw hope in the possibility of affecting policy makers:

OT   I felt that this part of the book was brilliant on theory but how about translating it into practice? For example about policy makers. People who work 'hands on' in the profession don't get listened to, people who make decisions may have little idea of what the job involves.

OT   There is a potential for people to have some kind of voice in making policies but what is necessary is for people to be asked in the first place and if the 'powers-that-be' aren't interested in asking they are not going to have that forum.

The need to be listened to, whatever form their expressions take (verbal, non-verbal, drama, visual art, etc.), was a major theme for the group of people with learning difficulties. It was finally reflected in their expression of pleasure at being involved in this particular project:

PLD   Thank you for your concern about us.

Index